D0812546

Immunotherapy with intravenous immunoglobulins

Immunotherapy with intravenous immunoglobulins

Proceedings of a conference held at Interlaken
6–9 May 1990

---

edited by

P. IMBACH

co-editors

Part I: U. E. NYDEGGER
Part II: A. MORELL
Part III: P. DE HAES
Part IV: B. A. PERRET
Part V: U. E. NYDEGGER

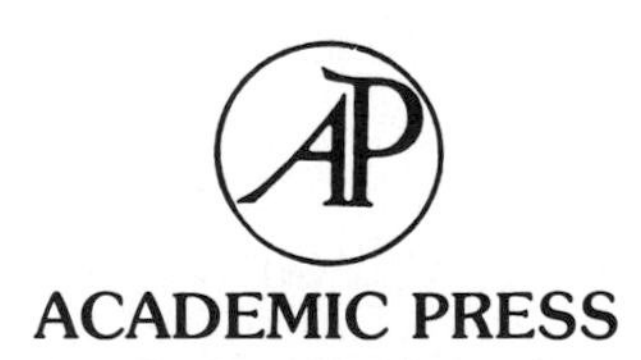

ACADEMIC PRESS

Harcourt Brace Jovanovich, Publishers

London · San Diego · New York · Boston · Sydney · Tokyo · Toronto

This book is printed on acid-free paper.
ACADEMIC PRESS LTD
24–28 Oval Road, London NW1 7DX

United States Edition published by
ACADEMIC PRESS, INC.
San Diego, CA 92101

A catalogue record for this book is available from the British Library

ISBN: 0–12–370725–0

Phototypeset by
J&L Composition Ltd, Filey, North Yorkshire

Printed in Great Britain at the University Press, Cambridge

Contributors

D. V. ABLASHI *International Institute of Immunopathology eV, Cologne–Washington, Hohenzollernring 14, 5000 Cologne 1, Federal Republic of Germany*

G. ANTONY *Department of Paediatric Endocrinology, Prince of Wales Children's Hospital, High Street, Randwick, New South Wales, Australia 2031*

R. BABINGTON *Sandoz Pharmaceuticals, Hanover, New Jersey 07936, USA*

C. J. BAKER *Myers–Black Section of Infectious Diseases, Departments of Pediatrics, Microbiology & Immunology, Baylor College of Medicine, 1 Baylor Plaza, Houston, Texas 77030, USA*

L. J. BEARD *Department of Immunology & University Department of Pediatrics, Adelaide Children's Hospital, South Australia 5006*

A. BENEVENTO *Department of Surgery, Ospedale Multizonale di Varese, Viale Borri 57, 21100 Varese, Italy*

E. M. BENSON *Department of Clinical Immunology, Prince Henry Hospital, University of New South Wales, Sydney, Australia*

P. BERCHTOLD *Department of Medicine, University of Bern, Inselsital, 3010 Bern, Switzerland*

E. BERNTOP *Department for Coagulation Disorders, University of Lund, Malmö General Hospital, 21401 Malmö, Sweden*

M. C. BESOZZI *Department of Surgery, Ospedale Multizonale di Varese, Viale Borri 57, 21100 Varese, Italy*

C. R. BOUGHTON *Departments of Immunology and Infectious Diseases, Division of Medicine; and the Mood Disorders Unit, Division of Psychiatry, Prince Henry Hospital, University of New South Wales, Sydney, Australia*

A. BRAND *Department of Immunohematology and Bloodbank, University Hospital, Leiden, The Netherlands*

G. R. BURGIO *Department of Pediatrics, University of Pavia, 27111 Pavia, Italy*

J. B. BUSSEL *New York Hospital, 525 East 68th Street N 740, New York, NY 10021, USA*

F. CAFIERO *Divisione di Oncologia Chirurgica, Istituto Nazionale per la Ricerca sul Cancro, Via le Benedetto XV, 10, 16132 Genoa, Italy*

H. CHAPEL *Department of Immunology, John Radcliffe Hospital, Oxford OX3 9DU, UK*

G. CHIRICO *Division of Neonatal Intensive Care, IRCCS Policlinico, S. Matteo, Italy*

D. L. CHRISTIE *Department of Pediatrics, University Washington School of Medicine, Seattle, Washington 98195, USA*

J. B. COFER *Transplantation Services, Baylor University Medical Center, 3500 Gaston Avenue, Dallas, Texas 75246, USA*

S. COLAGIURI *Department of Medicine, Prince of Wales Hospital, University of New South Wales, Sydney, Australia*

A. CORVETTA *Department of Internal Medicine, Ancona University, Medical School, Ancona, Italy*

C. COULAM *Center for Reproduction & Transplantation Immunology, Methodist Hospital of Indiana Inc., Indianapolis 46206, USA*

J. N. CURRIE *Department of Clinical Immunology, Prince Henry Hospital, University of New South Wales, Sydney, Australia*

G. DANIELI *Department of Medicine, Ancona University Medical School, Ancona, Italy*

G. DIETRICH *Unité d'Immunopathologie, INSERM U28, Hôpital Broussais, Paris, France*

R. DIONIGI *Department of Surgery, Ospedale Multizonale di Varese, Viale Borri 57, 21100 Varese, Italy*

L. DOMINIONI *Department of Surgery, Ospedale Multizonale di Varese, Viale Borri 57, 21100 Varese, Italy*

P. A. VAN DOORN *Department of Neurology, University Hospital Dijkzigt, Rotterdam, The Netherlands*

M. DUSE *Department of Pediatrics, University of Brescia, 25100 Brescia, Italy*

J. M. DWYER *University of New South Wales, P.O. Box 1, 2033 Kensington, New South Wales, Australia*

G. ELFENBEIN *The University of South Florida, Tampa, Florida 33624, USA*

W. FAULK *Center for Reproduction & Transplantation Immunology, Methodist Hospital of Indiana Inc., Indianapolis 46206, USA*

A. FERRANTE *Department of Immunology, Adelaide Children's Hospital, South Australia 5006*

G. W. FISCHER *Uniformed Services University of The Health Sciences, F. Edward Hébert School of Medicine, 4301 Jones Bridge Road, Bethesda, Maryland 20814, USA*

S. H. FISCHER *Department of Pediatrics, University of Washington School of Medicine, Seattle, Washington 98195, USA*

R. FISHER *Department of Medicine, Prince of Wales Hospital, University of New South Wales, Sydney, Australia*

E. W. GELFAND *Department of Pediatrics, National Jewish Center for Immunology & Respiratory Medicine, University of Colorado, Denver, Colorado 80206, USA*

R. GENNARI *Department of Surgery, Ospedale Multizonale di Varese, Viale Borri 57, 21100 Varese, Italy*

M. GIPPONI *Divisione di Oncologia Chirugica, Istituto Nazionale per la Ricerca sul Cancro, Via le Benedetto XV, 10, 16132 Genoa, Italy*

D. GOH *Department of Immunology & University Department of Pediatrics, Adelaide Children's Hospital, South Australia 5006*

R. M. GOLDSTEIN *Transplantation Services, Baylor University Medical Center, 3500 Gaston Avenue, Dallas, Texas 75246, USA*

T. A. GONWA *Transplantation Services, Baylor University Medical Center, 3500 Gaston Avenue, Dallas, Texas 75246, USA*

J. GRAHAM-POLE *The University of Florida, Gainesville, Florida 32610, USA*

H. GRIFFITHS *Department of Immunology, John Radcliffe Hospital, Oxford OX3 9DU, UK*

R. HAGGITT *Department of Pathology, University Washington School of Medicine, Seattle, Washington 98195, USA*

S. C. HARTH *Mater Children's Hospital, South Brisbane, Queensland, Australia*

V. G. HEMMING *Department of Pediatrics, The Uniformed Services University of the Health Sciences, Bethesda, Maryland 20814, USA*

I. B. HICKIE *Departments of Immunology and Infectious Diseases, Division of Medicine; and the Mood Disorders Unit, Division of Psychiatry, Prince Henry Hospital, University of New South Wales, Sydney, Australia*

R. HONG *The University of Wisconsin, Madison, Wisconsin 53792, USA*

M. HOURCADE *Department of Surgery, Ospedale Multizonale di Varese, Viale Borri 57, 21100 Varese, Italy*

B. S. HUSBERG *Transplantation Services, Baylor University Medical Center, 3500 Gaston Avenue, Dallas, Texas 75246, USA*

P. IMBACH *Central Laboratory of the Swiss Red Cross, Blood Transfusion Service, Wankdorfstrasse 10, CH–3000, Bern, Switzerland*

J. JANSEN *Indiana University, Indianapolis, Indiana 46202, USA*

N. KAPOOR *The Ohio State University, Bone Marrow Transplantation Division, Columbus, Ohio 43210, USA*

S. KAVERI *Unité d'Immunopathologie, INSERM U28, Hôpital Broussais, Paris, France*

M. KAZATCHKINE *Unité d'Immunopathologie, INSERM U28, Hôpital Broussais, Paris, France*

W. KIDSON *Department of Medicine, Prince of Wales Hospital, University of New South Wales, Sydney, Australia*

D. D. KIPROV *San Francisco Children's Hospital, San Francisco, California, USA*

G. B. KLINTMALM *Transplantation Services, Baylor University Medical Center, 3500 Gaston Avenue, Dallas, Texas 75246, USA*

A. L. D. KOBAYASHI *University of Nebraska, College of Medicine, Omaha, Nebraska, USA*

R. H. KOBAYASHI *Department of Pediatrics, UCLA School of Medicine, Los Angeles, California, USA*

J. KRISCHER *The University of Florida, Gainesville, Florida 32610, USA*

G. R. F. KRUEGER *International Institute of Immunopathology eV, Cologne–Washington, Hohenzollernring 14, 5000 Cologne 1, Federal Republic of Germany*

G. L. LARSEN *Department of Pediatrics, National Jewish Center for Immunology & Respiratory Medicine, University of Colorado, Denver, Colorado 80206, USA*

H. LAZARUS *Case Western Reserve University, Cleveland, Ohio 44106, USA*

M. LEE *Baxter Healthcare Corporation, California, USA*

N. LEE *Department of Pediatrics, UCLA School of Medicine, Los Angeles, California, USA*

U. LEMBKE *International Institute of Immunopathology eV, Cologne–Washington, Hohenzollernring 14, 5000 Cologne 1, Federal Republic of Germany*

G. M. LEONG *Department of Paediatric Endocrinology, Prince of Wales Children's Hospital, University of New South Wales, Sydney, Australia*

D. S. LEVINE *Department of Medicine, University of Washington School of Medicine, Seattle, Washington 98195, USA*

A. R. LLOYD *Departments of Immunology & Infectious Diseases, Division of Medicine; and the Mood Disorders Unit, Division of Psychiatry, Prince Henry Hospital, University of New South Wales, Sydney, Australia*

C. M. LOCKWOOD *Department of Medicine, Clinical School, Addenbrookes Hospital, Hills Road, Cambridge CB2 2QQ, UK*

R. L. LOH *Department of Immunology, Boston Children's Hospital, Boston, MA, USA*

M. M. LUCHETTI *Department of Internal Medicine, Ancona University Medical School, Ancona, Italy*

I. LUNDKVIST *Department of Immunohematology and Bloodbank, University Hospital, Leiden, The Netherlands*

M. G. MACEY *Department of Haematology, The London Hospital, Whitechapel, London E1 1BB, UK*

J. MCINTYRE *Center for Reproduction & Transplantation Immunology, Methodist Hospital of Indiana Inc., Indianapolis 46206, USA*

R. MCMILLAN *Department of Molecular and Experimental Medicine, Research Institute of Scripps Clinic, La Jolla, CA 92037, USA*

G. T. MAI *Department of Immunology & University Department of Pediatrics, Mater Children's Hospital, South Brisbane, Queensland, Australia*

B. D. MAZER *Department of Pediatrics, National Jewish Center for Immunology & Respiratory Medicine, University of Colorado, Denver, Colorado 80206, USA*

C. A. MORRIS *Transplantation Services, Baylor University Medical Center, 3500 Gaston Avenue, Dallas, Texas 75246, USA*

A. M. MUNSTER *Baltimore Regional Burn Center, Department of Surgery, Johns Hopkins University, Baltimore, Maryland 21205, USA*

A. C. NEWLAND *Department of Haematology, The London Hospital, Whitechapel, London E1 1BB, UK*

I. M. NILSSON *Department for Coagulation Disorders, University of Lund, Malmö General Hospital, 21401 Malmö, Sweden*

L. D. NOTARANGELO *Department of Pediatrics, University of Brescia, 25100 Brescia, Italy*

U. E. NYDEGGER *Division of Transfusion Medicine, Inselspital, CH 3010–Bern, Switzerland*

J. O'DAY *Department of Medicine, Alfred Hospital, Monash Medical School, Melbourne, Australia*

H. D. OCHS *Department of Pediatrics, University of Washington School of Medicine, Seattle, Washington, USA*

C. PEARSON *Department of Immunology & University Department of Pediatrics, Adelaide Children's Hospital, South Australia 5006*

A. PETERS *Center for Reproduction & Transplantation Immunology, Methodist Hospital of Indiana Inc., Indianapolis 46206, USA*

A. PLEBANI *Department of Pediatrics, University of Brescia, 25100 Brescia, Italy*

G. POMPONIO *Department of Internal Medicine, Ancona University Medical School, Ancona, Italy*

G. A. PRINCE *National Institute of Allergy and Infectious Diseases, Bethesda, Maryland 20892, USA*

A. RAMON *International Institute of Immunopathology eV, Cologne–Washington, Hohenzollernring 14, 5000 Cologne 1, Federal Republic of Germany*

D. ROBERTON *Department of Immunology & University Department of Pediatrics, Adelaide Children's Hospital, South Australia 5006*

G. RONDINI *Division of Neonatal Intensive Care, IRCCS Policlinico, S. Matteo, Italy*

F. ROSSI *Unité d'Immunopathologie, INSERM U28, Hôpital Broussais, Paris, France*

B. ROWAN-KELLY *Department of Immunology & University Department of Pediatrics, Adelaide Children's Hospital, South Australia 5006*

A. SA'ADU *Immune Deficiency Diseases Research Group, Clinical Research Centre, Watford Road, Harrow HA1 3UJ, UK*

U. B. SCHAAD *Divison of Pediatric Infectious Diseases, Department of Pediatrics, University of Bern, Bern, Switzerland*

Y. SHOENFELD *Department of Medicine B, Sheba Medical Center, Tel-Hashomer, Israel 52621*

S. T. SHULMAN *Department of Pediatrics, Northwestern University Medical School, Chicago, Illinois, USA*

P. J. SPAETH *Central Laboratory, Blood Transfusion Service of the Swiss Red Cross, Bern, Switzerland*

E. R. STIEHM *Division of Immunology, UCLA Department of Pediatrics, Los Angeles, CA 90024, USA*

R. B. STRICKER *San Francisco Children's Hospital, San Francisco, California, USA*

Y. SULTAN *Laboratoire d'Hemostase, Hôpital Cochin, Paris, France*

W. L. SUTKER *Department of Internal Medicine, Baylor University Medical Center, 3500 Gaston Avenue, Dallas, Texas, USA*

Z. THAYER *Department of Paediatric Endocrinology, Prince of Wales Children's Hospital, University of New South Wales, Sydney, Australia*

Y. H. THONG *University Department of Child Health, Mater Children's Hospital, South Brisbane, Queensland, Australia*

A. G. UGAZIO *Clinica Pediatrica dell' Università, Spedali Civili, 25100 Brescia, Italy*

M. VERMEULEN *Department of Neurology, University Hospital Dijkzigt, Rotterdam, The Netherlands*

P. VEYS *Department of Haematology, The Royal Free Hospital, Pond Street, London, UK*

V. VUDDHAKUL *University Department of Child Health, Mater Children's Hospital, South Brisbane, Queensland, Australia*

D. WAKEFIELD *Departments of Immunology & Infectious Diseases, Division of Medicine; and the Mood Disorders Unit Division of Psychiatry, Prince Henry Hospital, University of New South Wales, Sydney, Australia*

A. D. B. WEBSTER *Immune Deficiency Diseases Research Group, Clinical Research Centre, Watford Road, Harrow HA1 3UJ, UK*

R. J. WEDGWOOD *Department of Pediatrics, University of Washington School of Medicine, Seattle, Washington, USA*

L. E. WEISMAN *Uniformed Services University of The Health Sciences, F. Edward Hébert School of Medicine, 4301 Jones Bridge Road, Bethesda, Maryland 20814, USA*

E. WINTON *Emory University, Atlanta, Georgia 30322, USA*

M. ZANELLO *Istituto di Anestesia e Rianimazione, Universita di Bologna, Italy*

Contents

Part I
General aspects of IVIG

Part II
Neonatal infections

Part III
Secondary immunodeficiencies and infections

Part IV
Autoimmune disorders

Part V
New/prospective indications

Part VI
Closing Remarks

Part VII
Abstracts of poster sessions

Preface

This volume is the third in a series of proceedings of conferences on intravenous immunoglobulin, held in Interlaken, Switzerland, in 1981, 1985 and 1990.

The first volume, entitled "Immunotherapy" and edited by U. Nydegger, focused on biochemical and functional characteristics of the IgG molecule and on the then new aspect of intravenous versus intramuscular use of IgG (IVIG) in substitution therapy. In addition, a few articles already announced the efficacy of IVIG in patients with disorders other than hypogammaglobulinemia, i.e. in patients with ITP. Thc second volume, "Clinical Use of Intravenous Immunoglobulins" edited by A. Morell and U. Nydegger, again summarized recent experimental research on IgG molecules and antibody activity. However, most articles were devoted to the various new clinical indications of IVIG.

The present volume now updates the clinical experiences with IVIG treatment in several new indications as well as in situations which still have to be considered experimental.

A glance at the papers organized in the six sections and at the abstracts of the poster presentations in the final chapter reveals that IVIG therapy represents not simply an antibody replacement, but also a mediator of immunomodulatory and anti-inflammatory effects in a variety of disorders. The substitution of antibodies by IVIG in primary and secondary immunodeficiencies and in neonatal infections is described in Parts I, II and III. The immunomodulatory and anti-inflammatory effects of IVIG are discussed in Part IV on autoimmune disorders and in Part V on new prospective indications. Part VI contains a comprehensive update on the use of IVIG. Finally, the different effects of IVIG are again reflected in the abstracts of the poster sessions.

Ten years have elapsed since the original challenging observation of

IVIG treatment in ITP was made. The key observation was made in a 12-year-old boy who had suffered from severe chronic ITP with life-threatening bleeding episodes in the past and who had secondary hypogammaglobulinemia due to immunosuppressive treatment (vincristine and corticosteroids) prior to IVIG administration. The dramatic platelet response in this patient prompted us to perform additional clinical studies. A pilot study in 13 children with ITP and, later on, prospective and controlled clinical trials confirmed this observation. However, the discussion on the various possible mechanisms of action of IVIG in this new indication is still ongoing. Based on intensive laboratory research several modes of action of IVIG have been proposed as a rationale for the use of IVIG in treatment of patients with other immune-related disorders.

Today, the immunomodulatory and anti-inflammatory effects of IVIG may be explained by several possibilities within the complex immunological network, such as interference with Fc receptors on cells of the reticuloendothetial system; alterations in T-cell subsets and of B-cell functions; inhibition of mediator release, e.g. cytokine secretion; feedback inhibition of mediator synthesis and binding; and finally binding of anti-idiotypic antibodies to idiotypes on the target cells. Many of these possible mechanisms may be operative simultaneously and may lead to a new balance of the immune response. Details of possible mechanisms of action of IVIG are outlined in the first three articles of Part I, but are also given in various other contributions of this volume.

I would like to thank all the authors, the chairpersons and the workshop participants and all other contributors who helped to realize this exciting meeting. Special thanks are due to Professor H. J. Heiniger, chief executive officer and president of the Central Laboratory SRC, Dr B. Perret and the administrative secretaries at the Central Laboratory, the AKM Congress Service Basel, Miss A. Caplazi, my secretary, to Sandoz Ltd, Basel for financial support and Academic Press, represented by Dr S. King, for editorial work.

The editorial work has been carried out with several colleagues, namely Drs P. De Haes, A. Morell, U. Nydegger and B. A. Perret.

P. Imbach

Part I
General aspects of IVIG

IVIG and regulation of autoimmunity through the idiotypic network

G. DIETRICH[1], F. ROSSI[1], Y. SULTAN[2], S. KAVERI[1], U. E. NYDEGGER[3] and M. D. KAZATCHKINE[1]

[1] *Unité d'Immunopathologie, INSERM U28, Hôpital Broussais, Paris, France*
[2] *Laboratoire d'Hemostase, Hôpital Cochin, Paris, France*
[3] *Division of Transfusion Medicine, Inselspital, Bern, Switzerland*

The concept of an immunoregulatory effect of intravenous immunoglobulins (IVIG) on autoimmunity has been gaining increasing interest since the first observations of a beneficial effect of IVIG in idiopathic thrombocytopenic purpura (1) and in patients with autoantibodies to factor VIII (2). The suppressive effect of IVIG on autoimmune responses opens novel therapeutic prospects and provides a new approach for understanding the basic mechanisms underlying the emergence of pathological autoimmunity. IVIG has resulted in clinical improvement and/or decrease in autoantibody titer in a number of distinct human autoimmune diseases (Table 1). Early studies have suggested that IVIG may be effective in autoimmune disorders such as peripheral autoimmune cytopenias through reversible functional blockade of Fc receptor function on cells of the reticuloendothelial system (3–5). The present chapter focuses on studies which we have developed in the last 6 years, indicating that IVIG may exert their regulatory effect in autoimmune diseases by interfering with the function of the idiotypic network.

Immunotherapy with Intravenous Immunoglobulins
ISBN 0–12–370725–0

Table 1
Beneficial effect of IVIG in human autoimmune diseases[a]

Idiopathic thrombocytopenic purpura*
Autoimmune hemolytic anemias
Autoimmune neutropenia
Autoimmune erythroblastopenia*
Myasthenia gravis*
Chronic inflammatory demyelinating polyneuropathy*
Systemic vasculitis*
Kawasaki's disease
Birdshot retinopathy*
Recurrent abortions with anti-cardiolipin antibodies
Anti-factor VIII autoimmune disease*

[a] Autoimmune diseases in which a clinical improvement and/or decrease in autoantibody titer have been established or suggested.
The asterisk denotes diseases in which *in vitro* evidence indicates the presence in IVIG of anti-idiotypes against autoantibodies.

Evidence in animals and in humans has demonstrated the existence of a physiological autoreactivity and of an autonomous activity of the immune system which uses its own diversity to regulate the expression of the actual immune repertoire (6–8). Little is known, however, about the mechanism(s) of emergence and perpetuation of pathological autoimmunity. Pathological breakdown of self-tolerance could originate from defective idiotypic network regulation of autoimmunity. In this context, IVIG, which are prepared from large plasma pools of normal donors, may be considered as representing a wide spectrum of the idiotypes and anti-idiotypes that are expressed in normal individuals and participate in the prevention of expression of abnormal autoimmune responses under physiological conditions.

Remission or recovery from autoimmune diseases may correlate with the emergence of specific anti-idiotypes against autoantibodies

Auto-anti-idiotypes which inhibit the interaction between prerecovery autoantibodies and target autoantigens are found in the plasma of patients in remission or patients who have recovered from a variety of autoimmune diseases including systemic lupus erythematosus (9), Guillain-Barré syndrome (10), anti-factor VIII autoimmune disease (11, 12), anti-fibrinogen autoimmune disease (13), myasthenia gravis

(14) and systemic vasculitis with anti-neutrophil cytoplasmic antigen autoantibodies (15). Auto-anti-idiotypes are of the IgG and/or the IgM isotype (9–15). The antibodies may arise spontaneously or in patients receiving immunosuppressive therapy. Anti-idiotypes that occur in post-recovery sera from patients with Guillain-Barré syndrome and patients with anti-factor VIII autoimmune disease, recognize cross-reactive idiotypes on autoantibodies (10, 11). These observations suggest that remission of autoimmune diseases in which autoantibodies play a pathogenic role, may be associated with autologous suppression of autoantibodies through the idiotypic network. Regulatory auto-anti-idiotypes may preferentially be directed against cross-reactive idiotypes on autoantibodies.

Suppression of autoimmune responses by IVIG may depend on the presence in IVIG of specific anti-idiotypes against autoantibodies

Our initial studies involved patients with anti-factor VIII autoantibodies in whom infusion of IVIG resulted in a 95% decrease of autoantibody titer within 24–48 h (2). The suppressive effect of IVIG was observed for over 5 years, indicating that IVIG altered the synthesis of pathological autoantibodies. The rapid fall in autoantibody titer following infusion of IVIG suggested that IVIG could directly interact with circulating autoantibodies and led to the *in vitro* demonstration of the presence of specific anti-idiotypes against anti-factor VIII autoantibodies in IVIG (2, 11, 16, 17). The finding in IVIG of specific anti-idiotypes against autoantibodies was then extended to a number of disease-related autoantibodies, including antibodies to DNA, thyroglobulin, intrinsic factor (18, 19), peripheral nerve (10), neutrophil cytoplasmic antigens (15) and platelet gp IIb IIIa (20).

Four lines of evidence demonstrate the presence in IVIG of anti-idiotypes against autoantibodies:

1. $F(ab')_2$ fragments from IVIG inhibit the binding of autoantibodies to autoantigens and/or neutralize the functional activity of autoantibodies (22) (Table 2).
2. $F(ab')_2$ fragments containing autoantibody activity are specifically retained on affinity columns of Sepharose-bound $F(ab')_2$ fragments from IVIG (Table 3).
3. IVIG do not contain detectable anti-allotypes against the most common allotypic determinants expressed in the $F(ab')_2$ region of human IgG (16).

Table 2
Inhibition of autoantibody activity by $F(ab')_2$ fragments from IVIG[a]

Autoantibody	Maximal inhibition (%)	Autoantibody/$F(ab')_2$ of IVIG (mole/mole)[c]
Anti-factor VIII	100	0.450
Anti-thyroglobulin	61	0.090
Anti-DNA	96	2.900
Anti-peripheral nerve[b]	82	0.001
Anti-intrinsic factor	36	6.670
Anti-neutrophil cytoplasmic antigen	74	0.080

[a] $F(ab')_2$ fragments of IVIG (Sandoglobulin®) were incubated with $F(ab')_2$ fragments, IgG, or IgM containing autoantibody activity for 1 h at 37°C and overnight at 4°C. Residual anti-DNA anti-thyroglobulin, anti-intrinsic factor and anti-neutrophil cytoplasmic antigen activities were quantitated by an ELISA. Residual anti-factor VIII activity was measured using a functional coagulation assay. Anti-peripheral nerve activity was assessed by an indirect immunofluorescence.
[b] Antibodies against the NBL 108 cc 15 cell line (21).
[c] Molar ratio between autoantibody and $F(ab')_2$ from IVIG at maximal inhibition of autoantibody activity was observed.

Table 3
Chromatography of IgG or $F(ab')_2$ fragments containing autoantibody activity on Sepharose-bound $F(ab')_2$ fragments from IVIG[a]

Autoantibody	Specific autoantibody activity	
	Loaded	Acid-eluted
Anti-factor VIII $F(ab')_2$	0.8 BU[b]/mg	38.09 BU/mg
Anti-thyroglobulin $F(ab')_2$	1.26 U[c]/mg	18.20 U/mg
Anti-DNA IgG	0.31 U/mg	10.80 U/mg
Anti-intrinsic factor IgG	3.22 U/mg	4.32 U/mg
Anti-neutrophil cytoplasmic antigen IgG	1.12 U/μg	5.40 U/μg

[a] IgG or $F(ab')_2$ fragments containing autoantibody activity were chromatographed on Sepharose-bound $F(ab')_2$ fragments from IVIG. The columns were washed until no protein was found in the effluent and then eluted at pH 2.8. Autoantibody activity was measured in the loaded material and in the acid-eluted fractions. The finding of an enriched specific autoantibody activity in the acid-eluate as compared with the loaded material indicates that autoantibodies are specifically bound by IVIG through idiotypic determinants.
[b] Bethesda units.
[c] Arbitrary units.

4. Anti-idiotypes in IVIG recognize idiotypic determinants of autoantibodies that are also the targets of heterologous anti-idiotypic antibodies. Thus, IVIG were found to compete with monoclonal or polyclonal specific anti-idiotypic reagents for the binding to anti-factor VIII (17) and to anti-thyroglobulin (19) autoantibodies. The target idiotypes on autoantibodies were either binding-site related (17) or of the alpha type (i.e. outside the antibody combining site of antibodies (19) (Fig. 1).

We have recently found that IVIG recognize a cross-reactive α idiotype (termed T44) on anti-thyroglobulin autoantibodies from patients with Hashimoto's disease. The idiotype was defined by a

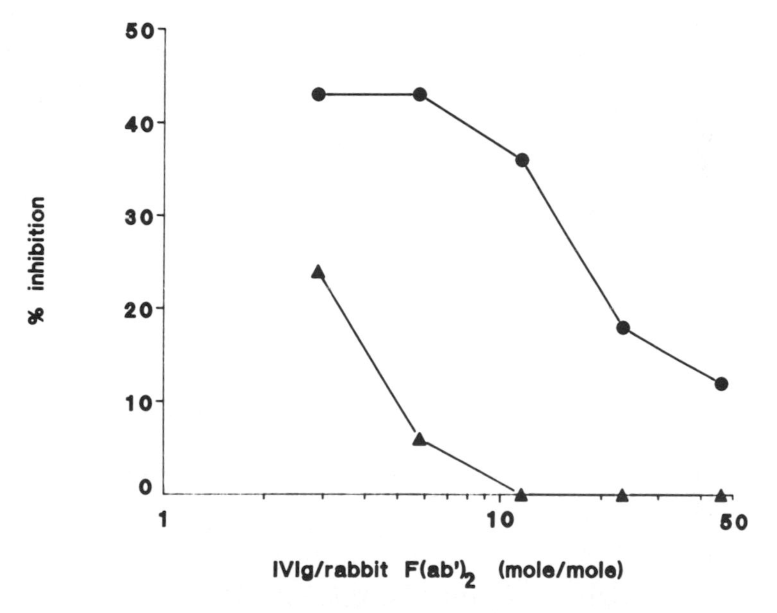

Figure 1. Increasing concentrations of F(ab')$_2$ fragments of rabbit anti-idiotypic IgG (anti-T44) directed against a human anti-thyroglobulin autoantibody from a patient with Hashimoto's disease, were incubated with IVIG (Sandoglobulin®) in microtiter wells coated with affinity-purified patient's anti-thyroglobulin F(ab')$_2$ fragments. Bound IVIG was detected using peroxidase-labeled goat anti-human Fcγ antibody. Dose-dependent inhibition of the binding of IVIG to anti-thyroglobulin F(ab')$_2$ fragments by rabbit anti-T44 F(ab')$_2$ fragments, indicates that anti-T44 antibody and IVIG share anti-idiotypic specificities against the same or overlapping determinants on patient's anti-thyroglobulin autoantibodies. Competitive binding with rabbit anti-T44 F(ab')$_2$ fragments: ●—●. Competitive binding with F(ab')$_2$ fragments of normal rabbit IgG: ▲—▲. (Reproduced from reference 19 by copyright permission of the American Society for Clinical Investigation.)

rabbit anti-idiotypic antibody raised against affinity-purified anti-thyroglobulin $F(ab')_2$ fragments of IgG from a patient with autoimmune thyroiditis (see Fig. 1 legend). The idiotype was expressed on anti-thyroglobulin IgG of eight out of nine patients with Hashimoto's disease but on no IgG of five healthy individuals that were tested. Anti-thyroglobulin autoantibodies expressing the T44 idiotype exhibited a restricted epitopic specificity against human thyroglobulin (23). The antigenic cluster of human thyroglobulin recognized by $T44^+$ autoantibodies was previously found to be the exclusive target of disease-associated anti-thyroglobulin autoantibodies, as opposed to anti-thyroglobulin antibodies from healthy individuals (24).

Cross-reactive idiotypes are expressed on human autoantibodies of various specificities (14, 25–28), suggesting that these idiotypes originate from a potential repertoire that is shared by a large number of non-related individuals, but which would not be expressed in healthy individuals, due to specific anti-idiotypic suppression. Cross-reactive idiotypes potentially represent the privileged targets for immunomodulatory therapy. The presence in IVIG of anti-idiotypes against disease-specific cross-reactive idiotypes of autoantibodies may indeed reflect the presence in normal human IgG of anti-idiotypes that control expression of the autoimmune repertoire.

Taken together the presence of anti-idiotypes against autoantibodies in therapeutic IVIG preparations and in remission sera from patients who recovered from autoimmune diseases, led us to speculate that the beneficial effect observed with IVIG in antibody-mediated autoimmune diseases mimicks the regulatory mechanisms leading to autologous suppression of autoimmunity in healthy individuals (22). In this respect, therapy with IVIG may be viewed as "immunorestoration" of a functional physiological idiotypic network (29).

Origin of anti-idiotypes in IVIG

IVIG contain $F(ab')_2$–$F(ab')_2$ dimers which are the consequence of idiotypic complementarity between immunoglobulins in the pool (30–32). As the number of donors participating in a pool of IVIG increases, the proportion of dimers also increases (30), indicating that the probability of a pool to express a given anti-idiotype increases with the size of the pool. Thus, it is likely that the idiotypic repertoire of IVIG from different commercial sources prepared from large pools of plasma from over 10 000 donors would be almost similar. The relative amount of anti-idiotypes directed against a private idiotype should, however, be lower in a given IVIG preparation than that of anti-idiotypes against cross-reactive idiotypes. Thus, IVIG preparations could differ in their relative ability to interact with specific idiotypes, which may be of clinical relevance in patients in whom infusion of a particular brand of IVIG has been inefficient.

We have also considered the possibility that some of the donors contributing to the pool of IVIG are privileged donors of specific anti-idiotypes against autoantibodies. These could be individuals who spontaneously recovered from overt or subclinical autoimmune disease. A relative predominance of specific anti-idiotypes against autoantibodies to factor VIII has also been found among aged donors (33).

Regulatory effect of IVIG on the function of the idiotypic network

The molecular and cellular basis and the dynamics of the interaction of IVIG with the idiotypic network are not yet fully understood. Idiotypic interactions occur between immunoglobulins in IVIG. IVIG also interacts through idiotypic interactions with natural human polyreactive IgM antibodies secreted by Epstein-Barr virus (EBV)-transformed normal human B cells (34), indicating that anti-idiotypic IgG originating from the normal actual repertoire may interfere with the expression of idiotypes belonging to the potential B cell repertoire (which is explored by studying EBV-transformed B cells). These observations indicate that IVIG do not act by simply providing the autoimmune patient with a source of neutralizing anti-idiotypes. Rather, IVIG may interfere with the function, the basic structure and the dynamics (see below) of the network.

It is still not known whether disease-associated autoantibodies represent an abnormal expansion of non-somatically mutated natural autoreactive clones or mutated clones. It is also unclear whether the basic perturbation in the network which allows the emergence of pathological autoimmunity is restricted to the regulatory mechanisms which control the expression of organ-specific autoantibodies or whether it affects the structure of the entire network. Preliminary evidence in humans and in mice supports the hypothesis of a generalized perturbation of the network in organ-specific and in systemic autoimmune conditions (35). In this regard, the intrinsic complexity of IVIG would provide a more logical rationale for immunoregulatory therapy of autoimmune disease than idiotype-specific suppression.

Summary

This chapter briefly reviews the evidence demonstrating the presence in intravenous immunoglobulins (IVIG) of anti-idiotypes directed against a variety of human disease-associated autoantibodies. Some of the target idiotypes are cross-reactive idiotypes. IVIG may also bind through idiotypic interactions to elements of the natural immune network, e.g. to natural IgM autoantibodies secreted by EBV-transformed normal peripheral blood B cells from healthy individuals and to "natural" IgG autoantibodies present in IVIG. We suggest that IVIG interferes with the structure and the function of the idiotypic network. IVIG may suppress pathological autoimmune responses by restoring a physiological immune network and imposing a normal behaviour on the pathological immune system of patients with autoimmune diseases.

Acknowledgements

The secretarial assistance of Nicole Levée and Annick Vioux is gratefully acknowledged.

References

1. Imbach, P., Barandun, S., d'Apuzzo, V. *et al.* High-dose intravenous gammaglobulin for idiopathic thrombocytopenic purpura in childhood. *Lancet* 1: 1228; 1981.
2. Sultan, Y., Kazatchkine, M. D., Maisonneuve, P. and Nydegger, U. E. Anti-idiotypic suppression of autoantibodies to factor VIII (antihaemophilic factor) by high-dose intravenous gammaglobulin. *Lancet* 2: 765; 1984.
3. Schmidt, R. E., Budde, V., Schäfer, G. and Stroehmann, I. High-dose intravenous gammaglobulin for idiopathic thrombocytopenic purpura. *Lancet* 2: 475; 1981.
4. Fehr, J., Hofmann, V. and Kappeler, U. Transient reversal of thrombocytopenia in idiopathic thrombocytopenic purpura by high-dose intravenous gammaglobulin. *N. Engl. J. Med.* **306**: 1254; 1982.
5. Saleh, M., Court, W., Huster, W. *et al.* Effect of commercial immunoglobulin G preparation on human monocyte Fc-receptor dependent binding of antibody coated platelets. *Br. J. Haemat.* **68**: 47; 1988.
6. Jerne, N. K. Towards a network theory of the immune system. *Ann. Immunol. (Inst. Pasteur)* 125C: 373; 1974.

7. Zanetti, M. Self-immunity and the autoimmune network: A molecular perspective to ontogeny and regulation of the immune system. *Ann. Immunol. (Inst. Pasteur)* 139: 619; 1988.
8. Coutinho, A. Beyond clonal selection and network. *Immunol. Rev.* 110: 63; 1989.
9. Zouali, M. and Eyquem, A. Idiotypic-anti-idiotypic interactions in systemic lupus erythematosus: demonstration of oscillating levels of anti-DNA antibodies and reciprocal anti-idiotypic activity in a single patient. *Ann. Immunol. (Inst. Pasteur)* 134C: 377; 1983.
10. Van Doorn, P. A., Rossi, F., Brand, A. *et al.* On the mechanism of high dose intravenous immunoglobulin treatment of patients with chronic inflammatory demyelinating polyneuropathy. *J. Neuroimmunol.* 29: 57; 1990.
11. Sultan, Y., Rossi, F. and Kazatchkine, M. D. Recovery from anti-VIII:C (antihemophilic factor) autoimmune disease is dependent on generation of anti-idiotypes against anti-VIII:C autoantibodies. *Proc. Natl. Acad. Sci. USA* 84: 828; 1987.
12. Tiarks, C., Pechet, L. and Humphreys, R. E. Development of anti-idiotypic antibodies in a patient with a Factor VIII autoantibody. *Am. J. Hematol.* 32: 217; 1989.
13. Ruiz-Arguelles, A. Spontaneous reversal of acquired autoimmune dys-fibrinogenemia probably due to an anti-idiotypic antibody directed to an interspecies cross-reactive idiotype expressed on anti-fibrinogen antibodies. *J. Clin. Invest.* 82: 958; 1988.
14. Lefvert, A. K. Idiotypes and anti-idiotypes of human autoantibodies to the acetylcholine receptor in myasthenia gravis. *Monogr. Allergy* 22: 57; 1987.
15. Rossi, F., Jayne, D. R. W., Lockwood, C. M. and Kazatchkine, M. D. Anti-idiotypes against anti-neutrophil cytoplasmic antigen autoanti-bodies in normal human polyspecific IgG for therapeutic use and in the remission serum of patients with systemic vasculitis. *Clin. Exp. Immunol.* (In press.)
16. Rossi, F., Sultan, Y. and Kazatchkine, M. D. Anti-idiotypes against autoantibodies and alloantibodies to VIII:C (anti-haemophilic factor) are present in therapeutic polyspecific normal immunoglobulins. *Clin. Exp. Immunol.* 74: 311; 1988.
17. Dietrich, G., Pereira, P., Algiman, M. *et al.* A monoclonal anti-idiotypic antibody against the antigen-combining site of anti-factor VIII autoantibodies defines an idiotope that is recognized by normal human polyspecific immunoglobulins for therapeutic use (IVIG). *J. Autoimmunity* (In press.)
18. Rossi, F. and Kazatchkine, M. D. Anti-idiotypes against autoantibodies in pooled normal human polyspecific Ig. *J. Immunol.* 143: 4104; 1989.
19. Dietrich, G. and Kazatchkine, M. D. Normal immunoglobulin G (IgG) for therapeutic use (intravenous Ig) contain antiidiotypic specificities

against an immunodominant, disease-associated, cross-reactive idiotype of human anti-thyroglobulin autoantibodies. *J. Clin. Invest.* **85**: 620; 1990.
20. Berchtold, P., Dale, G. L., Tani, P. and McMillan, R. Inhibition of autoantibody binding to platelet glycoprotein IIb/IIIa by anti-idiotypic antibodies in intravenous gammaglobulin. *Blood* **74**: 2414; 1989.
21. Van Doorn, P. A., Brand, A. and Vermeulen, M. Anti-neuroblastoma cell line antibodies in inflammatory demyelinating polyneuropathy. *Neurology* **38**: 1592; 1988.
22. Rossi, F., Dietrich, G. and Kazatchkine, M. D. Anti-idiotypes against autoantibodies in normal immunoglobulins: Evidence for network regulation of human autoimmune responses. *Immunol. Rev.* **110**: 135; 1989.
23. Dietrich, G., Piechaczyk, M., Pau, B. and Kazatchkine, M. D. Restricted idiotypic and epitopic specificity of anti-thyroglobulin autoantibodies in patients with autoimmune thyroiditis. *Eur. J. Immunol.* (In press.)
24. Piechaczyk, M., Bouanani, M., Salhi, S. L., Baldet, L., Bastide, M., Pau, B. and Bastide, J. M. Antigenic domains on the human thyroglobulin molecule recognized by autoantibodies in patients' sera and by natural autoantibodies isolated from sera of healthy subjects. *Clin. Immunol. Immunopathol.* **45**: 114; 1987.
25. De la fuente, B. and Hoyer, L. W. The idiotypic characteristics of human antibodies to factor VIII. *Blood* **64**: 672; 1984.
26. Shoenfeld, Y., Isenberg, D. A., Rauch, J. *et al.* Idiotypic cross-reactions of monoclonal human lupus autoantibodies. *J. Exp. Med.* **158**: 718; 1983.
27. Matsuyama, T., Fukumori, J. and Tanaka, H. Evidence of unique idiotypic determinants and similar idiotypic determinants on human anti-thyroglobulin antibodies. *Clin. Exp. Immunol.* **51**: 381; 1983.
28. Fong, S., Chen, P. P., Gilbertson, T. A. *et al.* Expression of three cross-reactive idiotypes on rheumatoid factor autoantibodies from patients with autoimmune diseases and seropositive adults. *J. Immunol.* **137**: 122; 1986.
29. Kazatchkine, M. D., Dietrich, G. and Rossi, F. Intravenous immunoglobulins and autoimmune disease. *Immunol. Today*. (In press.)
30. Tankersley, D. L., Preston, M. S. and Finlayson, J. S. Immunoglobulin G dimer: an idiotype-anti-idiotype complex. *Mol. Immunol.* **25**: 41; 1988.
31. Gronski, P., Bauer, R., Bodenbender, L. *et al.* On the nature of IgG dimers. I and II. *Behring Inst. Milt.* **82**: 127; 1988.
32. Roux, K. H. and Tankersley, D. L. A view of the human idiotypic repertoire: Electron microscopic and immunologic analyses of spontaneous idiotype-anti-idiotype dimers in pooled human IgG. *J. Immunol.* **144**: 1387; 1990.

33. Dietrich, G., Algiman, M., Rossi, F., Sultan, Y. and Kazatchkine, M. D. Origin of antiidiotypes in normal polyspecific immunoglobulins for therapeutic use. Joint meeting of the Dutch and French Societies of Immunology, Abstract p 200; 1990.
34. Rossi, F., Guilbert, B., Tonnelle, C., Fumoux, G., Avrameas, S. and Kazatchkine, M. D. Idiotypic interactions between normal human polyspecific IgG and natural IgM antibodies. *Eur. J. Immunol.* 20: 2089–2094; 1990.
35. Varela, F., Anderson, A., Dietrich, G., Sundblat, A., Holmberg, D., Kazatchkine, M. D. and Coutinho, A. The population dynamics of antibodies in normal and autoimmune individuals. *Proc. Natl Acad. Sci. USA*. (In press.)

Discussion

G. Gaedicke

If you treat a child with autoimmune thrombocytopenia with an Fab-fragmented preparation you won't experience any increase of thrombocyte count in your patient. Using an intact gammaglobulin, however, you'll observe a dramatic response. If the anti-idiotype mechanism plays an important role I would expect a response to therapy with a Fab-fragmented preparation as well.

M. D. Kazatchkine

There is *in vivo* and *in vitro* evidence that IVIG may, at least in part, be effective in peripheral autoimmune cytopenias through functional and reversible blockade of Fc receptors on splenic macrophages. Autoimmune thrombocytopenias are heterogeneous. Few examples so far have been reported in which an autoantibody should be characterized as being directed against (a) platelet membrane antigen(s) and as being prevented from binding to its autoantigen by $F(ab')_2$ fragments from IVIG. Thus, although anti-idiotypic suppression by IVIG may be operative in immune thrombocytopenia, or subgroups of ITP, this disease may indeed not be the best *in vivo* model to illustrate the regulatory effect of IVIG on the idiotypic network. In our experience, patients with ITP frequently respond to veinoglobulin, a preparation of IVIG which contains fragmented IgG.

R. Seger

1. After a single dose of IVIG to a patient with anti-factor VIII, how long does the inhibition of autoantibody activity last? Which cellular processes explain this period? Is the length of the period dose-dependent?
2. Can high-dose IVIG block autoantibody synthesis as opposed to autoantibody activity? For how long?

M. D. Kazatchkine
The duration of autoantibody suppression and of the clinical improvement that may be seen following infusion of IVIG varies with the nature of the disease and with the individual patient. In the two patients with anti-factor VIII antibodies whom we had treated in 1984, the autoantibody titer has now remained below 10% of pretreatment titer for over 6 years. In patients treated with IVIG for chronic inflammatory demyelinating polyneuropathy, the improvement is usually observed for periods of time ranging between 10 days and 3 weeks (van Doorn, 1990). I would not expect the length of duration of suppression to be related to the amount of infused IVIG.
We believe that IVIG interferes with autoantibody synthesis since suppression of autoimmune response following infusion of IVIG may indeed be prolonged and since evidence that I have discussed suggests that IVIG interferes with the function of the immune network. There is, however, only little evidence so far that IVIG may down-regulate auto-antibody synthesis *in vitro*.

R. Schiff
Is there evidence that IVIG has antibody that interacts with idiotypic sites on T-cell receptors? This could be a mechanism of specifically interacting with T-helper cells.

M. D. Kazatchkine
There is no direct evidence yet that IVIG recognizes idiotypic determinants on T-cell receptors.

Intravenous immunoglobulin: mechanisms of action and their clinical application

A. C. NEWLAND,[1] M. G. MACEY[1] and P. A. VEYS[2]

[1] *Department of Haematology, The London Hospital, Whitechapel, London, UK*
[2] *Department of Haematology, The Royal Free Hospital, Pond Street, London, UK*

Background

The accepted use of intravenous immunoglobulin (IVIG) is for antibody replacement in immunodeficiency states for the prevention and treatment of infectious disease. The availability of sufficient quantities of safe IgG preparations has established their importance and superiority over intramuscular preparations in the primary immunodeficiencies (1), and current studies suggest that they may have equal importance in the secondary immunodeficiency states (2) as well. Their value in the prevention and treatment of infection in the non-immune-suppressed host remains to be established, although anecdotal reports and studies on experimental septicemia in laboratory animals suggests that this may be the case (3).

The increasing clinical use of IVIG for immune modulation is more controversial and harder to justify. In the immune cytopenias a clinical response is seen in the majority of patients treated and in certain disorders of platelet destruction, for example post-transfusion purpura

Immunotherapy with Intravenous Immunoglobulins
ISBN 0–12–370725–0

and neonatal alloimmune thrombocytopenia, IVIG is arguably the treatment of choice (4). However, in others, particularly the immune thrombocytopenias (ITP), although there is an undoubted clinical effect, lack of controlled studies have obscured its role in early elective treatment. In the other immune cytopenias, hemolytic anemia and neutropenia, a response is usually less common and more transient than in ITP but in some clinical settings may be of value. In the organ-specific antibody-mediated disorders the response is often purely a laboratory phenomenon, reflected in a change in antibody level, and may lack clinical relevance (5).

Such a diversity of clinical responses does allow, however, close study of the mechanisms of action. Preliminary observations suggest several diverse and independent effects including impaired phagocyte function, reduced natural killer function and depression of antibody formation. The identification of the elements in IgG responsible for the activity may lead to the development of more specific products from IVIG with more utility in the treatment of this group of disorders.

Thrombocytopenic purpura

A brief review of the response of ITP to IVIG illustrates the diversity of effect. Imbach originally reported the response in seven children with chronic and six with acute ITP to 2 g/kg of IgG over 5 days. All responded within 24 h with normalization of the count. Six (including one with chronic disease) maintained normal counts without further treatment. Six of the remainder could be maintained with further infusions. These results were subsequently confirmed in adults, who were much less likely than children to develop spontaneous remission and in whom, therefore, the result could be directly related to the infusion of IgG (6). In addition, in this group of adults nine out of nineteen with steroid refractory disease within six months of presentation had a long-term remission (greater than 20 months). This was not seen in the group with chronic disease (greater than six months) in whom the response was little more than 20 days.

Studies in chronic adults, however, suggest that continuing exposure to IVIG may eventually lead to a long-term response. In a study of 37 patients in whom long-term maintenance therapy was given 17 (46%) eventually achieved a remission and no longer required therapy but received in the process a mean total dose of 515 g of IVIG (7).

A similar observation was made in children by Imbach in a

multicenter study of 108 previously untreated children with acute ITP. Although the initial response to steroids or IVIG was identical, in those requiring more than the initial course fewer proceeded to chronicity in the group receiving IgG. In addition, in a further 42 with steroid-resistant disease 50% ultimately responded long term to IVIG (8). These and other studies suggest a dual method of response, the initial reaction which commences within 24–48 h of the infusion and is often transient, and a longer term response that may last months but often requires recurrent infusions over a 3–6 month period to achieve. This accords with the suspected mechanisms of action and can be utilized in considering optimum treatment schedules.

Although the results are striking and reflect an alteration in the natural history of the disease, considerable debate as to which patients should be given IVIG remains. There are certain indications where it is useful, such as severe ITP when the count needs to be rapidly elevated; pre-operatively; in the third trimester of pregnancy and in the thrombocytopenic neonate. In contrast, its use in the child with acute ITP and in the adult with long-standing ITP remains unclear. An understanding of the mechanisms of action, however, may allow IgG to be incorporated in first-line protocols in a more rational manner. In addition it may also aid the development of specific product that is more precise in its effects and less cumbersome to administer. The apparent effect on the natural history of the disease with the long-term reduction in chronicity should encourage further studies.

Mononuclear phagocyte system blockade

Blockade with down-regulation of phagocyte function appears to be important in the short-term rapid increase in the platelet count in ITP. Fehr and co-workers (9) infused radiolabeled, antibody-coated autologous erythrocytes before and after IVIG and were able to show that clearance of their opsonized cells was inhibited. They suggested that mononuclear phagocyte system (MPS) blockade with subsequent inhibition of the binding and destruction of antibody/immune complex-coated platelets was mediated via the Fc receptor system. Subsequent studies using a monoclonal antibody to the Fc receptor (10) (FcRIII) confirmed that specific Fc blockade was responsible for the platelet increment. IVIG contains small amounts of dimers and aggregates (11) and it is also probable that following interaction with circulating antigen immune complexes will be produced. These, after binding to Fc receptors, are phagocytosed, because of multipoint attachment, with internalization and loss of Fc receptor expression contributing to, if not causing, the blockade.

In vitro studies of the binding of IVIG to paraformaldehyde-fixed granulocytes reveals that IgG binds specifically and that it is aggregates rather than monomeric IgG that is bound. With the specific binding, there is a reduction in expression of membrane FcRIII; FcRII expression is not altered. FcRIII is known, however, to have only a low affinity for monomeric IgG, binding complexed or aggregated IgG, and ultracentrifugation at 80 000 *g*, while not altering the total protein content of the IVIG, reduces the complexed IgG and subsequent binding to granulocytes (12). Observations *in vitro* show that patients with ITP receiving IVIG have a transient margination neutropenia in proportion to the degree of platelet increment (13). Results using monoclonal blocking show that FcRIII bind the majority of these aggregates without activation of the neutrophil. Once these have been completely blocked with reduced expression, binding to FcRII occurs which activates the cell causing expression of adhesive molecules and margination (14).

The role of the neutrophil in removal of antibody-coated platelets *in vivo*, however, remains uncertain. As the neutrophil mass is a large proportion of the MPS the neutropenia *per se* may be important or the reduced Fc expression may be a marker to a similar phenomenon in the remainder of the phagocyte system. That this is reflected in the function of the cells is demonstrated by *in vitro* studies of neutrophil phagocytosis. Following IVIG impaired function is invariably demonstrated with reduced uptake of antibody-coated platelets and opsonized bacteria (15). Thus there is a demonstrable qualitative and quantitative defect in MPS. This effect is short-lived, however, and most studies suggest it rarely extends beyond 4 weeks.

Immune modulation

The clinical response observed in many of the reports of IVIG, particularly those relating to adult immune thrombocytopenia, point to an alteration in the natural history of the disease (6, 7) following the infusion. The effects outlast those of MPS blockade and suggest a down-regulation of immunological reactivity; the subsequent reduction in autoantibody production may herald a return to immune "homeostasis". This regulation may be multifactorial, as many different events have been observed, including stimulation of suppression (16), reduced natural killer function, interference with antigen presntation by down-modulaton of Fc receptors (17) and regulation of the idiotype network (18).

Which of these mechanisms is predominant in immunomodulation is unclear although it is likely that each contributes. It is also unclear which element of the IVIG infused mediates the effect, although there are several candidates. The Fc portion of the molecule is known to non-specifically induce suppressor cell function (16) but lymphocyte subset studies suggest this may not be relevant. Similarly, certain types of immunoglobulin preparations contain antibodies that bind to HLA class II bearing cells and may block their activity (19). It is doubtful, however, whether currently available commercial products contain sufficient antibody of these specificities to be effective.

Apart from the modulation of Fc function with its global effect of the immune system, the most convincing *in vivo* evidence lies in the manipulation of the idiotype network. The importance of anti-idiotypic activity has been shown most clearly in acquired hemophilia (10) where Kazatchkine and his colleagues have examined idiotype–anti-idiotype interactions. Using two different preparations of IVIG they were able to suppress anti-factor VIII (VIII:C) activity and anti-factor VIII-C antibodies *in vivo* and *in vitro*. More importantly the $F(ab')_2$ fragments from the polymeric IgG inhibited the $F(ab')_2$ portion of the anti-factor VIII-C obtained from the plasma of the patients. In those patients in whom the activity was not suppressed no binding of anti-factor VIII-C to Sepharose-bound IgG was demonstrated. These results suggested that the IVIG contained anti-idiotype activity against both allo- and autoantibodies to VIII-C. These observations have been confirmed by several groups. The same group has also demonstrated anti-idiotype activity in IVIG against the immunodominant, disease-associated autoantibodies in eight out of nine patients with autoimmune thyroiditis (20), confirming that this is not an isolated phenomenon. Similar mechanisms have been postulated for the response seen in other antibody-mediated disorders, such as myasthenia gravis, Guillain-Barré syndrome and pemphigus, in addition to the immune cytopenias.

The effector mechanism by which the anti-idiotype antibodies modulate the immune process is unclear. It may be via Ag–Ab neutralization, but there is convincing evidence of an effect on lymphocyte numbers and function directly.

Several studies have examined the effect on lymphocyte subsets. In general these demonstrate a reduction in the CD4/CD8 ratio with an increase in the relative proportion of CD8-positive cells (21, 22). In the same studies the secretion of IgG *in vitro* by pokeweed mitogen was decreased as well as a non-specific decrease *in vivo* of various autoantibodies. The variable change in the ratio correlated significantly with the clinical response to IVIG. A more detailed study of CD4 subsets during treatment showed a closer correlation with a reduction in the $CD4^+$ $CD32^+$ (helper/inducer) subset, suggesting that the reduction in specific antibody synthesis may be a result of reduced T-cell help for B-cell immunoglobulin synthesis (13). Similar observations have been made in the acute febrile illness of childhood, in which coronary artery aneurysms occur, known as Kawasaki syndrome. It is associated with characteristic abnormalities of immune regulation, and following IVIG fever is reduced with alteration in T-cell subsets and down-regulation of the polyclonal B-cell activation (23).

The activity of natural killer (NK) cells may also be increased in ITP as well as in several other autoimmune disorders. IVIG will reduce NK activity in normal donors in a dose-dependent fashion and our studies show that in ITP, following an infusion of 2 g over 5 days NK cell numbers drop from a pretreatment mean of 0.19 to 0.11×10^9/l with a concomitant fall-off in function. This effect may be due to the presence of FcRIII on NK cells which may be activated following IVIG, affecting cell migration and consequently circulating numbers. The effect of this in disease activity is unknown.

Discussion

The use of IVIG is now established in the management of immunodeficiency syndromes for straightforward antibody replacement. In the primary deficiencies early use will prevent the chronic sinopulmonary infections that are responsible for much of the morbidity and early mortality in the group (1). There is also increasing evidence that adequate replacement is beneficial in the secondary immunodeficiencies, including chronic lymphatic leukemia (CLL) (24), bone marrow transplantation (2) and in children with AIDS (25), although this is by no means a universal finding. In some of these latter conditions changes may be seen in the cellular elements of the blood in addition to the improvement in infection rate. In CLL this may be simply a reduction in absolute B-cell numbers but following HIV infection immune-modulation may be seen with restoration of T-suppressor function (26).

These observations reflect the fact that the intravenous infusion of large amounts of polymeric immunoglobulin achieves more than simple antibody replacement and may have a profound influence on the cellular elements within blood and the lympho-reticular system. In part this may only reflect shifts of cells within the body compartments but often also reflects qualitative changes in cellular function. These in their turn affect the body's ability to capture, process and respond to antigenic stimuli and are associated with subtle changes in the immune response which may be beneficial, although often transient, in antibody-mediated autoimmune disorders. In those disorders which manifest a peripheral cytopenia there may also be a rapid cessation in peripheral cellular destruction with normalization, or near-normalization, of the clinical defect. It is possible that these effects are due to different mechanisms and may, therefore, be additive and could be exploited in future treatment strategies and in the development of new therapeutic materials.

Disordered immune function has been described as the underlying abnormality in autoimmune disease and some workers have demonstrated T-cell dysfunction in ITP which may be corrected by IVIG (27). As discussed, however, it remains unclear which element in IgG is responsible for the effects, and whether it is a non-specific effect of the molecule or whether it reflects direct anti-idiotype activity. Both B- and T-lymphocyte function may be affected by intact IgG, an effect that is not reproduced by $F(ab')_2$ fragments alone. However, the work of Kazatchkine clearly demonstrates the effect of $F(ab')_2$ fragments in two disorders of autoimmunity (18, 20). These responses may be due *in vivo* to either neutralization of antibody or a direct cellular effect causing reduced antibody synthesis. Our own observations (13) confirm that the T independent response of B lymphocytes is impaired by IgG, suggesting a direct cellular effect, and Moffatt and co-workers (28) have shown that in acquired hemophilia response is sometimes but not always accompanied by the neutralization described by Kazatchkine. These observations suggest that the response may be humoral or cellular and in the latter it may be via the T-cell system or a direct B-cell effect.

Between 4000 and 6000 donors are used to prepare each batch; 1 g of IgG having approximately 10×10^6 different antibody specificities. The data presented suggest that such pooled product contains naturally occurring anti-idiotype activity and this may be exploited in correcting the defect that has arisen in the development of diseases of autoantibody formation. Such described responses fulfil Jernes' network theory of autoimmunity (29) and are in keeping with the observation that autoantibodies from many patients with autoimmune disease react with IgG in pooled donor immunoglobulin (30).

The postulated idiotype–anti-idiotype reaction cannot, however, explain the immediate response seen in the cytopenias and it is likely that the mechanism is completely different. The concept of Fc blockade and modulation is now clearly proven and is the likely candidate for the immediate response. FcRIII blockade closely follows the clinical response and is primarily due to the binding of dimers and immune complexes (14). The effect lasts until the blockade is overcome, which following a 5-day course of IVIG rarely exceeds 24 days. Any long-term response will be due to concurrent, but separate, immune modulation. These two basic mechanisms can account for the majority of the clinical effects described; the influence of the effect on NK function and the suppression of the inflammatory response with reduced IL1 production remains unclear.

Such observation can be exploited in planning treatment strategies and perhaps in the development of new therapeutic materials. In the reversal of peripheral cytopenia due to immune destruction, short intense courses need to be devised, perhaps employing product that is dimeric rather than monomeric. The analogy is seen in the response following intramuscular IgG or anti-D immunoglobulin when these are diluted and given intravenously, as these contain significant quantities of polymerized IgG. The polymeric products, with their ability to activate complement, in general, need to be avoided. However, in the organ-specific antibody-mediated disease the need is for long-term immune suppression with restoration of "immune homeostasis". In the short term, intense treatment may be ineffective, or at best transient, and long-term infusions may be needed as has been demonstrated in ITP (7). The production for these of a product with anti-idiotype activity with intra-species cross-reactivity would be of value, reducing the complexity if not the expense of treatment.

In summary we are now much clearer as to the mechanisms of action of IVIG and their associations with the response in the different disease states. Unfortunately, except in the role of antibody substitution, we are no nearer either exploiting these for therapeutic gain or understanding the place of IVIG as an early, specific treatment in autoimmune disease.

Summary

Over the last decade the mechanisms of action of intravenous immunoglobulin (IVIG) have become much clearer. Several mechanisms are important and appear to operate simultaneously. In particular, there is a rapid, short term blockade of phagocyte function with a later down-regulation of immunological activity. The observations on the clinical effects of IVIG have developed independently of these studies. Although IVIG has developed empirically an established place in the management of the immune thrombocytopenias (ITP), it does not have a clear role in the early management of either ITP or the other autoimmune disorders. A clearer understanding of the mechanisms of action may, however, allow us to exploit IVIG in a more sensible and rational manner in the management of not only the immune-mediated cytopenias, but also autoantibody mediated diseases in general.

References

1. Cunningham-Rundles, C., Siegal, F. P., Smithwick, E. M. *et al.* Efficacy of intravenous immunoglobulin in primary immunodeficiency disease. *Ann. Intern. Med.* 101: 435–439; 1984.
2. Petersen, F. B., Bowden, R. A., Thornquist, M. *et al.* The effect of prophylactic intravenous immune globulin on the incidence of septicaemia in marrow transplant recipients. *Bone Marrow Transpl.* 2: 141–148; 1987.
3. Pennington, J. E., Small, G. J. and Hahn, H. Polyclonal and monoclonal antibody therapy for experimental pseudomonas aeruginosa pneumonia. *Infect. Immun.* 54: 239–244; 1984.
4. Newland, A. C. The use and mechanisms of action of intravenous immunoglobulin. *Br. J. Haemat.* 72: 301–305; 1989.
5. Eibl, M. M. and Wedgwood, R. J. Intravenous immunoglobulin: a review. *Immunodeficiency Rev.* 1(Suppl.): 1–42; 1989.
6. Newland, A. C., Treleaven, J. G., Minchinton, R. M. and Waters, A. H. High dose intravenous IgG in adults with autoimmune thrombocytopenic purpura. *Lancet* i: 84–87; 1983.
7. Bussell, J. B., Pham, L. C., Aledort, L. and Nachman, R. Maintenance treatment of adults with refractory immune thrombocytopenic purpura using repeated intravenous infusions of gamma globulin. *Blood* 72: 121–127; 1988.
8. Imbach, P., Berchtold, W., Hirt, A. *et al.* Intravenous immunoglobulin versus oral corticosteroids in acute immune thrombocytopenic purpura in childhood. *Lancet* ii: 464–468; 1985.

9. Fehr, J., Hofmann, V. and Kappeler, U. Transient reversal of thrombocytopenia in idiopathic thrombocytopenic purpura by high dose intravenous gamma globulin. *N. Engl. J. Med.* **306**: 1254–1258; 1982.
10. Clarkson, S. B., Bussel, J. B., Kimberley, R. P. *et al.* Treatment of refractory immune thrombocytopenic purpura with an anti FcG receptor antibody. *N. Engl. J. Med.* **314**: 1236–1239; 1986.
11. Romer, J., Morganthaler, J.-J., Scherz, R. and Skvaril, F. Characterisation of various immunoglobulin preparations for intravenous application. *Vox Sang.* **42**: 62–73; 1982.
12. Veys, P. A., Macey, M. G., Owens, C. M. and Newland, A. C. Neutropenia following intravenous immunoglobulin. *Br. Med. J.* **296**: 1800; 1988.
13. Newland, A. C., Macey M. G. and Veys, P. A. Cellular changes during the infusion of high dose intravenous immunoglobulin. *Blut* **59**: 82–87; 1989.
14. Veys, P. A., Macey, M., Newland, A. C. and Hoffbrand, A. V. Neutrophil Fc receptors in clinical disease. *Br. J. Haemat.* **74** (Suppl. 1): 24; 1990 (abstract).
15. Newland, A. C., Macey, M. G., McAvinchey, R. and Jones, L. The effect of intravenous IgG on reticulo-endothelial function and auto immune thrombocytopenia. *Br. J. Haemat.* **58**: 178; 1984 (abstract).
16. Sinclair, N. R. and Panoskaltsis, A. Immunoregulation by Fc signals. *Immunol. Today* **8**: 76–79; 1987.
17. Mannhalter, J. W., Ahmad, R., Wolf, H. M. and Eibl, M. M. Effect of polymeric IgG on human monocyte functions. *Int. Arch. Allergy Appl. Immunol.* **82**: 159–167; 1987.
18. Sultan, Y., Maisonneuve, P., Kazatchkine, M. D. and Nydegger, U. E. Anti idiotypic suppression of autoantibodies to factor VIII by high dose intravenous gammaglobulin. *Lancet* i: 765–768; 1984.
19. Maynier, M., Cosso, B., Brochier, J. and Clot, J. Identification of class II HLA alloantibodies in placenta-eluted gamma globulin used for treating rheumatoid arthritis. *Arthr. Rheumat.* **30**: 375–381; 1987.
20. Dietrich, G. and Kazatchkine, M. D. Normal IgG for therapeutic use contains anti-idiotypes against an immunodominant, disease associated, cross-reactive idiotype of human antithyroglobulin autoantibodies. *Br. Soc. Immunol. Proc.* 41 (Abstract 30); 1990.
21. Tsubakio, T., Kurato, Y., Katageri, S. *et al.* Alteration in T cell subsets and immunoglobulin synthesis in vitro during high dose gammaglobulin therapy in patients with idiopathic thrombocytopenic purpura. *Clin. Exp. Immunol.* **53**: 697–702; 1983.
22. Macey, M. G. and Newland, A. C. Modulation of T and B cell subpopulations during high dose intravenous immunoglobulin therapy. *Plasma Ther. Transfus. Technol.* **9**: 139–147; 1988.

23. Newburger, J. W., Takahaski, M., Burns, J. C. *et al.* The treatment of Kawasaki syndrome with intravenous gamma globulin. *N. Engl. J. Med.* 315: 341–347; 1986.
24. Cooperative Group for the Study of Immunoglobulin in Chronic Lymphocytic Leukaemia. Intravenous immunoglobulin for the prevention of infection in chronic lymphocytic leukaemia: a randomised, controlled clinical trial. *N. Engl. J. Med.* 319: 902–907; 1988.
25. Yap, P. L. and Williams, P. E. Immunoglobulin preparations for HIV infected patients. *Vox Sang.* 55: 65–74; 1988.
26. Gupta, A., Novick, B. E. and Rubinstein, A. Restoration of suppressor T-cell functions in children with AIDS following intravenous gammaglobulin treatment. *Am. J. Dis. Childh.* 140: 143–146; 1986.
27. Mylvaganam, R., Garcia, R., Ahn, S. *et al.* Depressed functional and phenotypic properties of T but not B lymphocytes in idiopathic thrombocytopenic purpura. *Blood* 71: 1455–1460; 1988.
28. Moffat, E. H., Furlong, R. A., Dannatt, A. H. G. *et al.* Anti-idiotypes to Factor VIII antibodies and their possible role in the pathogenesis and treatment of Factor VIII inhibition. *Br. J. Haemat.* 71: 85–90; 1989.
29. Jerne, N. K. Toward a network theory of immunity. *Ann. Immunol.* 125C: 373–389; 1974.
30. Rossi, F., Sultan, Y. and Kazatchkine, D. Anti-idiotypes against autoantibodies and alloantibodies to VIII-C are present in therapeutic polyspecific normal immunoglobulin. *Clin. Exp. Immunol.* 74: 311–316; 1988.

Hypothetic and established action mechanisms of therapy with immunoglobulin G

URS E. NYDEGGER

Central Laboratory of Haematology, University of Bern and Regional Red Cross Blood Transfusion Service, Bern, Switzerland

Introduction

We have come a long way in the understanding of the mechanisms of action at work upon infusion of intravenous immunoglobulin (IVIG) since the days when crude Cohn fraction II of human plasma was administered intramuscularly to patients suffering from Bruton's agammaglobulinemia, up to modern times, when biologists attempt to substitute IVIG with monoclonal antibodies or with genetically engineered heavy chains. In this contribution, an update of the present state of knowledge about how polyclonal polyspecific IgG may become operative once introduced into the recipient is presented (Table 1, Fig. 1). A distinction should be made between action mechanisms at the level of the disease-provoking pathogen and those at the level of a given disease provoked by the reaction of the host against that pathogen. Should a number of autoimmune diseases be caused by infectious agents (1), then the effects of IVIG are likely to be dual—anti-infectious as well as anti-(auto)-immune response. A

Immunotherapy with Intravenous Immunoglobulins
ISBN 0-12-370725-0

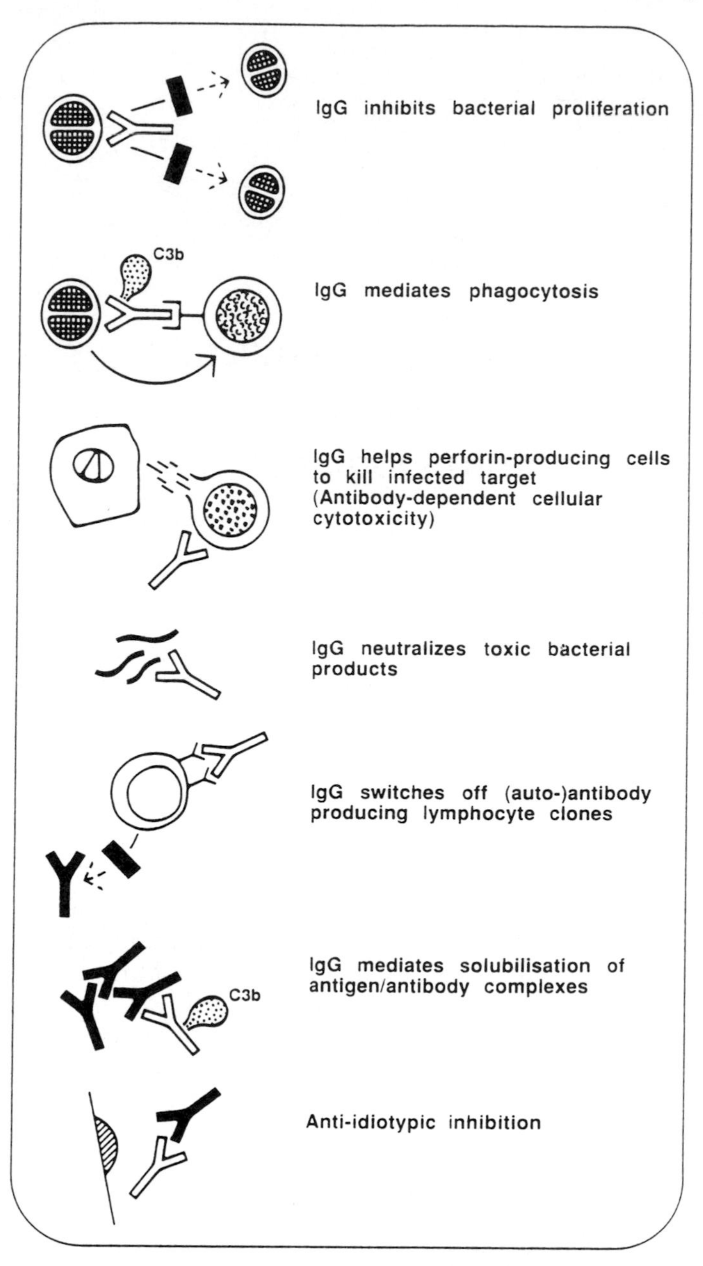

*Figure 1. Synoptic representation of selected action mechanisms ascribed to i.v. immunoglobulin therapy in infectious and autoimmune diseases. Closed "**Y**" symbols represent the host's own pathogenic IgG; open "Y" symbols represent therapeutic IgG.*

Table 1
Action mechanisms of i.v. immunoglobulins in selected human diseases

Type of action mechanism	What IVIG recognizes in the host	Which effector system is engaged
Anti-infectious		
Bacteriostatic	Epitope on microbial organism	Antiproliferative
Anti-toxic	Epitope on bacterial toxin	Neutralization
Pro-removal	Epitope on microbial organism	Opsonophagocytosis
Anti-inflammatory		
Fc receptor down-regulation	Fc fragment interacts with Fc receptor	Fc receptor engaged with monomeric therapeutic IgG not available for immune complex carrying targets
Improvement of immune complex disposal	Non-specific interaction of IVIG with immune complexes; non-polar groups stick to complex	Shift of antigen/antibody ratio facilitates the reticuloendothelial and complement system's capacity to dispose of immune complexes
Prevention of complement target cell binding	Complement components C3 and C4	Complement activation attenuated
Anti-idiotypic modulation	Idiotypes	Pathogenic autoantibodies

typical example of a disease recognized as being caused by the host's immune-response rather than by the infectious agent is hepatitis B viral infection which may remain a latent viral colonization of the hepatocytes only to be followed by clinically overt hepatitis when T cytotoxic lymphocytes attack the virus-infected cell. Similarly, Epstein-Barr virus infection is rarely pathogenic but may be so in patients with overt infectious mononucleosis and/or neoplasia.

Anti-infectious immunoglobulin G

A comprehensive review on this topic by this author has appeared earlier (2). Specific antibodies towards a large spectrum of microbial antigens present in IVIG are the hallmark of any substitutive prophylaxis for infectious diseases in the immunodeficient host. Significant reduction of infectious episodes in patients suffering from hypo- or agammaglobulinemia when substituted to half-normal, or when clinically relevant, to normal plasma levels of IgG is proof of the efficiency of IVIG against bacterial infections (3, 4). The types of microorganisms that may infect the compromised host include acquired and colonizing pyogenic as well as opportunistic organisms such as *Listeria monocytogenes*, *Candida*, herpes simplex and zoster viruses, *Pneumocystis carinii*, *Toxoplasma gondii* and legionella.

While it is now acknowledged beyond doubt that IVIG is effective for prophylaxis, we still debate its effectiveness in the treatment of overt bacterial or viral infection. Attempts to specifically prevent septic shock or at least attenuate its consequences using antibodies against the core glycolipid of endotoxin have so far failed to give encouraging results (5). One might speculate about such failure. Manifest infectious disease has reached a stage at which exhaustion of specific antimicrobial antibody is but one element of impaired immune response: insufficiency of the phagocytic system, deficient innate resistance to viruses (6), consumption upon overreaction of the complement system that may have immunosuppressive consequences (7) are other elements, and these will not be corrected by infusion of IVIG. In fact, many microbial organisms are a threat for the reticuloendothelial system and they are effective activators of complement. Although activation of complement by bacterial organisms allows the host to kill or opsonophagocytose these microorganisms, we must not forget that this very same mechanism allows bacteria and viruses to enter cells. If intracellular killing (suicidal or not for the cell) fails, viruses in particular will exploit their intracellular state to proliferate. It has been speculated that it is by opsonophagocytosis that human immunodeficiency virus antibodies would favor infection rather than prevent it.

Activators of the alternative pathway of complement have a diverse range of surface physical and biochemical properties. For example, soluble and particulate polysaccharides, lipopolysaccharides, various fungi, bacteria, parasites, viruses, as well as IgA bound to the antigen, and virus-infected mammalian cells, all may lead to exhaustion of the anti-infectious capacity of complement (8). By introducing IVIG, acquired complement deficiencies will not be corrected, which for certain patients means failure of therapeutic activity with IVIG. Further evidence for this situation is provided for patients suffering from chronic lymphocytic leukemia (CLL). Extensive clinical studies have demonstrated a prophylactic efficacy of IVIG for infections in CLL patients (9, 10) due to correction by IVIG of the well-known hypogammaglobulinemia/selective antibody deficiency in this disease. However, these patients also may suffer from granulocytopenia and recently, reduced levels of C1 and C4 as well as a reduced capacity of C3b to bind to *Streptococcus pneumoniae* have been described in CLL patients (11). Therefore, CLL patients not responding to IVIG prophylaxis may well suffer from such additional, complement-dependent immunodeficiencies and alternative procedures will have to be sought as a means for anti-infectious prophylaxis. Emphatically, each patient receiving IVIG for presumed humoral immunodeficiency should have the easy-to-perform and cheap hemolytic assays for total hemolytic complement activity (CH50) and alternative pathway hemolytic activity (AP50) done on his/her plasma in order to rule out deficiency(-ies) of one or more of the major complement proteins (12). The special situation with hypo-C1q-emia in hypogammaglobulinemia is addressed in an abstract (Spaeth, Engler, Scherz *et al.*). In addition, the finding of avoiding reductions of C3 and C4 plasma levels after therapeutic plasma exchange when supplementing patients with IVIG is unexplained so far (13). Similarly the mechanism of reversal of neutropenia present in newborn rats by IVIG is unclear (14).

Finally, we have speculated earlier that some patients suffering from infectious disease and who by *in vitro* testing exhibit sufficient amounts of specific antibody against the pathogenic microbial organism, would have the bactericidal function of that antibody suppressed, perhaps by core reactive anti-idiotypic antibodies. Until proof is shown to the contrary, such an ANTIS (anti-idiotypic suppression) may therefore compromise the primary antibodies' efficiency (15) independently on its isotype. Upon infusion of IVIG such patients may experience improvement of their infection because the idiotypes carried by the infused specific anti-microbial IgG are no longer recognized by the patient's anti-idiotypes and because the therapeutic IVIG is non-immunosuppressive since it recognizes a large spectrum of idiotypes as it is prepared from non-vaccinated healthy blood donors (16). The effect of antitoxic and bactericidal activity of IgG specific for microbial organisms and their products have been reviewed elsewhere (17).

Action mechanisms in chronic inflammatory diseases

That IVIG may become a therapeutic option for patients suffering from chronic inflammatory and autoimmune diseases, with the receptive antigen for IVIG known or unknown, was hardly conceivable 10 years ago. A rationale to try IVIG in autoimmunity was also lacking; perhaps the belief that many autoimmune diseases are triggered by viral infections (1) would have provided for attempts to combat such viruses with specific antibodies and consequently relieve autoimmune disease. But this is likely not the case in most autoimmune disorders responsive to IVIG, among them diseases far from disclosing causative agents. Several reviews and annotations have appeared in the meantime to analyze the possible action mechanisms of IVIG therapy in autoimmune disorders. With natural autoantibodies now known to occur in healthy subjects, we begin to envision IVIG administration as conferring a part of humoral immunity from healthy donors to deficient recipients. An analysis of the single mechanisms proposed so far that make such conferral possible is appropriate.

Antigen-non-specific down-regulation of Fc receptor (FcR)-mediated immune adherence

Shortly after description of the beneficial effect of i.v. infusions of intact 7S but not 5S $F(ab')_2$-fragmented IgG in children suffering from idiopathic thrombocytopenic purpura (ITP), the efficacy of IVIG was confirmed in adults and suggested to be based on down-regulation of FcR-bearing reticuloendothelial cells. In the meantime this finding has become the subject of extensive *in vitro* studies involving anti-FcR monoclonal antibodies and leading to elucidation of the heterogeneity of FcR types I, II and low affinity III. FcR down-regulation lasts for $\leq$ 30 days; the FcRs are rapidly restored; FcR down-regulation, therefore, only accounts for initial responses to IVIG but not for any alteration in the disease natural history. The finding that IVIG are active in alloimmunized thrombocytopenic patients for a rather short time only is further evidence that disease non-specific FcR-down-regulating activity is only transient (18).

Increased solubilization/enhanced elimination of immune complexes

A distinction must be made between physiological/beneficial and pathological/pathogenic antigen–antibody complexes. The former efficiently fix C3b and C4b and serve to expedite removal of antigen from the circulation by binding to complement receptors on red blood cells and presenting antigen to the reticuloendothelial system for disposal. Not so the latter type complexes, which circulate chronically, fix complement badly or, if they do, are not removed by a deficient complement receptor apparatus and/or deficient reticuloendothelial system. Such complexes become deposited in tissues and there trigger inflammation. It appears that IVIG favorably influences such immunopathological processes by facilitating immune complex solubilization and removal. The molecular mechanisms at work have been discussed in the previous book of this series and in a more recent review (19). Finally, IVIG may prevent further attack of target cells by continuously formed immune complexes (20). Very recently yet another type of preventive activity for immune complex-induced inflammation by IVIG has been proposed.

Prevention of complement component target cell binding

Using the model of Forssman shock that consists of injecting lethal doses of anti-Forssman antiserum into laboratory animals, IVIG was recently seen to increase survival and frequently prevent death when administered in sufficient dosage (21). The Forssman antigen is a blood group P-system-related globoside, is found in one of five people's bodily tissues (22) and may be expressed on mast cells. A significant positive correlation was found between IgG plasma levels and survival time in guinea-pigs treated with incremental amounts of IVIG. Infusions of IVIG had no effect on C3 and C4 levels; however, in *in vitro* experiments, uptake of C3 by guinea-pig red blood cells sensitized with rabbit anti-guinea pig red cell antibody was almost completely blocked by supraphysiologic levels of IVIG present in the system. This indicated that high levels of ambient IVIG may divert C4b and/or C3b from target membranes and suppress localized complement-mediated pathology, perhaps through non-covalent interaction of C3 and C3b with IgG (23).

Anti-idiotype (Id) modulation

The evidence of efficient provision of anti-idiotypic reactivity contained in IVIG is now complete and has been reviewed recently in detail (24, 25). Anti-Id are known to bind to autoantibodies, either in core or frame-reactive manner. By so fixing, they will either prevent reactivity of the accepting antibodies with their cognate antigen or they will shift the antigen/antibody ratio towards antibody excess providing for differential deposition of C3b and/or C4b on the immune complex lattice, which profoundly affects the capacity of immune complexes to interact with target/bystander cells. Binding of anti-Ids to B/T lymphocyte surface-associated immunoglobulins M and G will modulate the rate by which B lymphocytes synthesize antibody. An *in vitro* noticeable reduction of immunoglobulin production by B lymphocytes purified from peripheral blood of patients suffering from ITP treated with IVIG has been noted earlier and was ascribed to an absolute increase in T suppressor lymphocytes with a reversal of the helper/suppressor ratio and reduced B-cell activity (26).

Acknowledgement

The art work by Mr Ch. Langenegger, AUM, University of Bern, is kindly acknowledged.

References

1. Talal, N., Daupinee, M. J., Dang, H., Alexander, S. and Garry, R. Evidence suggesting a retroviral etilogy for human autoimmune disease. *In* "Progress in immunology" (Eds Melchers, F. *et al.*), Vol. VII, pp. 837–841. Springer, Berlin; 1989.
2. Nydegger, U. E. Pathophysiological aspects of bacterial infection. Towards a rationale for prophylaxis and treatment with intravenous immunoglobulins. *Clin. Immunol. Allergy* 5: 105–120; 1985.
3. So, A., Brenner, M. K., Hill, I. D., Asherson, G. L. and Webster, A. D. B. Intravenous gammaglobulin treatment in patients with hypogammaglobulinemia. *Br. Med. J.* **298**: 1177–1179; 1984.
4. Bernatowska, E., Madalinski, K., Janowicz, W., Weremovicz, R., Gutkovski, P. *et al.* Results of a prospective controlled two-dose crossover study with intravenous immunoglobulin and comparison (retrospective) with plasma treatment. *Clin. Immunol. Immunopathol.* **43**: 153–162; 1987.
5. Calandra, T., Glauser, M. P., Schellekens, J., Verhoef, J. and the Swiss-Dutch J5 Immunoglobulin Study Group. Treatment of gram negative septic shock with human IgG antibody to *Escherichia coli* J5: a prospective, double-blind, randomized trial. *J. Infect. Dis.* **158**: 312–319; 1988.
6. Sarmiento, M. and Kleinerman, E. S. Innate resistance of herpes simplex virus infection. Human lymphocyte and monocyte inhibition of viral replication. *J. Immunol.* **144**: 1942–1953; 1990.
7. Ambus, J. L., Peters, M. G., Fauci, A. S. and Brown, E. J. The Ba

fragment of complement factor B inhibits human B lymphocyte proliferation. *J. Immunol.* **144**: 1549–1553; 1990.
8. Kolb, W. P., Morrow, P. R. and Tamerius, S. D. Ba and Bb fragments of factor B activation: fragment production, biological activities, neoepitope expression and quantitation in clinical samples. *Complement Inflamm.* **6**: 175–204; 1989.
9. Intravenous immunoglobulin for the prevention of infection in chronic lymphocytic leukemia. Cooperative group for the study of immunoglobulin in chronic lymphatic leukemia. *N. Engl. J. Med.* **319**: 902–907; 1988.
10. Chapel, H. M., Griffiths, H., Lea, J., Brennan, V., Bunch, C. and Lee, M. Studies of immunoglobulin replacement therapy in patients with low-grade B-cell tumors. *In* "Proc. IIIrd Symposium on Immune Deficiency, Children's Memorial Hospital, Warsaw" (Ed. Madalsinski, K.). Immunological Invest. (In press.)
11. Varga, L., Clas, F., Füst G., Paloczi, K., Szegedi, G., Loos, M. and Hollan, S. R. Patients with CLL and hypocomplementaemia have an impaired serum bactericidal activity against the *Salmonella minnesota* Re mutant. *Complement Inflamm.* 5: 40–45; 1988.
12. Bird, A. G. Diagnosis of antibody deficiency states. *In* "IgG Subclass Deficiencies" (Ed. Levinsky, R. J.), pp. 3–12. Royal Soc Med Sv Ltd, London; 1989.
13. Zielinski, C. C., Preis, P. and Eibl, M. M. Effect of immunoglobulin substitution during plasmapheresis on serum immunoglobulin and complement concentrations. *Nephron* **40**: 253–254; 1985.
14. Redd, H., Christensen, R. D., and Fischer, G. W. Circulating and storage neutrophils in neonatal rats treated with immune globulin. *J. Infect. Dis.* 157: 705–712; 15.
15. Nydegger, U. E., Blaser, K. and Hässig, A. Anti-idiotypic immunosuppression (ANTIS) and its treatment with human immunoglobulin preparations. *Vox Sang.* **47**: 92–95; 1984.
16. Lucas, A. H. and Granoff, D. M. A major crossreactive idiotype associated with human antibodies to the *Haemophilus influenzae* b Polysaccharide. Expression in relation to age and immunoglobulin G subclass. *J. Clin. Invest.* **85**: 1158–1166; 1990.
17. Yap, P. L. Intravenous immunoglobulin for secondary immunodeficiency. *Blut* **60**: 8–14; 1990.
18. Kickler, T., Braine, H. G., Piantadosi, S., Ness, P. M., Herman, J. H. and Rothko, K. A randomized, placebo-controlled trial of intravenous gammaglobulin in alloimmunized thrombocytopenic patients. *Blood* **75**: 313–316; 1990.
19. Nydegger, U. E., Rieben, R. and Jungi, T. W. Synergy between plasma exchange and intravenous immunoglobulin. *Curr. Stud. Hematol. Blood Transfus.* **57**: 31–50; 1990.
20. Borradori, L., Castelli, D. Flueckiger, E. and Nydegger, U. E., Clinical significance of platelet-associated immunoglobulins in narcotic

addicts with human immunodeficiency virus infection. *Clin. Immunol. Immunopathol.* 54: 256–265; 1990.

21. Basta, M., Kirshbom, P., Frank, M. M. and Fries, L. F. Mechanism of therapeutic effect of high-dose intravenous immunoglobulin. Attenuation of acute, complement-dependent immune damage in a guinea pig model. *J. Clin. Invest.* **84**: 1974–1981; 1989.
22. Hakomori, S. Glycosphingolipids. *Sci. Am.* 254: 32–44; 1986.
23. Kulics, J., Rajnavolgy, I. E., Fust, G. and Gergely, J. Interaction of C3 and C3b with immunoglobulin G. *Molec. Immunol.* **20**: 805–810; 1983.
24. Dietrich, G., Rossi, F. and Kazatchkine, M. D. Modulation of autoimmune responses with normal polyspecific IgG for therapeutic use. *In* "Progress in Immunology", Vol. VII, pp. 1221–1227. Springer-Verlag, Berlin; 1989.
25. Nydegger, U. E., Sultan, Y. and Kazatchkine, M. D. The concept of anti-idiotypic regulation of selected autoimmune diseases by intravenous immunoglobulin. *Clin. Immunol. Immunopathol.* **53**: S72–S82; 1989.
26. Dammacco, F., Iodice, G. and Campobasso, N. Treatment of adult patients with ITP with intravenous immunoglobulin: effect on T-cell subsets and PWM induced antibody synthesis *in vitro*. *Br. J. Haemat.* **62**: 125–135; 1986.

The distribution and catabolism of IVIG preparations in immunodeficient patients

RALPH J. WEDGWOOD

Department of Pediatrics, University of Washington School of Medicine, Seattle, Washington, USA

Background

In 1970 Morell, Terry and Waldmann published a classical paper on the catabolism and distribution of IgG and IgG subclasses in man (1). Myeloma proteins of the four IgG subclasses were purified, labeled and injected into 12 patients with neoplastic (and other) diseases. By using two different radioactive labels they were able to measure two subclasses in the same patient simultaneously. Both urinary excretion and plasma levels were quantitated. Calculation of the volume of distribution and catabolism was thus possible. *In vivo* and *in vitro* labeling were compared. I know of no subsequent study that has paid such attention to such niceties.

The authors noted "considerable variation ... in different individuals". They found (Table 1) the half-life for IgG_1, IgG_2 and IgG_4 to approximate 21 days and the fractional catabolic rate 7.35% per day. For IgG_3 the half-life was 7.1 days and the catabolic rate 16.8% per day. The catabolism of IgG_3 was identical for exogenously and endogenously labeled protein.

Volumes of distribution showed the proportion of IgG_1, IgG_2 and

Immunotherapy with Intravenous Immunoglobulins
ISBN 0–12–370725–0

Table 1
The half-life and fractional catabolic rate (FCR) of IgG subclasses in non-immunodeficient patients

	Half-life (days)	FCR	Distribution (% intravascular)
IgG_1	21.2 (5.4)	0.080 (0.020)	51 (4)
IgG_2	20.2 (1.9)	0.069 (0.003)	53 (6)
IgG_3	7.1 (0.7)	0.168 (0.006)	64 (6)
IgG_4	20.6 (2.6)	0.069 (0.014)	54 (5)

All data as arithmetic mean (standard deviation).

IgG_4 remaining in the intravascular space to be similar (53%) but significantly different from IgG_3 (64%). The catabolic rate for IgG was concentration-dependent.

The Brambell model

These data confirmed findings dating back to the 1950s for IgG (2) and extended them to the IgG subclasses. They fit the model for IgG metabolism proposed by Brambell, Hemmings and Morris (3). This model posits that each day half the intravascular IgG passes from the capillaries and returns to the bloodstream by way of the lymphatics. In transit through the extravascular space, some of the IgG is trapped on Fc receptors in the reticuloendothelial system, internalized and destroyed. The lost IgG is replaced by synthesis. At steady state in normal persons, degradation and replacement (in this case, synthesis) are equal; the rate approximates 35 mg/kg/day. Fc receptors are the rate-determining factor. Morell's data showed no Fc receptor subclass specificity; all subclasses competed equally for receptor binding. The shorter half-life of IgG_3 was presumed to be due to differences in molecular stability.

The concentration dependence of IgG catabolism is explicable on the basis of the model; the higher the concentration of IgG, the greater the chance of random interaction with the limited number of Fc receptors.

Fc receptors for IgG (FcγR)

The Brambell model views Fc receptors as inert, non-selective molecular sponges. Knowledge of Fc receptors has expanded enormously

Table 2
Characteristics of human Fc receptors for IgG

	FcγRI	FcγRII	FcγRIII
Monomer affinity	High	Low	Low
Distribution	Macrophages Monocytes "Activated" neutrophils	Macrophages Monocytes Granulocytes B Lymphocytes Platelets Trophoblasts	Macrophages Granulocytes NK-Cells T Lymphocyte Subset
IgG subclass specificity	IgG_1, IgG_3 $>IgG_4>>>IgG_2$	$IgG_1>IgG_2=$ $IgG_4>>IgG_3$	IgG_1, IgG_3
Recycling	No	Yes	?
Polymorphism	Minimal	Marked	Marked

From references 4 and 5.

in the last few years. They are neither inert nor non-selective (4, 5). There are at least three varieties of receptors (Table 2) that bind the Fc domain of human IgG (huFcγR). All are members of the immunoglobulin super-gene family; like many other receptors they have integral membrane glycoprotein and an extracellular portion with two or three IgG-like disulfide-looped domains. They have structural similarity to the poly-Ig receptor for IgM and IgA transport in the gut and the Fcε receptor.

Human FcγRI has high affinity for monomeric IgG. It is found on macrophages, monocytes and activated neutrophils. It shows IgG subclass preference for IgG_1 and IgG_3; IgG_4 is bound with much lower affinity; IgG_2 is bound little or perhaps not at all. At rest there are around 10^4 receptors on each cell. When cultured with IFN-γ granulocytes develop high numbers of the receptor; monocytes and macrophages increase receptor expression 10–20-fold. The receptor is thus highly sensitive to regulation by this and (as noted later) other mediators. Because of its high affinity for monomeric IgG, the receptor is the prime candidate for the normal catabolism of IgG. However, receptor-mediated catabolism of monomeric IgG by the pinocytosis of coated pits has not been shown, and the receptor does not appear to recycle. While polymorphisms at the DNA level appear to be minimal, there may be differences in tissue-specific expression.

The second Fc receptor (huFcγRII) is strikingly different. It has only low affinity for monomeric IgG. It is distributed on a wider variety of cell types—including platelets and trophoblasts. In contrast to FcγRI, FcγRII has strikingly lower affinity for IgG_3 than IgG_1. FcγRII is capable of cycling between the plasma membrane and the endocytic vesicle compartment, which would be most important for a major role in IgG transport and catabolism. It plays a major role in triggering cell activation and the metabolic burst. Interpretation of studies is complicated by at least three known allotypic and probably significant tissue specific variations.

The third receptor, huFcγRIII, also has only low affinity for monomeric IgG. It is present on macrophages but not monocytes, on granulocytes and on a subset of T lymphocytes, including NK cells. It binds IgG_1 and IgG_3 but not IgG_2 or IgG_4. In neutrophils the receptor is membrane-linked by a phophatidylinositol glycan, rather than the usual transmembrane polypeptide found in NK cells and macrophages, and is thus easily cleaved, perhaps explaining the functional differences between cell types. There are 5–10 times more huFcγRIII per neutrophil than other Fc receptors; it is probably the major player in removal of immune complexes. Once the receptor has been saturated and cleared it does not reappear for weeks; recycling seems unlikely, down-regulation by saturation is easy.

Both direct and indirect studies indicate that both up- and down-regulation of huFcγR occurs readily. For example, INF-γ induces expression on granulocytes and increases expression in monocytes *in vitro*; this must also occur *in vivo* with infections and inflammation. Fc expression is also modulated by C1q (6): C1q levels are diminished in hypogammaglobulinemia (7). Immune clearance, presumably FcγR-mediated, is diminished in many diseases including rheumatoid arthritis (8) and may be affected by steroids (9) or components of the clotting system (10). Fc receptors are also down-regulated by IVIG preparations (11). Genetically controlled differences in huFcγR expression between individuals also probably exist. Thus Fc expression is both individual- and state-dependent. Considerable variation in IgG clearance among persons and patients would be expected.

The measurement of IgG catabolism

The usual approach to the measurement of IgG catabolism is based on the assumption of a steady state. With this assumption the simple measurement of serum levels can provide a reasonable estimate of both volume of distribution and catabolism. The idealized first-order kinetics give a two-phase curve; the first phase equates with distribution to the extravascular space, the second "linear" phase equates with catabolism, and the slope of the exponential line reflects clearance—catabolism or "half-life". If the steady state is not perturbed the calculated distribution and catabolism concur with total body measures. This method has been used in virtually all studies on the "half-life" of IVIG.

We have conducted several such studies (12–15). In these studies immunodeficient patients were equilibrated by administration of 400 mg/kg IVIG every 28 days for 6 months prior to study. By that time pre-infusion serum IgG trough levels had become constant; in this regard the patients were "in steady state". The results for three different products are given in Table 3.

Table 3
The half-life of IgG and IgG subclasses in immunodeficient patients following infusion of IVIG

	Immunoglobulin half-life (days) Product		
	A	B	C
IgG	26	32	40
IgG_1	30	35	34
IgG_2	27	40	45
IgG_3	16	24	30
IgG_4	ND	36	38

The half-lives for IgG, IgG_1, IgG_2 and IgG_4 were longer than those for IgG_3. The half-lives for antibody generally approximated those for IgG. Any differences observed probably related more to procedure than to product. We noted, as have others (16, 17), wide variation in clearance rates between individuals. While the calculated half-lives had statistical validity and "significance", they are, however, on simple inspection, biologically and therapeutically absurd.

The repeated administration of any substance at intervals more frequent than its half-life must result in a systematic increase in trough levels. A basic criterion for the studies was that the serum trough levels were stable. During the half-life study period serum trough levels before and at the end of study (28 days) were by measurement essentially identical. Thus effectively the catabolism must have approximated the dosage of 400 mg/kg/month: the net catabolism of

100% IVIG catabolism in 28 days is not compatible with the calculated half-lives. One must conclude that the data do not "fit" first-order kinetics.

The steady-state assumption required for first-order kinetic calculations simply does not pertain to IVIG infused in immunodeficient patients. The infusion itself perturbs the state. The sudden increase in serum levels (often an actual doubling) creates a dramatic disequilibrium between the vascular and extravascular spaces; high IgG levels will increase diffusion rates. IVIG will also down-regulate Fc receptor expression. IVIG itself contains dimers. These, with complexes formed by interaction of infused antibody with antigen, will interact with and may saturate Fc receptors and modulate their expression. From this alone it appears that the situation is not "steady state".

Additionally, the serum IgG levels do not merely measure the disappearance of IVIG just infused, but also the reducing amounts of IgG carried over from the previous infusion—and indeed of all preceding infusions. The levels also reflect the intrinsic (or baseline) synthesis of IgG in the patient. The disappearance curve is the net result of all of these factors. It is not a simple exponential function.

Correction of serum IgG values for the contribution of previous infusions and baseline production requires a great many assumptions and is inherently inaccurate. The resulting numbers are non-linear. Concentration dependence of the catabolic rate appears as the limiting factor. There is no single half-life when serum levels change.

Therapeutic implications

Since the catabolism of IVIG is both state- and concentration-dependent, dosage cannot be based on half-life values. Furthermore, the variation of catabolism among individuals requires dosage to be individualized. Adequacy of dosage must be assessed by serum levels and clinical response. Diminished intervals between injections, permitting smaller amounts of IVIG for each infusion, decreases peak and trough differences and diminishes the potential magnitude of the Fc-mediated metabolic perturbations. More constant IgG levels may result and may reduce catabolism because the rate is so concentration-dependent at high IgG concentrations.

Summary

IgG is normally distributed equally between the intra- and extravascular spaces. In steady-state conditions, catabolism of IgG follows first order kinetics and is concentration dependent, limited by Fc receptor availability. Immunodeficient patients receiving IVIG are not in the steady state required for calculation of distribution and catabolic rate. Reported half-lives, while statistically sound, may be biologically absurd. Thus therapy must be individualized and assessed on the basis of carefully monitored serum levels and clinical response. More consistent serum levels may be obtained by decreasing the interval between infusions, dampening the metabolic perturbations resultant from extreme peak and trough levels.

References

1. Morell, A., Terry, W. D. and Waldmann, T. A. Metabolic properties of IgG subclasses in man. *J. Clin. Invest.* 49: 673–680; 1970.
2. Janeway, C. A., Rosen F. S., Merler E. and Alper, C. A. "The Gammaglobulins". Little, Brown and Co., Boston; 1966.
3. Brambell, F. W. R., Hemmings, W. A. and Morris, I. G. A theoretical model of gammaglobulin catabolism. *Nature (Lond.)* 203: 1352; 1964.
4. Unkeless, J. C. Human Fc receptors for IgG. *Int. Rev. Immunol.* 5: 165–171; 1989.
5. Anderson, C. L. Human IgG Fc receptors. *Clin. Immunol. Immunopathol.* 53: S63–71; 1989.
6. Leu, R. W., Zhou, A., Rummage, J. A. *et al.* Exogenous C1q reconstitutes resident but not inflammatory mouse peritoneal macrophages for Fc receptor-dependent cellular cytotoxicity and phagocytosis. *J. Immunol.* 143: 3250–3257; 1989.
7. Kohler, P. F. and Müller-Eberhard, H. J. Metabolism of human C1q. *J. Clin. Invest.* 51: 868–875; 1972.
8. Lobatto, S., Daha, M. R., Westedt, M. L. *et al.* Diminished clearance of soluble aggregates of human immunoglobulin G in patients with rheumatoid arthritis. *Scand. J. Rheumatol.* 18 (2): 89–96; 1989.
9. Schreiber, A. D., Nettl, F. M., Sanders, M. C. *et al.* Effect of endogenous and synthetic sex steroids on the clearance of antibody-coated cells. *J. Immunol.* 141 (9): 2959–2966; 1988.
10. Chien, P., Pixley, R. A., Stumpo, L. G. *et al.* Modulation of the human monocyte binding site for monomeric immunoglobulin G by activated Hageman factor. *J. Clin. Invest.* 82: 1554–1559; 1988.

11. Mannhalter, J. W. and Eibl, M. M. Down regulation of Fc receptors by IVIgG. *Int. Rev. Immunol.* 5: 173–179; 1989.
12. Ochs, H. D., Morell, A., Skvaril, F. *et al.* Survival of IgG subclasses following administration of intravenous gammaglobulin in patients with primary immunodeficiency diseases. *In* "Clinical Use of Intravenous Immunoglobulins (Eds Morell, A. and Nydegger, U. E.). Academic Press, London; 1986.
13. Mankarious, S., Lee, M., Fischer, S. *et al.* The half-lives of IgG subclasses and specific antibodies in patients with primary immunodeficiency who are receiving intravenously administered immunoglobulin. *J. Lab. Clin. Med.* 112: 634–640; 1988.
14. Fischer, S. H., Ochs, H. D., Wedgwood, R. J. *et al.* Survival of antigen-specific antibody following administration of intravenous immunoglobulin in patients with primary immunodeficiency diseases. *Monogr. Allergy* 23: 225–235; 1988.
15. Fischer, S. H. and Ochs, H. D. (personal communication).
16. Schiff, R. I. and Rudd, C. Alterations in the half-life and clearance of IgG during therapy with intravenous γ-globulin in 16 patients with severe primary humoral immunodeficiency. *J. Clin. Immunol.* 6: 256–264; 1986.
17. Lever, A. M. L., Yap, P. L., Cuthbertson, R. *et al.* Increased half-life of gammaglobulin after prolonged intravenous replacement therapy. *Clin. Exp. Immunol.* 67: 441–446; 1987.

Discussion

R. van Furth

We are filling up the extracellular compartment by giving IgG subcutaneously. In a number of these patients we found that after 4–6 years the levels hardly increase after subcutaneous (s.c.) IgG infusions, while earlier they reacted normally and had an estimated normal half-life of IgG in the plasma. Would it be possible that after many years of s.c. IgG administration, local fibrosis as well as exudated monocytes and polymorphonuclear leukocytes could increase catabolism at the site of infusion?

R. J. Wedgwood

If, as I understand, the catabolism of IgG following intravenous infusions in these patients is normal, the problems must relate to local changes in the subcutaneous tissues following prolonged s.c. administration. Sixteen per cent IgG is potentially locally irritating. Thus local reactions after long-term subcutaneous use might be expected. With this, there might be either decreased absorption (local sequestration) and/or increased local catabolism—perhaps related to increased local expression of tissue-fixed Fcγ receptors. Comparison of catabolism with subcutaneous versus intravenous infusion could prove this point. Parenthetically, one wonders whether local accumulation of mercurial preservatives might play a role in the problem of tissue damage.

A. D. B. Webster
Chronic inflammatory bowel disease is common in both X-LA and CVID patients. Protein loss from the bowel may explain differences in catabolic rate for IgG between patients. Some of these patients do not have overt diarrhea and the diagnosis can be missed.

R. J. Wedgwood
Increased catabolic rates for IgG could be predicted to occur with any inflammatory process through cytokine-mediated up-regulation of Fcγ receptors. As noted, expression of the high-affinity FcγRI is induced by IFN-γ and expression on monocytes and macrophages is increased 10–20-fold. Increased catabolism in inflammatory bowel disease may be due to this as well as (or rather than) to protein-losing enteropathy. That is why perhaps it is important to eradicate all foci that may induce an inflammatory response—whether sino-pulmonary or gut-associated. The diagnosis of inflammatory bowel diseases—or any bowel disease in patients with X-LA or CVID can be difficult. Giardia lamblia can often only be identified by duodenal biopsy and can be very hard to eradicate.

The home administration of IVIG in children with primary immunodeficiency

ROGER H. KOBAYASHI[1], AI LAN D. KOBAYASHI[2], NAPOLEON LEE[1], SUSANNA FISCHER[3], and HANS D. OCHS[3]

[1] *Department of Pediatrics, UCLA School of Medicine, Los Angeles, California, USA*
[2] *Department of Pediatrics, University of Nebraska College of Medicine, Omaha, Nebraska, USA*
[3] *Department of Pediatrics, University of Washington School of Medicine, Seattle, Washington, USA*

Introduction

The use of intravenous immunoglobulin (IVIG) has expanded widely to include a variety of immune deficiency disorders, autoimmune diseases and inflammatory states (1–3). In the case of primary antibody deficiency diseases, IVIG is infused in an outpatient setting. Generally, this is done in a hospital outpatient clinic or in a doctor's office. Occasionally, health care nursing teams may infuse IVIG to patients in their homes. While the benefits (frequently life-saving) are unquestioned, there are several major disadvantages which limit the use of IVIG. These include: (1) very high costs for the product, (2) considerable infusion expenses, (3) technical difficulties which may be encountered, particularly in children, (4) serious reactions which may occur, (5) a time-consuming and inconvenient procedure which is particularly the situation when patients and their families must travel

Immunotherapy with Intravenous Immunoglobulins
ISBN 0–12–370725–0

to a medical facility to have infusions given over a 3–6 h period on a regular basis.

Several researchers have demonstrated that home self-administration of IVIG is feasible and safe (4–7). While self-infusion in adults is technically simpler, infusions in children can be much more difficult and also require the active support and participation of the parents.

The primary purpose of this study was to determine whether long-term home self-infusion in children was both possible and safe. We were especially interested in determining whether home IVIG therapy was feasible in very young children. The second aspect of the study was to do a limited survey of representative costs in three settings where a relatively large number of patients were receiving IVIG. For convenience, this was limited to Omaha, Nebraska.

Methods

Twelve children with primary antibody deficiency, ages 2–17 years old (mean + SD = 9.8 + 5.3) from two centers (University of Nebraska and University of Washington) participated in a 9-month study, in which the child or his/her parents were taught how to self-infuse IVIG and how to manage potential adverse reactions. Prior to the study, all children had been receiving IVIG in an outpatient clinic setting for several months to several years. Excluded from the study were children with a history of adverse reactions to IVIG, significant T-cell defects, impaired renal/liver function, diabetes or poor compliance. The protocol was approved by both Investigational Review Boards of the Universities of Nebraska and Washington and consent forms were signed by parents and children (if older than 7 years).

There were four phases during the 9-month study: (1) Phase I—teaching phase involving 1–5 days of teaching regarding techniques of IVIG preparations, i.v. infusion techniques, recognition and management of untoward effects. (2) Phase II—supervisory phase lasting 2–3 months where patients returned to the study site every 2 weeks for supervised self-infusions, blood collection and reinforcement. (3) Phase III—home infusion phase lasting 6 months where the children or their parents infused IVIG at prescribed intervals (6–18 infusions). Two children from the Nebraska study site had a nurse present in the home in order to comply with IRB requirements. These nurses did not assist or advise the parents during the infusion. (4) Phase IV—summary phase where examination and collection of final data took place. Eight children received IVIG every 2 weeks, two children

Table 1
Children receiving IVIG every 2 weeks

Initials	Age (years)	DX	GG (mg/kg/2 weeks)	Trough (mg/dl)	Peak (mg/dl)	Difference (mg/dl)
J.MCD.	2	CVI	200	561	836	275
S.L.	2	THI	285	722	1080	358
M.C.	6	CVI	280	773	1128	354
J.L.M.	11	XLA	200	624	1005	381
A.S.	15	CVI	184	624	888	264
J.C.	15	CVI	200	585	850	265
C.S.	16	HGM	126	490	884	394
S.S.	17	CVI	157	596	863	267
Summary	10.5 +/− 6.3		204 +/− 12.5	627 +/− 16.6	946 +/− 20.2	319 +/− 14.3

Table 2
Children receiving IVIG on a different schedule

Initials	Age (years)	DX	GG (mg/kg)	Trough (mg/dl)	Peak (mg/dl)	Difference (mg/dl)
S.A.S.⋆	7	CVI	400	512	1172	660
K.M.B.⋆	12	CVI	400	402	1039	639
J.A.B.+	11	XLA	250	476	823	347
M.A.B.+	6	XLA	240	630	857	227

⋆ Receives IVIG every 4 weeks.
+ Receives IVIG every 10 days.

received IVIG every 10 days and two other children received IVIG every 4 weeks. Infusion pumps were not utilized and the rate of infusion (100–150 mg/kg/h) was adjusted by counting the number of drops per minute in the drip chamber. Laboratory studies were performed on a monthly basis to monitor serum IgG levels, blood chemistries and blood counts. In the case of determining costs, data were collected directly from the health care providers in Omaha.

Results

The 12 children finished the study without technical difficulties or significant adverse reactions. In the eight children who received IVIG every 2 weeks, the average biweekly dose was 204+12.5 mg/kg (Table 1). The mean peak and trough levels of IgG were 946+20.2 mg/dl and 627+16.6 mg/dl, respectively. The peak–trough difference was 319 + 14.3 mg/dl. Because of rapid metabolism, two children received IVIG every 10 days (240–250 mg/dl/kg) and their peak and trough levels and peak–trough differences were 840+24 mg/dl, 553+109 mg/dl and 287 mg/dl, respectively. Two other children received 400 mg/kg per month and had a peak and trough level of 1105+94 mg/dl and 457+78 mg/dl (Table 2). The peak–trough difference was 648 mg/dl. Laboratory parameters monitored during the study did not change from baseline values (data not shown).

During the supervisory phase, there were two minor reactions manifested by irritability in an 18-month-old infant. These reactions were transient and resolved quickly after the rate was decreased. No adverse reactions were observed during the home infusion phase. Two hundred and twenty-four infusions were given, resulting in an adverse reaction rate of 0.9% (2 reactions out of 224). At the start of the study, the parents of the two youngest children (ages 18 months and 2 years) experienced some technical difficulties; however, these were overcome by the time the home infusion phase started (Phase III) and the parents became quite proficient at starting i.v.s. There was no difference in the frequency of illness, antibiotic usage or school absences when comparing the home infusion phase with the previous phase when IVIG was administered in a medical setting by health care professionals.

A survey of the costs of IVIG and its administration yielded major differences depending on the source of care giver and supplier. While the wholesale cost of the major brands ranged from $30–45 per g, the retail cost varied considerably from $55 to 115 per g (Table 3). In a

Table 3
Comparative costs of IVIG treatment

	Wholesale	Retail
1. IVIG product:	Wholesale	Retail
Sandoglobulin®	$41.00/g	$55–115/g
Amer. Red Cross	$30.00/g	$55–115/g
Gamimune N	$45.00/g	$55–115/g
2. Supplies:		$30–85
3. Facility charge:		$60–90/h
4. Professional charges:		
Doctor		$45–100
Visiting nursing charge (if given at home)		$100–300
Pharmacy mixing fee		$50–75

Table 4
Comparative costs for treating a 12-year-old child with 10 g IVIG

1. Hospital example	
Supplies ($115/g)	$1150.00
Facilities	225.00
Pharmacy fees	75.00
Nursing fees	105.00
IV supplies	85.00
(Doctor's fees)	(85.00)
	$1640.00
2. Doctor's office	
Supplies ($55/g)	$550.00
Facilities	40.00
IV supplies	30.00
Doctor's fees	180.00
	$800.00
3. Home nursing service	
Supplies ($95/g)	$950.00
Nursing services	300.00
IV supplies	75.00
	$1325.00
4. Self-infusion at home	
Supplies ($55.00/g)	$550.00
IV supplies	30.00
	$580.00

hypothetical example of a 12-year-old youngster receiving 10 g of immunoglobulin once a month, the cost ranged from a high of $1640 per infusion (hospital outpatient setting) to a low of $580 (self-infusion at home). While home nursing services are convenient, the costs are not necessarily inexpensive (Table 4). These costs tend to become magnified over a period of one year. For example, monthly infusions in a hospital outpatient setting may be as much as $1060 per month or $12 720 per year more than home self-infusion (Table 5). Over a period of a year, infusion in a hospital outpatient setting could cost $10 080 more than if given in a doctor's office and $3780 more than the home health care nursing services.

Table 5
Comparative costs of IVIG treatment: differences between sites

Site	Cost	per month	per year
Hospital	$1640.00	$1060.00	$12 720.00
Doctor's office	800.00	220.00	2 640.00
Nursing team	1325.00	745.00	8 940.00
Self-infusion	580.00	N.A.	N.A.

Discussion

This study demonstrates that it is possible to have children or their parents administer IVIG to themselves at home. Additionally, it is safe procedure provided careful patient selection is adhered to (Table 6). Except for two minor reactions in an infant during the supervisory phase, there were no adverse reactions. None of our patients had a previous history of adverse reactions to IVIG in a hospital or outpatient setting and this was a very important selection criteria.

Table 6
Patient selection criteria

a. Children must have received IVIG in the past without adverse reactions
b. Parents/patients must be reliable
c. Parents/patients must be supportive of home infusion
d. Children must be cooperative
e. Parents/patients must possess self-confidence
f. Children should be older than 2 years of age and preferably over 5 years
g. Patients must be willing to return for periodic evaluation

In the majority of children, IVIG was infused every 2 weeks and trough levels were maintained above 600 mg/dl. Nevertheless, peak–trough fluctuations were still considerable (greater than 300 mg/dl), but less than the large fluctuations seen when administered once a month (greater than 600 mg/dl). This study also demonstrated that it is possible to self-infuse IVIG every 10 days as was the case in two children (J.A.B. and M.A.B.). Earlier studies established the feasibility of home self-infusion. Ashida and Saxon (4) treated seven adult patients with primary antibody deficiency with monthly infusion using an autosyringe pump. No adverse reactions were observed after as long as 25 months of treatment. In another study by Ochs *et al.* (6) seven patients, including three under 18 years of age, were treated by self-infusion every 9–14 days. Minor reactions occurred in 6 out of a total of 277 infusions (reaction rate of 2.2%). Sorensen *et al.* (5) treated nine patients, two of which were children. Adverse reactions occurred in 2 out of 171 infusions (1.2%). It can therefore be seen that in these patients, the incidence of adverse reactions is 2% or less. The cost savings of home IVIG can be substantial. Ochs *et al.* (6) estimated a cost savings of $355 per infusion when compared to clinic based infusions. Ryan *et al.* (7) also suggested significant savings when IVIG was administered at home, which he felt was important in the British health care system. We also estimated substantial savings if IVIG were administered at home. In addition to the medical cost savings, savings from lost wages and transportation costs may also be a factor. Additionally, several studies have alluded to patient preference and convenience for home self-infusion (4, 6, 8). However, with the economic competition and incentive for performing IVIG service, hospitals, doctors and home nursing care services may not be enthusiastic about supporting self-infusion (Table 7). In the case of doctors, significant income could be lost if patients were to infuse IVIG at home. The physician would not be reimbursed for overseeing the patient's care and could potentially face legal liability should the patient suffer adverse reactions at home. These economic and legal hurdles need to be addressed before home IVIG infusion becomes a more widely accepted practice.

Table 7
Comparative costs for IVIG treatment: factors working against home self-infusion of IVIG

Economic incentives
Legal disincentives
Insurance company disincentives
Patient participation
Doctor resistence
Health services competition

Summary

Twelve children with primary immunodeficiency, ages 2–17 years of age (9.8 ± 5.3, mean ± 1 SD) were enrolled in a 9-month study to determine the safety and feasibility of home self-infusion of IVIG. The study was divided into four phases including a training phase, a supervisory phase (2 months), home infusion phase (6 months) and a summary phase. Children or their parents administered IVIG in a home setting and a total of 224 infusions were given with only two minor reactions (reaction rate 0.9%). Eight children received IVIG (200 mg/kg) every 2 weeks, while 4 other children received treatments every 10 days or 1 month. Except for initial technical difficulty in starting i.v.s in the two youngest children (ages 18 months and 2 years), no problems were encountered and all 12 children completed the study. Potential cost savings are considerable, however legal and economic factors need to be resolved before home IVIG therapy becomes an acceptable practice. In summary, our study shows that home self-infusion of IVIG can be safe and feasible.

References

1. Stiehm, E. R. Human gammaglobulin as therapeutic agents. *Adv. Pediatr.* **35**: 1–72, 1988.
2. Berkman, S. A., Lee, M. L. and Gale, R. P. Clinical uses of intravenous immunoglobulins. *Seminars Hemat.* **25**: 140–158, 1988.
3. Stiehm, E.R. Intravenous immunoglobulins as therapeutic agents. *Ann. Intern. Med.* **107**: 367–382, 1987.
4. Ashida, E. R. and Saxon, A. Home intravenous immunoglobulin in therapy by self-administration. *J. Clin. Immunol.* **6**: 306–309, 1986.
5. Sorensen, R. U., Kallick, M. D. and Berger, M. Home treatment of antibody deficiency syndromes with intravenous immune globulin. *J. Allergy Clin. Immunol.* **80**: 810–815, 1987.
6. Ochs, H. D., Lee, M. L., Fischer, S. H., *et al.* Self-infusion of intravenous immunoglobulin by immunodeficient patients at home. *J. Infect. Dis.* **156**: 652–654, 1987.
7. Ryan, A., Thomson, B. and Webster, A. D. B. Home intravenous immunoglobulin therapy for patients with primary hypogammaglobulinaemia. *Lancet* **2**: 793 (letter); 1988.
8. Evans, J. H., Daly, P. V., Kobayashi, R. H. and Kobayashi, A. D. Quality of life correlates and psychological effects of home-base intravenous IgG infusion therapy. *J. Allergy Clin. Immunol.* **81**: 288 (abstract); 1988.

Discussion

R. van Furth

Another way of home treatment of agammaglobulinemic patients is self-infusion by the subcutaneous route with the intramuscular preparations. We use a similar training and follow-up program as you do. Trained patients are seen only every 3–4 months by the doctor. The only problem we encounter in a small number of patients (over 30 patients older than 14 years are in the Leiden program) is a decreased absorption from the subcutaneous space. This is probably due to fibrosis or local catabolism. In such cases we give IgG intravenously for 4–6 months. Thereafter they tolerate subcutaneously infused IgG better. In general, subcutaneous IgG is well accepted without any side effects.

R. H. Kobayashi

Thank you for your comment. It is certainly less expensive to infuse immunoglobulin in the fashion you describe; also it would be technically simpler. Whether sufficiently high serum levels would be achieved and whether it is as efficacious need to be considered. This was a practice tried in the US but abandoned in favor of intravenous immunoglobulin.

M. Haney

We have an adolescent boy who self-infuses IVIG. He deliberately infuses at an excessively fast rate because he experiences an intensely pleasurable "electric buzz" throughout his body. This can last for up to 5 min before he develops an atypical phlogistic reaction. Have you come across this in any of your patients?

R. H. Kobayashi

My colleagues and I have also received unsolicited comments from some patients suggesting a "pleasurable" sense of well-being from IVIG infusion. This observation has been seen at conventional infusion rates. Dr Pirovsky from the University of Oregon has conducted a trial where a 12% IVIG solution was infused in 15–30 min and also has noted patients' reports of a "pleasurable" sensation. Whether this is due to endorphin release or not, I am not sure. I suspect someone could do a study to look at endorphin levels before, during and after IVIG infusion to see if there are any changes.

H. Chapel

The experience in the UK is very similar to yours. There are over 85 patients in the UK home therapy register set up 4 years ago. There are now four centers for training with three more in the process of being set up. What proportion of patients receiving IVIG in the US do you expect to do self-infusion eventually?

R. H. Kobayashi

Thank you for letting us know about your experience in Great Britain. A letter to the editor from Dr Ryan (UK) in the *Lancet* suggested significant cost savings in England. In the United States, the economic, social and political forces, not to mention legal forces, make centralized coordination difficult. There are economic and legal disincentives to home self-infusions. I suspect that even government recommendations will not alter this. Only if the private insurance companies lower their reimbursements for facility and health care personnel charges, will it become economically unfeasible for the health care providers, thus encouraging self-infusion. Once the private insurance companies realize they can save money by altering their reimbursement programs, I believe they will change. Until then it will be difficult to guess what percentage of patients will self-infuse, but it will be small.

Part II
Neonatal infections

IVIG can save many preterm infants

G. ROBERTO BURGIO

Pediatrics Clinic, University of Pavia, Pavia, Italy

Immunoglobulins are a "finished" product of the immunocompetent system and constitute the fundamental humoral protagonist in specific defenses.

B and T lymphocytes and their products

Not many years ago, with reference to the physiological need for the cooperative function of the two immune defense cell lines, namely T lymphocytes and B lymphocytes, R. Good, with a colorful allegory, expressed the concept that "it takes two to tango". However, there is a deep difference between these two lines: at least at the present time, only the "finished product" of B lymphocytes (or at least the main one, IgG) is largely employed. On the other hand, many "products" of T lymphocytes and their functions are essentially known. Consider cytokines and their role in the regulation not only of the immune response but also, more generally, of growth and cell differentiation. Some of them, made available in large amounts by molecular biology techniques, have therapeutic applications in specific conditions. For example, alpha interferon is used in the therapy of hairy cell leukemia (1), of other myelo- and lymphoproliferative disorders (2, 3, 4) and of some

Immunotherapy with Intravenous Immunoglobulins
ISBN 0–12–370725–0

viral diseases (especially chronic hepatitis B (5)); and interleukin 2 is used in the therapy of renal carcinoma and melanomas (6, 7). But who could conceive of compensating a severe deficit of T lymphocytes by administering this or that product of their activities? From this point of view, even the most active (and welcome) thymic hormones have scored, as a whole, only partial success. Due to all these issues, a severe T-lymphocyte deficit remains the field of application of bone marrow transplantation (BMT) or, for certain prospects, of fetal liver cell transplantation. In other words, cell-mediated immunity, being a direct function of the lymphocytes themselves with their complex antigen–receptor apparatus, remains a field of application of these cells and therefore it is their progenitors which must be transplanted, with all the reservations concerning the take and/or the risk of graft versus host disease (GVHD).

This is obviously not true for humoral (antibody-mediated) immunity, for which we acknowledge IgG to be the "finished product" which solves the problem. In fact, the organism is severely—and thus also very precociously—threatened by infections (by the most diverse pathogens) not only if the two cell lines are lacking but even if only one is deficient. Thus, for T-lymphocyte deficit, infections (predominantly viral and mycotic ones, but bacterial ones as well) have an easy onset soon after birth, whereas in B-lymphocyte deficit (a classic prototype, almost an "*experimentum naturae*", being Bruton's agammaglobulinemia), infections, which are bacterial to an overwhelming extent, predominantly start from the second semester of life onward. This is true, at least to a significant extent, for infants affected by Bruton's disease, since the finished product, generated by the B-cell system of the mother (in other words, maternal IgG, not—as is known—IgA and IgM), passes to the fetus and protects the newborn and, for many months, the infant. However, the chronology of this transplacental passage of IgG is rather limited: it is confined mainly (and not equally for all subclasses) to the last six weeks of gestation. Therefore every fetus born preterm risks having a deficit of this important immune resource (8, 9). The earlier the pregnancy is interrupted, the higher the risk (10).

IVIG in preterm infants

The natural history of the preterm infant includes, among several functional limitations related to the immaturity of various organs and systems, the serious threat of sepsis starting from the intestine, the navel, the skin in general, and from the mucosa of the respiratory system, particularly if instrumental respiration by intubation has been necessary. It has been calculated that especially for infants born before the 34th week of prenatal life the prevalence of infections is between 24 and 32%, with a mortality which oscillates between 11 and 33% (11, 12).

Certainly one must not underestimate the fact that other immune functions particularly orientated toward anti-bacterial defense are also suppressed in preterm infants. We mention, for example, that in these infants the classical pathway of complement activation and the alternate pathway are both highly deficient (13) and that, among granulocyte functions, chemotaxis and bactericidal activity are highly suppressed. Whereas this suppression lasts approximately 1 week in the full-term neonate (14, 15), in the preterm neonate, especially if born from a pregnancy interrupted before the 34th week, it lasts up to one and a half months (16–18).

In any case, there are specific and highly significant data which have reasonably motivated the use of IgG in the preterm neonate, especially in view of the fact that this use is extraordinarily facilitated by modern intact IgG preparations for i.v. injection (19).

Chirico *et al.* (20) demonstrated that the half-life of IgG infused in the neonate is 7–10 days. On this basis, treatment schedules have been designed with weekly injections of 0.5 g/kg body weight of IVIG. This treatment in preterm infants allows prompt achievement of serum IgG levels similar to those observed in term newborns and was found to reduce significantly morbidity and mortality due to infections in a group of severely preterm neonates (gestational age < 34 weeks). These results have been subsequently confirmed by other groups (21–23).

A detailed proposal for differentiated dosages depending on whether the neonates weigh < 1 kg or > 1 kg has been formulated by Kyllonen *et al.* (24): 700 mg/kg at least every 2 weeks for infants > 1 kg and 900 mg/kg for infants below 1 kg are proposed, with monitoring on the 6th and 12th day after infusion to allow individualization of the dosage.

It is not difficult to conclude that the conceptual premises valid for the proposal of IVIG treatment of preterm infants have been significantly confirmed by the results obtained, although even recently this use has been cautiously included among those considered a matter of debate (19). This will be, for us, a debate which will certainly have the merit of stimulating, perhaps even initiating, new studies and researches; on the other hand we are far from imagining that this debate may really leave doubts on the objective criteria for the application of IVIG in preterm infants in the prevention of many infections.

Summary

Immunoglobulins (Ig) can be judged and therefore presented as a "finished product" of B lymphocytes. As regards IgG, the industry has made this product available with a high degree of purity and in large amounts for clinical use. Besides true diseases related to "immunodeficiencies" caused or characterized by B lymphocyte deficit, in which the use of IgG is to be considered as an indispensable replacement therapy, other indications are known. In particular it does not seem irrelevant to consider that preterm infants are deficient in Ig to an extent which is directly related to how early the pregnancy was interrupted. Therefore they constitute a category of infants at risk for menacing sepses, and for these infants the prophylactic use of IgG is now extensively and reasonably considered as a possible precious resource.

References

1. Quesada, J. R., Reuben, J., Manning, J. T. *et al.* Alpha interferon for the induction of remission in hairy cell leukemia. *N. Engl. J. Med.* 15: 310; 1984.
2. Talpaz, M., Kantarjian, H. M., McCredie, K. *et al.* Hematologic remission and cytogenetic improvement induced by recombinant human interferon alpha A in chronic myelogenous leukemia. *N. Engl. J. Med.* 314: 1065; 1986.
3. Foon, K. A., Sherwin, S. A. and Abrams, P. G. Treatment of advanced non-Hodgkin lymphoma with recombinant leukocyte A interferon. *N. Engl. J. Med.* 311: 1148; 1984.
4. Mandelli, F., Tribalto, M. and Avvisati, G. Recombinant interferon alpha 2B as post-induction therapy for responding multiple myeloma patients. M84 protocol. *Cancer Treat. Rev.* 15: 43; 1988.
5. Lock, A. S. F., Lai, C. L. and Wu, P. C. Long term follow-up in a randomized controlled trail of recombinant alpha 2 interferon in Chinese patients with chronic hepatitis B infection. *Lancet* i: 298; 1988.
6. Rosenberg, S. A., Packard, B. S., Aebersold, P. M. *et al.* A progress report on the treatment of 157 patients with advanced cancer using

lymphokine-activated killer cells and interleukin 2 or high-dose interleukin 2 alone. *N. Engl. J. Med.* **316**: 889; 1987.
7. Rosenberg, S. A., Packard, B. S., Aebersold, P. M. *et al.* Use of tumor infiltrating lymphocytes and interleukin 2 in the immunotherapy of patients with metastatic melanoma. A preliminary report. *N. Engl. J. Med.* **319**: 1676; 1988.
8. Morell, A., Skvaril, F., Van Loghen, E. *et al.* Human IgG subclasses in maternal and fetal serum. *Vox Sang* **21**: 481; 1971.
9. Pitcher-Wilmott, R. W., Hinducha, P. and Wood, C. B. S. The placental transfer of IgG subclasses in human pregnancy. *Clin. Exp. Immunol.* **41**: 303; 1980.
10. Pilgrim, U., Fontanellaz, H. P., Evers, G. *et al.* Normal values of immunoglobulins in premature and in full-term infants, calculated as percentiles. *Helv. Paediatr. Acta* **30**: 121; 1975.
11. Usher, R. H. The special problems of the premature infant. In "Neonatology" (Ed. Avery, G. B.). Pathophysiology and management of the newborn. J. B. Lippincott, Philadelphia; 1981.
12. Hemming, V. G., Overal, J. C. and Britt, M. R. Nosocomial infections in a newborn intensive-care unit: results of forty-one months of surveillance. *N. Engl. J. Med.* **10**: 1310; 1976.
13. Notarangelo, L. D., Chirico, G., Chiara, A. *et al.* Activity of classic and alternative pathways of complement in preterm and small for gestational age infants. *Pediatr. Res.* **18**: 281; 1984.
14. Miller, M. E. Phagocytosis in the newborn infant: humoral and cellular factors. *J. Pediatr.* **74**: 225; 1969.
15. Miller, M. E. Chemotactic function in human neonate: humoral and cellular aspects. *Pediatr. Res.* **5**: 487; 1971.
16. Hill, H. R. H. and Sacchi F. Mechanism of abnormal neutrophil function in the human neonate: prospects for therapy. In "Immunology of the neonate" (Eds Burgio, G. R., Hanson, L. A. and Ugazio, A. G.). Springer-Verlag, Heidelberg, Berlin, New York; 1987.
17. Sacchi, F., Rondini, G., Stronati, M. *et al.* Different maturation of neutrophil chemotaxis in term and preterm newborn infants. *J. Pediatr.* **101**: 273; 1982.
18. Chirico, G., Marconi, M., De Amici, M. *et al.* Deficiency of neutrophil bactericidal activity in terms and preterm infants. *Biol. Neonate* **47**: 125; 1985.
19. Ugazio, A. G., Duse, M. and Notarangelo, L. D. Intravenous immunoglobulin and immunodeficiency in children. *Current Opinion in Pediatrics* **1**: 5; 1989.
20. Chirico, G., Rondini, G., Plebani, A. *et al.* Intravenous gammaglobulin therapy for prophylaxis of infection in high-risk neonates. *J. Pediatr.* **110**: 437; 1987.
21. Stiehm, E. R. The use of human intravenous immune globulin in

immunoregulatory disorders and in the newborn period. *Immunol. Allergy Clin. North. Am.* **8**: 39; 1988.
22. Ruderman, J. W., Gall, R. L., Pomerance, J. J. *et al.* Use of intravenous immunoglobulin in hypogammaglobulinemia of prematurity disorders. *Pediatr. Res.* **33**: 488; 1988.
23. Clapp, D. W., Kliegman, R. M., Baley, J. E. *et al.* Use of intravenously administered immune globulin to prevent nosocomial sepsis in low birth weight infants: Report of a pilot study. *J. Pediatr.* **115**: 973; 1989.
24. Kyllonen, K. S., Clapp, D. W., Kliegman, R. M. *et al.* Dosage of intravenously administered immune globulin and dosing interval required to maintain target levels of immunoglobulin G in low birth weight infants. *J. Pediatr.* **115**: 1013; 1989.

Neonatal sepsis: an overview

CAROL J. BAKER

Myers-Black Section of Infectious Diseases, Departments of Pediatrics, Microbiology & Immunology, Baylor College of Medicine, Houston, Texas, USA

Neonatal sepsis is a clinical syndrome occurring in infants 28 days of age or younger which is characterized by systemic symptoms and signs of infection *and* isolation of a pathogenic organism (usually a bacterium) from the blood (bacteremia) (1). While sepsis may be accompanied by focal infections such as meningitis, cellulitis or osteoarthritis, for example, bacteremia is the usual prelude. Despite this strict definition by age, it is clear that some infants, especially those born before 30–32 weeks gestation, develop "neonatal" sepsis, as defined by etiology, clinical pattern and mode of transmission, at ages beyond 28 days. Two epidemiologically and clinically distinct patterns, designated as early and late onset sepsis, characterize these infections (1) and are salient to any discussion of new modalities, such as intravenous immunoglobulin (IVIG), for their treatment or prevention. Other significant issues include the distribution of etiologic agents associated with neonatal sepsis, the relative importance of IgG as an opsonin-promoting effective attachment, ingestion and killing of a specific organism by polymorphonuclear leukocytes within the bloodstream, and the proposed use of IVIG as adjunctive therapy (2, 3) or prophylaxis (2, 4–7).

Immunotherapy with Intravenous Immunoglobulins
ISBN 0–12–370725–0

Age at onset and modes of transmission

Early onset (≤ 5 days of age) neonatal sepsis (Table 1) often has its onset *in utero* with symptoms appearing at or within a few hours after birth in up to two-thirds of cases. Its incidence has been estimated to be 1–5 per 1000 live births, the attack rate being inversely related to birthweight (1). The range in incidence mirrors the prevalence of maternal risk factors associated with infant sepsis, especially premature onset of labour, premature rupture of membranes or chorioamnionitis (1). These risk factors, especially in the term infant, may be the only clue to bacteremia prior to the onset of often rapidly progressive symptoms. The etiology reflects the vertical mode of transmission. Maternal genital flora either are aspirated *in utero*, as in prolonged rupture of membranes or chorioamnionitis, or during passage through the birth canal intrapartum. Neonates with an *in utero* onset frequently have pneumonia, circulatory collapse, neutropenia and a fatal outcome despite institution of antimicrobial therapy at birth (1). Signs of infection, by contrast, may be delayed as long as 2–3 days in the term infant when fever, apnoeic episodes and grunting, poor feeding and lethargy appear. Some of these infants have no identifiable maternal risk factors.

For nearly 20 years, group B *Streptococcus* (GBS) has been the single most frequent etiologic agent causing early onset sepsis. Other agents include *Escherichia coli* and other enterics, other streptococci (the viridans group, *Enterococcus*, and Lancefield groups A, C, and G), *Listeria monocytogenes* and non-typable *Haemophilus influenzae*. Both prompt detection and improvement in supportive care have produced a significant reduction in mortality rates from more than 50% in the 1970s to approximately 20% currently (1, 2).

Late onset sepsis (> 5 days of age) in the term or larger preterm neonate is less common, often presents clinically as fever with non-specific symptoms, and may or may not be associated with focal findings, such as respiratory signs (pneumonia), bulging fontanelle or seizures (meningitis), or soft tissue inflammation (abscess, septic arthritis or osteomyelitis) (1). For the neonate discharged home without complications, the mode of transmission may be vertical, in association with agents such as GBS, *E. coli* or *Listeria monocytogenes*, or community acquisition, with such infecting agents as *S. aureus* or group A *Streptococcus*. However, for very low birth weight (VLBW) infants requiring prolonged hospitalization for the medical complications of prematurity as well as nutritional support, late onset sepsis has a high incidence, multiple episodes may occur in the same infant, and

Table 1
Patterns of sepsis in term, premature and very low birth weight (VLBW) neonates

Feature	Early onset (term, premature)	Late onset (term, premature)	Late onset (VLBW)
Mean onset (days)	1 ($\leqslant 5$)	21 ($\geqslant 6$)	10–28[a]
Incidence (per 1000)	1–5	1	200[b]
Mode of transmission	Vertical (intrapartum)	Vertical/community	Nosocomial/vertical
Maternal complications[c]	Common	Unusual	Common
Clinical features	Symptoms at birth; pneumonia common (RDS,[d] apnoea, neutropenia, poor perfusion, fever)	Variable: insidious to fulminant onset; fever without focal signs or meningitis, cellulitis, pneumonia	Usually non-specific (A & B,[e] poor feeding, abdominal distention, lethargy, etc.)
Etiologic agents	GBS[f]	GBS	CONS;[g] *S. aureus*
	E. coli (enterics)	*S. aureus*	*Enterococcus*
	Other streptococci	*Listeria monocytogenes*	*Klebsiella* (enterics)
	Listeria monocytogenes	*E. coli*	*Pseudomonas*/*Serratia*
	Haemophilus influenzae		*Candida* species
Mortality (%)	20	10	5

[a] Often appears beyond 28 days; multiple episodes may occur.
[b] Estimate based on 90% survival of infants and 30% rate during neonatal hospitalization.
[c] Premature onset of labor or rupture of membranes, prolonged rupture of membranes > 24 hours, chorioamnionitis, UTI in third trimester, postpartum endometritis ± bacteremia.
[d] Respiratory distress syndrome.
[e] Apnoea and bradycardia.
[f] Group B *Streptococcus*.
[g] Coagulase negative staphylococci (*S. epidermidis* and other species).

onset may occur after the first month of life (1). The mode of transmission either may be vertical (*E. coli*, *Candida* species, GBS and *Enterococcus*) or nosocomial via the hands of personnel (coagulase negative staphylococci, methicillin-susceptible and resistant *S. aureus*, *Klebsiella pneumoniae*, *Pseudomonas aeruginosa*, *Serratia marcescens*, etc.). Because of immaturity, symptoms in these infants often are subtle, early inflammatory response with focal infections is meager, and certain associated conditions which are rare in term infants are common (necrotizing enterocolitis, intravascular catheter-related infected thrombi, scalp abscesses at intravenous needle sites, etc.) (4, 5).

Distribution of etiologic agents

Historically, changes in the etiology of neonatal sepsis are common. For vertically transmitted infections caused by maternal genital flora, changes occur every 2–3 decades for some organisms (i.e. *E. coli* and GBS), while for nosocomially transmitted agents, shifts in etiology vary from hospital-to-hospital and from year-to-year within a given neonatal intensive care unit (1). For nearly 20 years, the etiology of early onset and late onset sepsis in term infants has been stable (Table 1). GBS and *E. coli* are the predominant, but not exclusive, causative pathogens. New agents reported during the past two decades include viridans group streptococci and non-typable strains of *Haemophilus influenzae*, but the number of these cases each comprises less than 15% of the total (1). However, "new pathogens" have emerged as causative agents of nosocomial sepsis, especially among VLBW infants. These include coagulase negative staphylococci, methicillin-resistant *S. aureus*, *Enterococcus*, *Candida* species and a myriad of other organisms (1, 4, 5). Some of these organisms are opportunists which are acquired from endogenous sources (for example, *Candida*) and sepsis occurs only when mucosal barriers are bypassed (indwelling intravascular catheters), normal flora are altered (prolonged broad spectrum antibiotic use), or in the setting of abnormal host defense (hypogammaglobulinemia, low levels of complement, abnormal neutrophil function). Others represent historically common nosocomial pathogens such as methicillin-susceptible *S. aureus*, strains of *Klebsiella* or other enterics, *Pseudomonas*, *Serratia*, etc. The single most frequent cause of infection in VLBW infants is the nosocomially acquired, opportunistic agent, coagulase negative *Staphylococcus* (CONS), the most frequent species of which is *Staphylococcus epidermidis* (1, 4, 5). Thus, age at onset, information concerning hospital flora causing nosocomial infection in the nursery, and knowledge of host factors predicting likelihood of sepsis with a specific pathogen all are required to appropriately select empiric antimicrobial therapy. This complex listing of potential pathogens serves to underscore the immensity of the task of developing pathogen-specific intravenous immune globulins or human monoclonal antibody reagents as adjunctive therapeutic agents for neonates with either early or late onset sepsis (2, 3, 6, 7).

Host defense interactions

A number of factors and their complex interaction determine whether a neonate will, assuming contact with a potential pathogen at mucous membrane sites, develop either early or late onset systemic infection. Defined maternal factors, listed previously, significantly increase risk for early onset sepsis and for GBS specifically also include maternal postpartum bacteremia. Low levels of antibody to the type-specific polysaccharide capsular antigens of these organisms also increase risk (3). Neonatal factors are represented by the entire spectrum of host defense mechanisms which are "physiologically" deficient, and these are exaggerated in the preterm infant who has, in addition, hypogammaglobulinemia (1). Bacterial factors also are important in the formula, determining interactions which produce or prevent invasiveness. For example, the capsular structures of GBS type III and *E. coli* K_1 are particularly efficient in avoiding opsonophagocytosis and activation of the alternative complement pathway, in invading the meninges, and at depleting the neutrophil storage pools of neonates with early and late onset sepsis (1, 3). However, for both agents a sufficient amount of capsular specific IgG antibody appears to overcome these virulence properties (3, 8). Unfortunately, it appears that most women lack sufficient amounts of GBS-specific antibodies to protect to their neonates, especially if they are born prior to 32 weeks gestation (9). Thus, use of IVIG to provide specific opsonins for early onset pathogens has been proposed as an adjunct to conventional therapy (2, 3, 6, 10). This proposal is based upon extensive *in vitro* data indicating that IVIG augments opsonization and phagocytosis of GBS by neonatal sera (3, 11, 12) and is protective, if given in sufficient amounts, in several animal models of lethal GBS or *E. coli* infection (3, 8). IVIG hyperimmune for GBS was produced by Gloser *et al.* (13) by immunizing adult plasma donors with GBS polysaccharide vaccines. This material is considerably more protective than is standard IVIG, an observation predicted by the very high titers of specific antibodies (3, 6, 13).

By contrast to what is known concerning human immunity of the neonate to GBS, little is known concerning the role of human IgG antibody in host defense against the pathogens causing late onset sepsis in VLBW infants. Table 2 is an attempt to summarize these pathogens, their clinical features, and the role of antibody and complement as opsonins promoting host defense. While much more research will be required to further define host defense interactions as they apply to VLBW infants, it appears that both antibody to surface and cell wall antigens as contained in IVIG *and* complement proteins are important in promoting opsonization and phagocytic ingestion of CONS (14–16). Similarly, for some strains of *Pseudomonas* both IgG and complement are probably important for opsonophagocytosis (2, 17). However, for other prominent causative agents, the information is limited.

Table 2
Late onset sepsis in VLBW infants

Pathogen	Sites of infection	Opsonins	
Coagulase negative staphylococci	Intravascular catheters; blood; soft tissue; NEC[a]	Antibody Complement	+++ ++
S. aureus[b]	Intravascular catheters; blood; bone; joint; heart; lungs; soft tissue	Antibody Complement	+++ +++
Enterococcus	Blood; NEC; intravascular catheters	Antibody Complement	? ?
Klebsiella	Blood; CSF;[c] lungs; NEC	Antibody Complement	+ +
Pseudomonas	Blood; CSF; lungs	Antibody Complement	+++ ++
Candida	Intravascular catheters; blood; CSF; kidneys; eye; bone; joint; soft tissue	Antibody Complement	+ +++

+++ = important; ++ = probably important; + minimal importance or poorly studied.

[a] Necrotizing enterocolitis.

[b] Both methicillin-susceptible and resistant strains.

[c] Cerebrospinal fluid.

IVIG for therapy or prophylaxis

Despite early diagnosis and prompt initiation of antimicrobials, the mortality and morbidity from neonatal sepsis remains formidable. This "irreducible baseline" has provoked interest in the development of adjunctive therapeutic modalities aimed at augmenting neonatal host defense which theoretically should improve outcome. Among those suggested is IVIG, employed either as a commercially available standard preparation or hyperimmune for a specific organism. While, as previously noted, there is considerable experimental data concerning the importance of human IgG antibody in host defense against GBS, and to a lesser extent *E. coli*, information for other neonatal pathogens is limited or non-existent. Several laboratories have reported that standard IVIG preparations contain only modest levels of GBS antibodies (3, 6), are variable in their effect on *in vitro* opsonophagocytosis by dose and preparative method (3), and are significantly less protective in experimental models of infection than is IVIG prepared from adults immunized with GBS (hyperimmune IVIG). Thus, is seems reasonable to suggest that IVIG preparations proposed for future adjunctive therapy of early onset neonatal sepsis should be hyperimmune for GBS, and perhaps other etiologic agents. However, large, multicenter, controlled clinical trials demonstrating the safety and efficacy of standard or hyperimmune preparations of IVIG will be required before any of these products can be recommended for routine therapy. As to the use of IVIG as therapy in late onset neonatal sepsis, the vast array of etiologic agents suggests that pathogen-specific therapy may be impractical. However, research regarding the importance, or lack thereof, of IgG as an opsonin for the most prominent of these late onset pathogens should be encouraged.

Another proposed use of IVIG for neonatal sepsis involves its administration for the prevention of late onset sepsis in VLBW infants who have the highest risk of acquiring one or more episodes of infection. This proposal is based on the observation that infants with gestations < 32 weeks are hypogammaglobulinemic at birth (mean IgG levels < 400 mg/dl) (18, 19) due to lack of placental transport of maternal IgG. This condition worsens for the next several weeks before endogenous production of IgG by the infant ensues. What constitutes "hypogammaglobulinemia" in these infants, however, is controversial. Sasidharan (18, 19) has suggested that serum IgG levels in excess of 200 mg/dl are "physiologic", while Clapp *et al.* (5) imply that levels less than 700 mg/dl are "pathologic". Any definition, however, is arbitrary until clinical trials verify the level below which risk for sepsis increases significantly. However, theoretical additional reasons for "replacement" IVIG in these VLBW infants are compelling: the high attack rate for late onset sepsis with its attendant mortality and morbidity, the poor neutrophil function and inflammatory response of these infants, and the unavailability of IgM, IgA or secretory IgA reagents (1–3). Finally, two recent reports suggest that the administration of a standard preparation of IVIG to preterm neonates at periodic intervals reduces the incidence of late onset sepsis (4, 5). In the study by Clapp *et al.* (5), each of the infections in the placebo group occurred when IgG levels were less than 400 mg/dl. While these preliminary results are encouraging, much more information will be required to establish the efficacy of IVIG as prophylaxis for late onset infection and whether the reduction in infection rate is broad or pathogen-specific, to determine the optimal and interval of IVIG by birthweight group, and to document the long-term safety of IVIG as a possible modulator of response to foreign antigens (i.e. vaccines) or endogenous synthesis of IgG. Until these issues are resolved, the routine use of IVIG for prophylaxis of late onset sepsis in VLBW infants should be discouraged, and its use in term infants should be considered to be contraindicated.

References

1. Klein, J. O. and Marcey, S. M. Bacterial sepsis and meningitis. *In* "Infections in the Fetus and Newborn Infant", 3rd edn (Eds Remington, J. S. and Klein, J. O.) pp. 601–656. W. B. Saunders, Philadelphia; 1990.
2. Gonzales, L. A. and Hill, H. R. The current status of intravenous gamma globulin use in neonates. *Pediatr. Infect. Dis. J.* 8: 315–322; 1989.
3. Baker, C. J. and Noya, F. J. D. Potential use of intravenous immune globulin for group B streptococcal infection. *Rev. Infect. Dis.* (Suppl.) 12: S476–482; 1990.
4. Baker, C. J. and the Neonatal IVIG Collaborative Study Group. Multicenter trial of intravenous immunoglobulin (IVIG) to prevent late-onset infection in preterm infants: preliminary results (Abstract). *Pediatr. Res.* 25: 275A; 1989.
5. Clapp, D. W., Kliegman, R. M., Baley, J. E. *et al.* The use of intravenously administered immune globulin to prevent nosocomial sepsis in low birth weight infants: report of a pilot study. *J. Pediatr.* 115: 973–978; 1989.

6. Fischer, G. W. Immunoglobulin therapy of neonatal group B streptococcal infections: an overview. *Pediatr. Infect. Dis. J.* (Suppl.) 7: 13–16; 1988.
7. Baker, C. J., Rench, M. A., Noya, F. J. D. and Garcia-Prats, J. A. Role of intravenous immunoglobulin in prevention of late-onset infection in low-birth-weight neonates. *Rev. Infect. Dis.* (Suppl.) 12: S463–469; 1990.
8. Harper, T. C., Christensen, R. D. and Rothstein, G. The effect of administration of Ig to newborn rats with *E. coli* sepsis and meningitis. *Pediatr. Res.* 22: 455–460; 1987.
9. Baker, C. J., Edwards, M. S. and Kasper, D. L. Role of antibody to native type III polysaccharide of group B Streptococcus in infant infection. *Pediatrics* 68: 544–549; 1981.
10. Sidiropoulus, D., Bohme, U., von Muralt, G., Morrell, A. and Barandun, S. Immunoglobulin-substitution bei der Behandlung der neonatalen Sepsis. *Schweiz med Wschr* 111: 1649–1655; 1981.
11. Givner, L. B., Edwards, M. S., Anderson, D. C. and Baker, C. J. Immune globulin for intravenous use: enhancement of *in vitro* opsonophagocytic activity of neonatal serum. *J. Infect. Dis.* 151: 217–220; 1985.
12. Kim, K. S., Wass, C. A., Kang, J. H. and Anthony, B. F. Functional activities of various preparations of human intravenous immunoglobulin against type III group B *Streptococcus*. *J. Infect. Dis.* 153: 1092–1097; 1986.
13. Gloser, H., Bachmayer, H. and Helm, A. Intravenous immunoglobulin with high activity against group B streptococci. *Pediatr. Infect. Dis.* (Suppl.) 5: S176–179; 1986.
14. Fleer, A., Gerards, L. J., Aerts, P. *et al.* Opsonic defense to *Staphylococcus epidermidis* in the premature neonate. *J. Infect. Dis.* 152: 930–937; 1985.
15. Verbrugh, H. A., Peterson, P. K., Nguyen, B. T., Sisson, S. P. and Kim, Y. Opsonization of encapsulated *Staphylococcus aureus*: the role of specific antibody and complement. *J. Immunol.* 129: 1681–1687; 1982.
16. Shaio, M. F., Yang, K. D., Bohnsack, J. F. and Hill, H. R. Effect of immune globulin intravenous on opsonization of bacteria by classic and alternative complement pathways in premature serum. *Pediatr. Res.* 25: 634–640; 1989.
17. Pennington, J. E., Pier, G. B., Sadoff, J. C. and Small, G. J. Active and passive immunization strategies for *Pseudomonas aeruginosa* pneumonia. *Rev. Infect. Dis.* (Suppl.) 8: S426–S433; 1986.
18. Ballow, M., Cates, K. L., Rowe, J. C., Goetz, C. and Desbonnet, C. Development of the immune system in very low birth weight (less than 1500 g) premature infants: concentrations of plasma immunoglobulins and patterns of infections. *Pediatr. Res.* 20: 899–904; 1986.

19. Sasidharan, P. Postnatal IgG levels in very-low-birth-weight infants. *Clin. Pediatr. (Phila.)* 27: 271–274; 1988.

Discussion

B. Wolach

Searching for the influence of polymorphonuclear cells (PMN) on neonatal immunity, we recently found that PMN plasma membrane fluidity was significantly increased in 25 healthy, 2–4-day-old newborns, compared to 23 healthy adults. Accordingly, cholesterol and the cholesterol/phospholipid ratios of plasma membranes were lower in neonatal PMNs than in the adult cells. Moreover, the addition of cholesterol to neonatal PMNs *in vitro* significantly improved the PMN chemotactic activity. We believe that membrane fluidity modulates the receptor distribution and accessibility. It seems that optimal levels of cholesterol are required for normal neutrophil function.

C. Baker

Your findings are interesting. Clearly, we have unraveled only a few of the many ways in which the neonate, especially the preterm infant, is immunodeficient. Much work remains to be done to define specific mechanisms relating to the bacterial (predominantly) and other pathogens which infect these infants.

M. Xanthou

You showed that opsonophagocytosis of GBS induced with serum from premature (<34 weeks) neonates diminishes very soon after administration of IVIG. How do you explain this while the immunoglobulin levels remain high for a much longer period?

C. Baker

While the total IgG levels remain high for many days post-infusion, the type III GBS-specific antibodies fall off somewhat more rapidly with a half-life of about 10 days. But more importantly, sera from these infants with very low levels of specific antibody (<2 μg/ml) pre-IVIG infusion, required a mean level of 12 μg/ml post-infusion to promote significant opsonophagocytosis of type III GBS. Only a dose of 750 mg/kg IVIG containing approximately 25 μg/ml of type III GBS-specific antibody at the 15-min post-infusion time resulted in this *in vitro* correlate; in the same sera, activity was 40% at 24 h and undetectable at 96 h. These observations suggest that higher levels of pathogen-specific antibody are necessary for optimal interactions with complement and neutrophils from premature infants, and that preparation of IVIG hyperimmune for GBS will be necessary to achieve adequate therapeutic or preventative activity.

Immunoglobulin treatment and prophylaxis in the neonate

A. G. UGAZIO[1], G. CHIRICO[2], M. DUSE[1], A. PLEBANI[1],
L. D. NOTARANGELO[1], G. RONDINI[2] and G. R. BURGIO[3]

[1] *Department of Pediatrics, University of Brescia, Italy*
[2] *Division of Neonatal Intensive Care, IRCCS Policlinico S. Matteo, Italy*
[3] *Department of Pediatrics, University of Pavia, Pavia, Italy*

Neonatal infections

Infections are still a major cause of infant morbidity and mortality during the first month of life despite development of broad-spectrum antimicrobial agents and technological advances in life-support therapy. In industrialized countries the overall risk of infections during the first month of life is up to 10% and the frequency of severe infections such as sepsis and meningitis ranges from 1 to 5 per 1000 live births (1). Between 20 and 50% of severely infected infants die. These figures are much higher (14–25% of infections) in developing countries. The relative rates of morbidity and mortality vary with gestational and chronological age. In very low birth weight (VLBW) infants (neonatal weight less than 1500 g) the incidence of systemic infections is very high (14–32%) with a mortality rate of about 30% (2).

The most common bacteria are group B *Streptococcus* (GBS), *Staphylococcus aureus* and *Escherichia coli*; less frequently other Gram-negative bacteria such as *Pseudomonas*, *Klebsiella* and *Aerobacter*

Immunotherapy with Intravenous Immunoglobulins
ISBN 0–12–370725–0

aerogenes may cause neonatal sepsis, while *Staphylococcus epidermidis* is found with increasing frequency, at least in preterm infants (1, 3).

Viruses, mainly cytomegalovirus (CMV), herpes virus (HSV), echovirus and rubella are frequently isolated in neonatal infections (4). Fungi such as *Candida albicans* and protozoa, mainly *Toxoplasma gondii* may also cause infections in the fetus and neonate (3).

The high susceptibility to infections is likely to result from several predisposing factors including maternal genital colonization—particularly when associated with prolonged rupture of membranes—traumatic delivery, prematurity, resuscitation maneuvers, treatment in intensive care units, and association with underlying diseases such as hyaline membrane disease and congenital heart diseases. Furthermore, the capacity of the neonate to get rid of the invading microrganisms is severely hampered by a physiological immunodeficiency that is particularly profound and long-lasting in preterm neonates (5–8).

Immunodeficiency of the neonate

Over the last two decades, a great number of studies have demonstrated that the immune function of the neonate is deficient as compared to later ages (5, 8–12).

The number of circulating T cells is comparable in adults and neonates (13) but neonatal T lymphocytes include a high percentage of cells with an "immature" (thymic-like) phenotype (6, 11, 14–17) and several studies have demonstrated that cord blood lymphocytes poorly support B cell activation and immunoglobulin production as a result of either excessive suppression (18) or deficient helper function (12).

Functional impairment of the cytokine network may also contribute to the increased susceptibility of the neonate to infections. Although preliminary studies had reported low IL-1 production by neonatal mononuclear cells, there is now substantial agreement that neonatal monocytes are competent for IL-1 production (19).

The term newborns secrete low but substantial amounts of tumor necrosis factor (TNF) (20), while TNF secretion is highly impaired in preterm neonates (19) as well as the production of IFN-γ (21–22). The natural killer (NK) activity—known to play an important role in antiviral immunity (23)—is also severely impaired (24–26). Several phagocyte functions are impaired, including chemotaxis, phagocytosis and bacterial killing (27–30). The opsonic activity of the serum is low, partly because of the antibody deficiency (see later), partly due to low levels of complement factors and activity (10, 31). All these functions and activities are by far more defective in preterm babies and for many of them a direct relationship has been demonstrated with gestational age (27). Furthermore, attainment of normal, adult-type function occurs much earlier in term than in preterm neonates (31).

With regard to humoral immunity, in healthy newborns nearly all serum immunoglobulins are IgG of maternal origin with only traces (less than 1%) of immunoglobulins synthesized by the fetus (5, 32). Because transplacental transfer of IgG occurs almost exclusively during the last 6 weeks of gestation, the level of serum IgG is directly related to gestational age: term newborns have adult levels of IgG

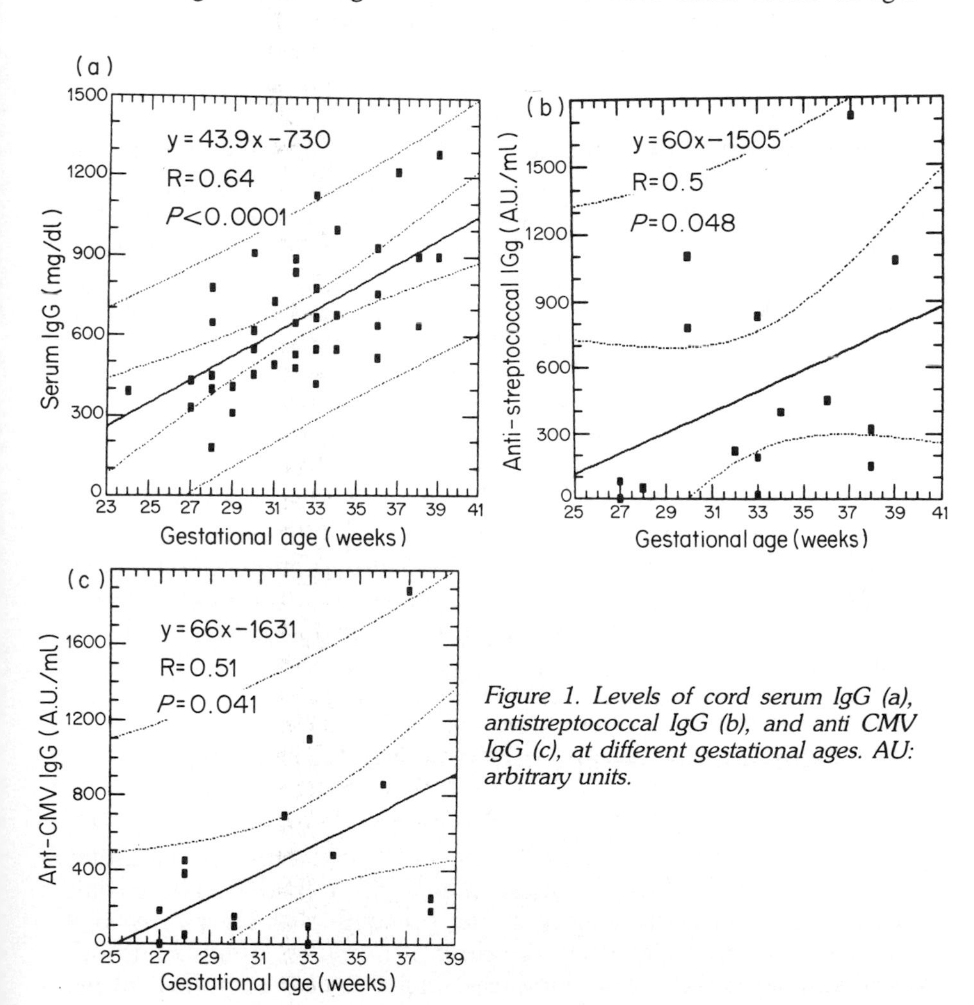

Figure 1. Levels of cord serum IgG (a), antistreptococcal IgG (b), and anti CMV IgG (c), at different gestational ages. AU: arbitrary units.

while preterm infants of about 25–32 weeks gestational age have extremely low total and specific serum IgG levels (5) (Fig. 1a, b, c).

Although all four IgG subclasses can cross the placenta (33–35), some studies (36, 37) indicate that IgG_1 are transported to a greater extent than are IgG_2. The latter are known to include most anti-polysaccharide antibodies while the former are mainly synthesized during the antibody response to protein antigens (9, 38). Therefore the preferential passage of IgG_1 over IgG_2 may account at least in part for the high susceptibility of the neonate to capsulated bacteria (39, 40).

Due to the half-life of maternally acquired IgG and to the slow onset of endogenous immunoglobulin synthesis, serum IgG levels decrease during the first months of life, to reach a nadir that, in preterm neonates, is comparable to that of agammaglobulinemic patients (5, 41, 42).

The capacity of the neonate to mount an antibody response is severely impaired. The percentage of circulating B lymphocytes is normal (18) but most neonatal B cells display an "immature" phenotype expressing simultaneously membrane IgM and IgD (18). Furthermore *in vitro* studies have demonstrated that the poor capacity of neonatal B cells to synthesize and secrete antibodies, particularly of the IgG and IgA isotypes is the result of an intrinsic defect of B cells (probably related to incomplete maturation) (9) as well as of defective helper activity (18) and/or excessive suppression (12) by neonatal T cells. Furthermore the antibody repertoire is defective with particular regard to anti-polysaccharide antibodies (9, 43, 44), while antibodies directed against protein antigens are produced but are restricted to the IgM isotype and their specific affinity is low (18). As a result, the humoral defense mechanisms of the neonate are almost completely accounted for by the immunological experience of the mother transmitted via transplacental passage of IgG during the last weeks of gestation.

Substitution therapy: pharmacological problems

Early observations of low serum IgG levels in preterm infants (45) prompted substitution trials with the immunoglobulin preparations available at that time, i.e. for intramuscular route (IMIG). These trials showed only moderate efficacy in the prevention of severe neonatal infections (45, 46). However, the dose of immunoglobulins administered did not result in a significant increase of serum IgG levels. Indeed, in their study on the administration of IMIG at the dose of

1.5 ml/kg at 1-month intervals during the first 8 months of life, Amer *et al.* found that serum IgG levels were not affected by IMIG injection. They also reported that 1 year after therapy was stopped, serum gammaglobulin levels were higher in the control group than in the group of infants treated with IMIG. However, the difference was not statistically significant.

IMIG are a 16% protein solution so that 1 ml of injected volume can provide a maximum of 160 mg of IgG. This figure is actually lowered by *in situ* proteolysis. Due to pain and tissue injury at the site of injection, only small volumes of IMIG can be administered to term neonates and even less to preterm infants, so that the lack of protective effects in these studies may well be accounted for by failure to increase significantly serum IgG levels (47).

The availability of immunoglobulin preparation for intravenous administration (IVIG) has opened a new era in the use of human immunoglobulins (48). High doses of IVIG can be safely administered in a very short period of time, thus allowing rapid attainment of normal or nearly normal IgG levels even in agammaglobulinemic patients (49). In fact, all patients with agammaglobulinemia are now under IVIG treatment with a well-documented improvement of their quality of life and resistance to infections as compared to the previous IMIG treatment (50).

IVIG contain all IgG subclasses with antibodies directed against most pathogens involved in neonatal infections (51–53). The reported side-effects in various patients treated with IVIG range from exceptional life-threatening anaphylactoid reactions to more common fever, chills, rash and vagous pain (54).

Their proven efficacy and relative safety have prompted preliminary trials in the neonate. Pharmacological studies in non-infected preterm neonates have given heterogeneous results with half-lives ranging from 10 (41) to 17 (55) or 22 days (56). On the whole, these figures are lower than those reported in older patients treated with the same IVIG preparations. However, careful evaluation of the half-life of IVIG in subjects with agammaglobulinemia has demonstrated striking heterogeneity among patients and in the same patient treated on different occasions (57). Indeed the differences found in the various pharmacokinetic studies of IVIG in neonates are likely to result from various factors including individual variability, type of IVIG preparation used and clinical status of the infant (42, 58–60).

As suggested by Kyllonen *et al.* (42), monitoring of serum IgG in the single neonate may allow individualization of the dosage and dosing intervals to obtain optimal target levels.

Animal models

In order to study the efficacy of IVIG preparations in the prevention and treatment of various neonatal infections, several experimental animal trials have been designed.

With regard to GBS infection, rabbit (61) and human (62) hyperimmune gammaglobulin preparations have been shown to protect lethally infected mice or chick embryos. Further studies have confirmed the protective role of IVIG in septic animals demonstrating that, in order to be effective, IVIG had to be administered within 6–12 h after GBS inoculation (63–66).

On the other hand, rat studies with hyperimmune IVIG obtained from pooled plasma of donors vaccinated with a GBS preparation (65, 67, 68) have demonstrated that these immunoglobulins are effective even if administered 24 h after infection.

However, Weisman and Lorenzetti (69) found a higher mortality in GBS-infected rats treated with penicillin plus high-dose IVIG (2.7 g/kg) than in rats treated with penicillin alone, and an enhanced survival and bacterial clearance with low-dose IVIG (0.68 g/kg). This apparently paradoxical phenomenon may result from the increasingly recognized immunosuppressive properties of IVIG at high doses (70) and suggests caution in the clinical use of very high-dose IVIG for the treatment of infected newborns.

The problem of GBS infection in the animal model has been recently approached by means of murine monoclonal antibodies (MoAb) directed against various GBS antigens. Mortality in GBS-infected mice was reduced by treatment with MoAb, IgM MoAb conferring greater protection than IgG or IgA MoAbs (71–73). The efficacy of MoAb of any isotype was significantly improved by simultaneous administration of fibronectin (74). This finding may be related to the reported fibronectin deficiency of the neonate (75).

Preparations of IVIG have low titres of antibodies directed against *E. coli* capsular antigens. Nevertheless they have been shown to provide opsonic activity and to prolong survival of newborn rats infected with *E. coli* (76–78). Comparative evaluation of antibiotics, antibiotics plus IVIG or IVIG alone, has demonstrated a higher efficacy of the combined therapy, provided that treatment is started within 22 h from infection (78). Similar results have been obtained in piglets (79). MoAb directed against *E. coli* 0111:B4 lipopolysaccharide antigen has been successfully employed in the treatment of *E. coli* sepsis in mice (80).

Hyperimmune IVIG preparations have been tested for prophylaxis and treatment of viral infections in animal models. In cotton rats, the combined use of IVIG and ribarivin aerosol was more efficient against RSV infection than use of either agent alone. The combined treatment significantly reduced histologic pulmonary lesions (81). Similarly, monkeys given IVIG 5 days after RSV infection, cleared viruses from the lung and did not develop pulmonary disease (82).

Immunoglobulin treatment and prophylaxis

Preterm neonates are far more susceptible than term neonates to severe infections and their levels of maternally acquired IgG is extremely low. However, as previously mentioned, early attempts at prophylaxis of neonatal infections by means of substitution treatment with IMIG were unsuccessful (45, 46). Only in one report, were IMIG

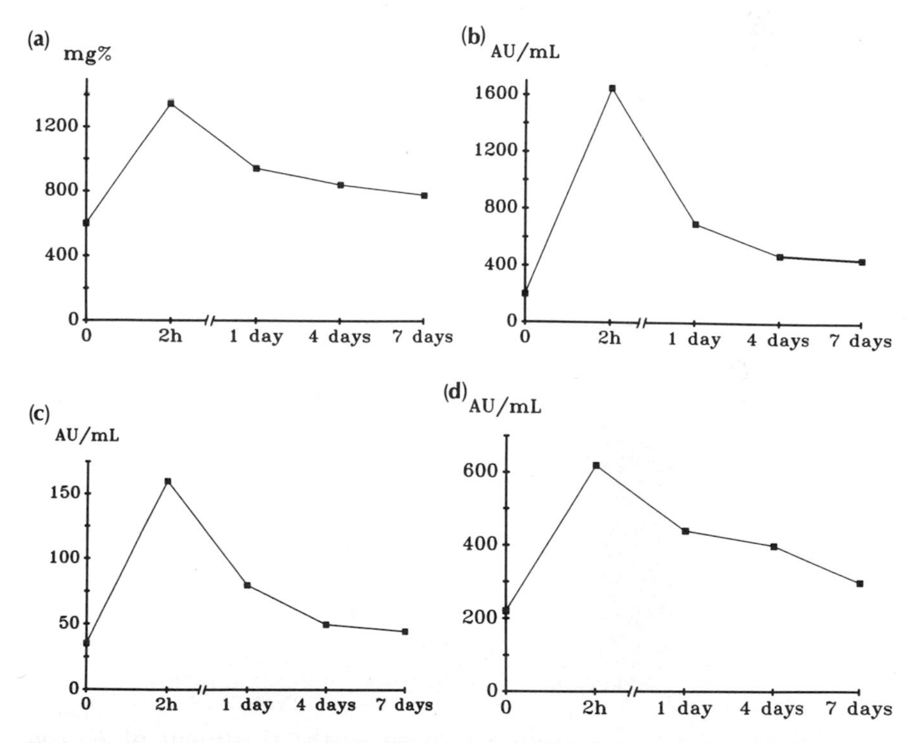

Figure 2. Levels of serum IgG (a), antistreptococcal IgG (b), anti E. coli *IgG (c) and anti-CMV IgG (d) in neonates of birth weight ⩽ 1500 g, gestational age ⩽ 34 weeks, following infusion of 400 mg/kg IVIG (Sandoglobulin®). AU: arbitrary units.*

used successfully to provide protection against an epidemic of echovirus 11 infection in an intensive care unit (83). IMIG were administered to 18 babies at the dosage of 250 mg after checking that the IMIG preparation contained neutralizing antibodies at reasonable titer. None of the treated children developed symptoms of infection.

With the availability of IVIG, new trials of substitution treatment of neonatal hypogammaglobulinemia have been carried out during the last decade. Chirico *et al.* (41, 84) studied 133 high-risk newborns stratified in two groups: babies of birth weight ⩽ 1500 g and gestational age ⩽ 34 weeks and infants with birth weight more than 1500 g under intensive care. Both groups were mainly composed of newborns under assisted ventilation (85% in the first group and 100% in the second group). Children in both groups were randomized to treatment or no treatment. IVIG (Sandoglobulin®) were given at a dose of 0.5 g/kg/week for 1 month in the first group and during the intensive care period in the second. Serum IgG levels were 616 ± 215 mg/dl and 948 ± 288 mg/dl in the two groups respectively.

Following IVIG infusion, serum IgG attained levels similar to those in term neonates in the first group with a significant enhancement of specific antibody titres (Fig. 2a, b, c, d). The results of the study clearly demonstrate that, in spite of the low number of severe infections in the study group, IVIG prophylaxis significantly reduced the occurrence of overall infections (51% versus 77%; $P < 0.02$) and

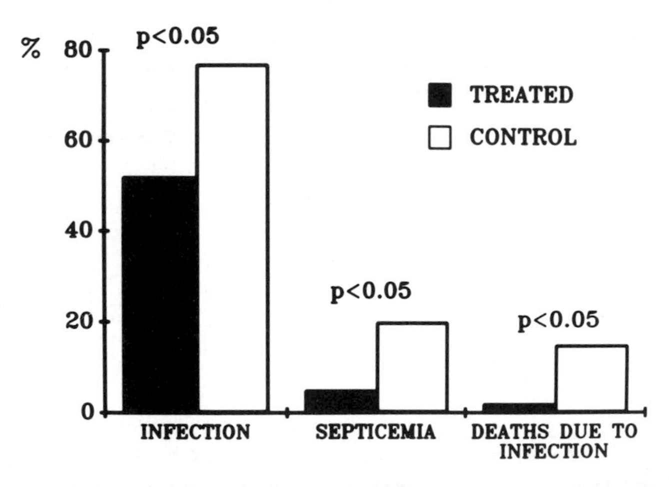

Figure 3. Prophylaxis with IVIG (Sandoglobulin®) in preterm neonates (birth weight ⩽ 1500 g, gestational age ⩽ 34 weeks) of infections, septicemia and mortality due to infection in the 43 treated and 40 control neonates.

sepsis (5% versus 20%; $P < 0.05$) in the first group of infants (Fig. 3). No significant differences were observed in the incidence of infections or sepsis in treated and control infants belonging to the group with birth weight $\geqslant$ 1500 g. A reduction, although statistically not significant, of the incidence of necrotizing enterocolitis (NEC) was observed in the treated low birth weight infants; this finding has been recently confirmed by a multicenter study (85). Interestingly, a preparation of oral IgG and IgA has also proven useful for prevention of NEC in low birth weight infants (86).

Although carried out in a different epidemiological setting, with different doses and different schedules of IVIG administration, the study by Haque *et al.* (87) has given similar results, demonstrating a significantly lower infection rate in the treated versus control group ($P < 0.005$).

No significant efficacy of IVIG in the prophylaxis of neonatal sepsis in premature infants was reported by Stabile *et al.* (88). This may be related to the high gestational age of the neonates included in the study.

In a recent double-blind controlled trial, Clapp *et al.* (89) reported a significant reduction of incidence of nosocomial sepsis in 56 preterm infants, treated with IVIG in a protocol designed to maintain a therapeutic serum target level of 700 mg/dl, as compared to 59 controls (0 vs. 7 episodes of sepsis, $P < 0.01$). All patients in the placebo group in whom sepsis developed had serum IgG levels < 400 mg/dl at the time sepsis developed.

Several other trials are in progress and preliminary data confirm the efficacy of IVIG administration in the prophylaxis of infections in preterm newborns (90–92). The possible *therapeutic* effect of IVIG in the treatment of neonatal sepsis has been studied by several groups (93–97). Von Muralt and Sidiropoulos (97) have analyzed the efficacy of IVIG (0.5–1 g/kg/day for 6 days) in two series of newborns with overt infections studied during the years 1976–1979 and 1980–1986: a significant increase of IgG serum levels was induced by IVIG treatment in infants of any gestational age. The most convincing result was the reduction of lethality resulting from sepsis in preterm babies treated with IVIG plus antibiotics (mortality rate: 8%) versus antibiotics alone (mortality rate: 44%).

A double-blind placebo-controlled study using IVIG in newborns with RSV pneumonia is in progress (98). Preliminary data suggest efficacy of the treatment with IVIG as indicated by improved oxygenation and significant reduction of viral shedding.

Finally, on the basis of successful treatment with IVIG in established echovirus, adenovirus and cytomegalovirus infections in older patients, IVIG trials will likely be attempted in the near future in infected neonates.

Summary

The high susceptibility of the newborn to infections is likely to result, at least in part, from a physiological immunodeficiency. In the neonate, nearly all immunoglobulins are IgG of maternal origin, passed across the placenta during the last 6 weeks of gestation. Therefore, during the first months of life, serum IgG of preterm infants decrease down to agammaglobulinic-like levels.

These observations prompted substitution trials, formerly with intramuscular immunoglobulin (IMIG) and, more recently, with intravenous preparations (IVIG). IMIG did not demonstrate a prophylactic effect against infections, mainly because their administration does not result in a significant increase of serum IgG levels. Conversely, large studies have demonstrated that the prophylactic use of IVIG significantly reduces the occurrence of severe infections in preterm babies.

The possible therapeutic effect of IVIG has been investigated in animal models. Most experiments have shown that normal, hyperimmune IVIG or monoclonal antibodies directed against specific pathogens, in combination with antibiotics, accelerate clearance of bacteria and protect lethally-infected animals.

Clinical trials have, therefore, been attempted in infected newborns, with an apparent reduction of lethality in preterm babies. On the basis of successful treatment with IVIG of viral infections in older patients, similar therapeutic trials are currently under way in the neonate.

References

1. Freedman, R. M., Ingram, D. L., Gross, I., Ehrenkranz, R. A., Warshaw, J. B. and Baltimore, R. S. A half century of neonatal sepsis at Yale: 1928–1978. *Am. J. Dis. Child.* 135: 140–144; 1981.
2. Uscher, R. Extreme prematurity. *In* "Neonatology Pathophysiology and Management of the Newborn" (Ed. Avery, G. B.) pp. 264–292. J. B. Lippincott, Philadelphia; 1987.
3. Miller, M. E. Immunodeficiency of Immaturity. *In* "Immunologic Disorders in Infants and Children" (Ed. Stiehm, E. R.), pp. 196–225. W. S. Saunders, Philadelphia; 1989.

4. Hanshaw, J. B., Dudgeon, J. A. and Marshall, W. C. "Viral Diseases of the Fetus and Newborn", pp. 287–300. W. B. Saunders, Philadelphia; 1985.
5. Ballow, M., Cates, K. L., Rowe, J. C., Goetz, C. and Desbonnet, C. Development of the immune system in very low birth weight (less than 1500 g) premature infants: concentration of plasma immunoglobulins and patterns of infections. *Pediatr. Res.* 20: 899–904; 1986.
6. Maccario, R. and Burgio, G. R. T and NK lymphocyte subpopulations in the neonate. *In* "Immunology of the Neonate" (Eds Burgio, G. R., Hanson, L. and Ugazio, A. G.), pp. 120–129. Springer-Verlag, Berlin; 1987.
7. Ugazio, A. G. Il neonato come immunodepresso. *In* "Il Bambino Immunodepresso: Perché lo é e Come va Difeso". Selecta Pediatrica. Vol IV, pp. 139–152. Edizioni Mediche Italiane; 1983.
8. Ugazio, A. G., Maccario, R. and Burgio, G. R. Ontogeny of T cell subsets in the neonatal period. *In* "Recent Advances in Primary and Acquired Immunodeficiencies" (Eds Aiuti, F., Rosen, F. and Cooper, M. D.), Vol 28, pp. 245–254. Raven Press, New York; 1986.
9. Andersson, U. Regulation of antibody synthesis in the neonate. *In* "Immunology of the Neonate" (Eds Burgio, G. R., Hanson, L. A. and Ugazio, A. G.), pp. 37–50. Springer-Verlag, Berlin; 1987.
10. Bellanti, J. A. and Zeligs, J. B. Immunity and infections in the neonate. *In* "Immunology of the Neonate" (Eds Burgio, G. R., Hanson, L. A. and Ugazio, A. G.), pp. 135–144. Springer-Verlag, Berlin; 1987.
11. Solinger, A. M. Immature T lymphocytes in human neonatal blood. *Cell Immunol.* 92: 115–122; 1985.
12. Tosato, G., Magrath, I. T., Koski, I. R., Dooley, N. J. and Blaese, R. M. B cell differentiation and immunoregulatory T cell function in human cord blood lymphocytes. *J. Clin. Invest.* 66: 383–388; 1980.
13. Ugazio, A. G., Altamura, D., Giraudi, V., Mingrat, G., Belloni, C. and Burgio, G. R. Peripheral blood T lymphocyte subpopulation in newborns. *Boll Ist Sieroter.* 55: 451–459; 1976.
14. Maccario, R., Notarangelo, L. D., Montagna, D., Vitiello, A., Porta, F. A., Lanfranchi, A., Marseglia, G. L. and Ugazio, A. G. Lymphocyte subpopulations in the neonate: *in vitro* proliferation, IL-1 and IL-2 productions by a subset of HNK–1^-, OKT3^-, OKT8^+ lymphocytes displaying NK activity. *Thymus* 3: 225–234; 1986.
15. Montagna, D., Ferrari, P., Alberini, C., Porta, F., De Amici, M., Astaldi-Ricotti, G. C. B. and Ugazio, A. G. Lymphocytes subpopulations in the neonate: high percentage of circulating B73.1+ HNK-1^- cells. *Thymus* 8: 171–178; 1986.
16. Notarangelo, L. D., Panina, P., Imberti, L., Malfa, P., Ugazio, A. G. and Albertini, A. Neonatal T4 lymphocytes: analysis of the expression of 4B4 and 2H4 antigens. *Clin. Immunol. Immunopath.* 46: 61–67; 1988.

17. Vitiello, A., Maccario, R., Montagna, D., Porta, F. A., Alberini, C. M., Mingrat, G., Astaldi Ricotti, G. C. B., Nespoli, L. and Ugazio, A. G. Lymphocyte subpopulations in the neonate: a subset of NK-1$^-$, OKT8+ lymphocytes displays natural killer activity. *Cell Immunol.* **85**: 252–257; 1984.
18. Butler, J. L., Suzuki, T., Kubagawa, H. and Cooper, M. D. Humoral immunity in the human neonate. *In* "Immunology of the Neonate" (Eds Burgio, G. R., Hanson, L. A. and Ugazio, A. G.), pp. 27–36. Springer-Verlag, Berlin; 1986.
19. Weatherstone, K. B. and Rich, E. A. Tumor necrosis factor/cachectin and interleukin–1 secretion by cord blood monocytes from premature and term monocytes. *Pediatr. Res.* **25**: 342–346; 1989.
20. English, B. K., Burchett, S. K., English, J. D., Ammann, A. J., Wara, D. W. and Wilson, C. B. Production of lymphotoxin and tumor necrosis factor by human neonatal mononuclear cells. *Pediatr. Res.* **24**: 717–722; 1988.
21. Virilizier, J. L. and Wakasugi, N. Analysis of the immunological dysregulation underlying defective interferon secretion in the human neonate. *In* "Immunology of the Neonate" (Eds Burgio, G. R., Hanson, L. A. and Ugazio, A. G.), pp. 130–134. Springer-Verlag, Berlin; 1987.
22. Panina, P., Notarangelo, L. D., Malfa, P., Imberti, L., Antonelli, G., Ugazio, A. G. and Dianzani, T. High responsiveness to hr IL-2 of newborn lymphocyte. *Eur. J. Pediatr.* **146**: 339A; 1987.
23. Kohl, S., Loo, L. S. and Goni, K. B. Analysis in human neonates of defective antibody dependent cellular cytotoxicity and natural killer cytotoxicity to herpes simplex. *J. Infect. Dis.* **150**: 14–19; 1984.
24. Chin, T. W., Murakami, D., Gill, M., Strom, S. and Stiehm, R. E. Cytotoxic studies in human newborns: lessened allogeneic cell-induced (augmented) cytotoxicity but strong lymphokine-activated cytotoxicity of cord mononuclear cells. *Cell Immunol.* **103**: 241–244; 1986.
25. Montagna, D., Maccario, R., Ugazio, A. G., Mingrat, G. and Burgio, G. R. Natural cytotoxicity in the neonates: high levels of lymphokine activation killer (LAK) activity. *Clin. Exp. Immunol.* 71: 177–181; 1988.
26. Nair, M. P. N., Schwartz, S. A. and Menon, M. Decreased natural and antibody-dependent cellular cytotoxicity is associated with decreased production of natural killer cytotoxic factors and interferon in neonate. *Pediatr. Res.* **19**: 279A; 1985.
27. Chirico, G., Marconi, M., De Amici, M., Gasparoni, A., Mingrat, G., Chiara, A., Rondini, G. and Ugazio, A. G. Deficiency of neutrophil bactericidal activity in term and preterm infants: a longitudinal study. *Biol. Neonate* **47**: 125–129; 1985.
28. Hill, H. R. H. and Sacchi, F. Mechanism of abnormal neutrophil function in the human neonate: prospects for therapy. *In* "Immunology

of the neonate" (Eds Burgio, G. R., Hanson, L. A. and Ugazio, A. G.), pp. 67–75. Springer-Verlag, Berlin; 1987.

29. Hill, H. R., Ashwood, E. R., Augustine, H. and Newton, J. A. Abnormality in membrane fluid properties of PMNs from neonates: pharmacologic correction. *Pediatr. Res.* **23**: 464A; 1989.
30. Smith, J. B., Campbell, D. E. and Douglas, S. D. Fetal neutrophils have distinct subpopulations which differ in complement and Fc receptor expression. *Pediatr. Res.* **23**: 468A; 1989.
31. Notarangelo, L. D., Chirico, G., Chiara, A., Colombo, A., Rondini, G., Plebani, A., Martini, A. and Ugazio, A. G. Activity of the classical and alternative pathway of complement in preterm and small for gestational age infants. *Pediatr. Res.* **18**: 281–285; 1984.
32. Pilgrim, V., Fontanellaz, H. P., Hitzig, W. H. and Evers, G. Normal values of immunoglobulin in premature and in full-term infants, calculated as percentiles. *Helv. Pediatr. Acta* **30**: 121–124; 1985.
33. Aucouturier, P., Berthie, R., Bonneau, D. and Preud'homme, J. L. Concentrations serique des sous-classes d'IgG chez l'enfant normal. *Arch. Fr. Pediatr.* **45**: 255–258; 1988.
34. Einhorm, M. S., Granoff, D. M., Nahm, M. H., Quinn, A. and Shackelford, P. Concentration of antibodies in paired maternal and infants sera: Relationship to IgG subclasses. *J. Pediatr.* **111**: 783–788; 1987.
35. Pitcher Wilmott, R. W., Hinducha, P. and Wood, C. B. S. The placental transfer of IgG subclass in human pregnancy. *Clin. Exp. Immunol.* **41**: 303–308; 1980.
36. Schur, P., Depert, E. and Alper, C. Gamma G subgroups in human fetal cord and maternal sera. *Clin. Immunol. Immunopathol.* **2**: 62–66; 1973.
37. Schur, P. H. IgG subclass: a review. *Ann. Allergy* **58**: 89–99; 1987.
38. Shackelford, P. G. and Granoff, Dan M. IgG subclass composition of the antibody response of healthy adults and normal or IgG2 deficient children to immunization with the Influenzae type B polysaccharide vaccine or Hib PS-protein conjugate vaccines. *Monogr. Allergy* **23**: 269–281; 1988.
39. Baker, C. J. and Kasper, D. L. Correlation of maternal antibody deficiency with susceptibility to neonatal group B streptococcal infection. *N. Engl. J. Med.* **294**: 753–757; 1976.
40. Bojer, K. H., Papierna, K. and Gadzola, R. N. Transplacental passage of IgG antibody to group B streptococcus serotype. *J. Pediatr.* **104**: 618–621; 1984.
41. Chirico, G., Rondini, G., Plebani, A., Chiara, A., Massa, M. and Ugazio, A. G. Intravenous gammaglobulin therapy for prophylaxis of infection in high-risk neonates. *J. Pediatr.* **110**: 437–442; 1987.
42. Kyllonen, K. S., Clapp, D. W., Kliegman, R. M., Baly, J. E., Shenker, N., Fanaroff, A. A. and Berger, M. Dosage of intravenously administered immunoglobulin and dosing interval required to

maintain target levels of immunoglobulin G in low birth weight infants. *J. Pediatr.* 115: 1013–1016; 1989.
43. Cowan, M. J., Amman, A. J., Wara, D. W., Howie, V. M., Schultz, L., Dayle, N. and Kaplan, M. Pneumococcal polysaccharide immunization in infants and children. *Pediatrics* **62**: 721–724; 1978.
44. Baker, C. J., Edwards, M. S. and Kasper, D. L. Role of antibody to neutralize type III polysaccharide of group B streptococcus in infant infection. *Pediatrics* **68**: 544–549; 1981.
45. Steen, J. A. Gammaglobulin in preventing infections in premature infants. *Arch. Pediatr.* 77: 291–298; 1960.
46. Amer, J., Ott, E., Ibbott, F. A., O'Brien, D. and Kempe, C. H. The effect of monthly gammaglobulin administration on morbidity and mortality from infection in premature infants during the first year of life. *Pediatrics* **32**: 4–9; 1963.
47. Hitzig, W. H. and Muntener, U. Conventional Immunoglobulin therapy. *In* "Immunodeficiency in Man and Animals" (Ed. Bergsma, D.), *Birth Defects.* (Original Article Series) **9**: 339–342; 1975.
48. Dwyer, J. M. Thirty years of supplying the missing link. History of gammaglobulin therapy for immunodeficient states. *Am. J. Med.* **76**: 46–57; 1984.
49. EGID. Intravenous gammaglobulin for immunodeficiency: Report from the European Group for Immunodeficiencies (EGID). *Clin. Exp. Immunol.* **65**: 683–690; 1986.
50. Amman, A. J., Ashman, R. F., Burckly, R. M., Nardie, W. R., Krantmann, H. J., Nelson, J., Ochs, M., Stiehm, E. R., Tiller, T., Wara, D. W. and Wedgwood, R. Use of intravenous immunoglobulin in antibody immunodeficiency: results of a multicenter controlled trial. *Clin. Immunol. Immunopathol.* 22: 60–67; 1982.
51. Duarte, F., Aucouturier, P. and Makuba, M. F. Subclass composition of a new intact intravenous IgG. Comparison with various available preparations. *In* "Proceedings of the 6th International Congress of Immunology", Toronto, Vol. 3, p. 52; 1986.
52. Romer, J., Morgenthaler, J. J., Scherz, R. and Skvaril, F. Characterization of various immunoglobulin preparations for intravenous application. I. Protein composition and antibody content. *Vox Sang.* **42**: 74–84; 1982.
53. Skvaril, F. and Gardi, A. Differences among available immunoglobulin preparation for intravenous use. *Pediatr. Infect. Dis. J.* 7 (Suppl.): 43–48; 1988.
54. Eibl, M. M. Adverse reactions to iv immunoglobulin: a critical review. *In* "Recent Advances in Primary and Acquired Immunodeficiencies" (Eds Aiuti, F., Rosen, F. S. and Cooper, M. D.) Vol. 28, pp. 383–394. Raven Press; 1986.
55. Ruderman, J. W., Gall, R. G., Pomerance, J. J., Peter, J. B., Stewart, M. E. and Stiehm, E. R. Use of intravenous immunoglobulin in hypogammaglobulinemia (hypoG) of prematurity. *Pediatr. Res.* **23**: 468A; 1989.

56. Noya, F. J. D., Rench, M. A., Garcia-Prats, J., Mc Jones, T., Baker, C. J. Disposition of an immunoglobulin intravenous preparation in very low birth weight neonates. *J. Pediatr.* 112: 278–283; 1988.
57. Pirofsky, B., Campbell, S. M. and Montanaro, A. Individual patient variation in the kinetics of intravenous immune globulin administration. *J. Clin. Immunol.* (Suppl.) 2: 7–15; 1982.
58. Nolan, B. H. and Kauffman, R. Pharmacokinetics and effectiveness of intravenous gammaglobulin in neonates (letter). *J. Pediatr.* 112: 325–326; 1988.
59. Stiehm, E. R. The use of human intravenous immune globulin in immunoregulatory disorders and in the newborn period. *Immunol. Allergy Clin. North Am.* 8: 39–50; 1988.
60. Weisman, L. E., Fischer, G. W., Henning, V. G. and Peck, C. C. Pharmacokinetics of intravenous immunoglobulin (Sandoglobulin) in neonates. *Pediatr. Infect. Dis.* 5 (Suppl.): 185–188; 1986.
61. Lancefield, R. C., McCarty, M. and Everly, W. Multiple mouse protective antibodies directed against group B streptococci. *J. Exp. Med.* 142: 165–169; 1975.
62. Vogel, L. C., Kretschmer, R. R. and Paduos, D. M. Protective value of gammaglobulin preparations against group B streptococcal infection in chick embryo and mice. *Pediatr. Res.* 14: 788–795; 1987.
63. Fischer, G. W., Hunter, K. W. and Wilson, S. R. Modified human immune serum globulin for intravenous administration: in vitro opsonic activity and in vivo protection against group B streptococcal disease in suckling rats. *Acta Paediatr. Scand.* 71: 639–644; 1982.
64. Fischer, G. W., Hemming, V. G. and Hunter, K. W. Intravenous immunoglobulin in the treatment of neonatal sepsis: Therapeutic strategies and laboratory studies. *Pediatr. Infect. Dis.* 5: 171–175; 1986.
65. Fischer, G. W. Immunoglobulin therapy for neonatal group B streptococcal infection: an overview. *Pediatr. Infect. Dis. J.* 7: 513–516; 1988.
66. Santos, J. I., Shigeoka, A. O., Rose, N. S. *et al.* Protective efficacy of a modified immune serum globulin in experimental group B streptococcal infection. *J. Pediatr.* 99: 873–877; 1973.
67. Givner, L. R. Human IgG hyperimmune for type III group B streptococcus (III GBS): efficacy in newborn rats. *Pediatr. Res.* 23: 473A; 1989.
68. Gloser, H., Bachmayer, H. and Helm, A. Intravenous immunoglobulin with high activity against group B streptococci. *Pediatr. Infect. Dis.* 5 (Suppl.): 176–179; 1986.
69. Weisman, L. E. and Lorenzetti, P. M. High intravenous doses of human immune globulin suppress neonatal group B streptococcal immunity in rats. *J. Pediatr.* 115: 445–450; 1989.
70. Sahmon, J. E., Kayur, S. and Kimberly, R. P. Gammaglobulin for intravenous use induces an Fc gamma receptor-specific decrement in phagocytosis by blood monocytes. *Clin. Immunol. Immunopathol.* 43: 23–31; 1987.

71. Christensen, R. D., Rothstein, G., Hill, H. R. and Pincus, S. H. Treatment of experimental group B streptococcal infection with monoclonal antibody. *Pediatr. Res.* 18: 315A; 1984.
72. Egan, M. L., Pritchard, D. G., Dillon, U. G. and Gray, B. M. Protection of mice from experimental infection with type III group B streptococcus using monoclonal antibodies. *J. Exp. Med.* 158: 1006–1011; 1983.
73. Harris, M. C., Douglas, S. D. and Kalski, G. B. Functional properties of anti streptococcus group B monoclonal antibodies. *Clin. Immunol. Immunopathol.* 24: 342–346; 1982.
74. Shigeoka, A. O., Pritchard, D. G., Egan, M. L., Sholly, L. and Hill, H. R. Monoclonal or polyclonal antibody-mediated protection against group B streptococci is markedly enhanced by fibronectin. *Pediatr. Res.* 23: 286A; 1988.
75. Hill, H. R. Shigeoka, A. O. and Augustine, N. Fibronectin deficiency: a correctable defect in the neonate's host defense mechanism. *Pediatr. Res.* 18 (4): 252A; 1984.
76. Bortolussi, R. Potential for intravenous gamma-globulin use in neonatal gram-negative infection: an overview. *Pediatr. Infect. Dis.* 5: (S): 198–200; 1986.
77. Bortolussi, K. S. and Fischer, G. W. Opsonic and protective activity of immunoglobulin, modified immunoglobulin and serum against neonatal *Escherichia coli* K1 infection. *Pediatr. Res.* 20: 175–178; 1986.
78. Harper, T. E., Christensen, R. D. and Rothstein, G. The effect of administration of immunoglobulin to newborn rats with *Escherichia coli* sepsis and meningitis. *Pediatr. Res.* 22: 455–460; 1987.
79. Griffin, P. M., Gore, D. C., Lobe, T. E., Reinarz, J. A., Roart, L., Hall, M. and Stein, D. Immunoglobulins (IgG) do not improve survival in gram-negative septic shock in piglets. *Pediatr. Res.* 23: 473A; 1989.
80. Dunn, D. L., Bogard, W. C. and Cerra, F. B. Enhancement of survival during murine gram-negative bacterial sepsis by use of a murine monoclonal antibody. *Arch. Surg.* 120: 50–56; 1985.
81. Gruber, W. C., Wilson, S. Z., Throop, B. J. and Wyde, P. R. Immunoglobulin administration and ribavirin therapy: efficacy in respiratory syncytial virus infection of the cotton rat. *Pediatr. Res.* 21: 270–274; 1987.
82. Hemming, V. G., Prince, G. A. and Harswood, R. L. Studies of passive immunotherapy for infections of respiratory syncytial virus in the respiratory tract of a primate model. *J. Infect. Dis.* 152: 1083–1087; 1985.
83. Nagtington, J., Gandy, G., Walker, J. and Gray, J. J. Use of normal immunoglobulin in an echovirus 11 out break in a special-care baby unit. *Lancet* 2: 443–446; 1983.
84. Chirico, G., Duse, M., Chiara, A., Rondini, G. and Ugazio, A. G. Neonatal immunodeficiency and new perspectives of prophylaxis of

infections with intravenous intact gammaglobulin. *In* "Proceedings of XVII International Congress of Pediatrics", Manila; 1983.
85. Baker, C. J. Multicenter trial of intravenous immunoglobulin to prevent late-onset infection in preterm infants: preliminary results. *Pediatr. Res.* **23**: 275A; 1989.
86. Eibl, M. M., Wolf, H. M., Furnkranz, H. and Rosenkranz, A. Prevention of necrotizing enterocolitis in low-birth-weight infants by IgA-IgG feeding. *N. Engl. J. Med.* **319**; 1–7; 1988.
87. Haque, K. N., Zaidi, M. H., Haque, S. K., Bahakim, H., El-Hazmi, H. and El-Swailam, M. Intravenous immunoglobulin for prevention of sepsis in preterm and low birth weight infants. *Pediatr. Infect. Dis.* **5**: 622–625; 1986.
88. Stabile, A., Miceli, S., Romanelli, V., Pastore, M. and Pesaresi, M. A. Intravenous immunoglobulin for prophylaxis of neonatal sepsis in premature infants. *Arch. Dis. Child.* **63**: 441–443; 1988.
89. Clapp, D. W., Kliegman, R. M., Baley, J. E., Shenker, N., Kyllonen, K., Fanaroff, A. A. and Berger, M. Use of intravenously administered immune globulin to prevent nosocomial sepsis in low birth weight infants: Report of a pilot study. *J. Pediatr.* **115**: 973–978; 1989.
90. Homan, S. E., Kurth, C. G., Meade, V. and Hall, R. T. Prophylactic intravenous immunoglobulin (IVIG) in the low birth weight (LBW) infant: infusion effects. *Pediatr. Res.* **23**: 464A; 1989.
91. Steele, R. N., Burks, A. W. and Williams, L. W. Intravenous Immunoglobulin: new clinical applications. *Ann. Allergy* **60**: 89–94; 1988.
92. Bussel, J. B., LaGamma, E. F. and Giuliano, M. Intravenous gammaglobulin (IVGG) prophylaxis of late sepsis in VLBW infants: a randomized placebo controlled trial. *Pediatr. Res.* **29**: 471; 1989.
93. Christensen, K. K. and Christensen, P. Intravenous gammaglobulin in the treatment of neonatal sepsis with special reference to group B streptococci and pharmacokinetics. *Pediatr. Infect. Dis.* **5** (Suppl. 3): 189–192; 1986.
94. Fischer, G. W. Therapeutic use of intravenous gammaglobulin for pediatric infections. *Pediatr. Clin. North Am.* **35**: 517–533; 1988.
95. Yoder, M. C. Immunotherapy of neonatal septicemia. *Pediatr. Clin. North Am.* **33**: 481–501; 1986.
96. Christensen, K. K., Christensen, P., Bucher, H. U., Duc, G., Kind, C. H., Mieth, D., Muller, B. and Seger, R. A. Intravenous administration of human IgG to newborn infants: changes in serum antibody levels to group B streptococci. *Eur. J. Pediatr.* **143**: 123–127; 1984.
97. Von Muralt, G. and Sidiropoulos, D. Prenatal and postnatal prophylaxis of infections in preterm neonates. *Pediatr. Infect. Dis.* **7**: S72–78; 1988.
98. Hemming, V. G., Prince, G. A., Rodriguez, W., Kim, H. W., Brand, C. D., Parrott, R. M., London, W. T., Fischer, G. W., Baron, P. A. and Henson, S. A. Respiratory syncytial infections and intravenous gammaglobulins. *Pediatr. Infect. Dis. J.* **7** (Suppl.): S103–106; 1988.

Discussion

R. van Furth
Is the high catabolic rate of IgG in immature neonates due to the same mechanism as in adults or due to loss via the intestinal tract?

L. D. Notarangelo
The reasons for the high catabolic rate soon after birth in premature babies are still largely unknown. Indeed, several drugs show reduced half-lives in the newborn. Intestinal losses alone probably do not represent the main causal factor for the high catabolic rate of IgG in premature infants. More studies should be performed on this; in particular, Fcγ receptor-mediated catabolism should be studied.

Note added in proof

Important new data on immunoglobulin treatment and prophylaxis in the neonate were communicated at the NIH Consensus Development Conference on Intravenous Immunoglobulin (May 21–23, 1990). In particular, Baker reported on the first multicenter, randomized, double-blind, placebo-controlled study in which 577 newborn infants (birthweight 500–1750 g) were randomly assigned to receive IVIG (500 mg/kg) or albumin (1). IVIG were administered (with no major side-effects reported) at age 3–7 days, one week later, and then every 14 days for a total of 5 infusions or until discharged. Infections, length of hospitalization, and duration of mechanical ventilation were significantly reduced in IVIG recipients weighing less than 1500 g, but not in those over this weight. Mortality was comparable in IVIG and placebo recipients.

Fischer reported on a multicenter, double-blind placebo-controlled trial to determine if IVIG improves survival in early onset sepsis (2). For this, 753 neonates were enrolled, including 31 babies with early onset sepsis and 7 deaths. IVIG were administered at 500 mg/kg; albumin served as placebo. Infection-related deaths occurred in 5/17 (29%) receiving antibiotics plus placebo and 1/14 (7%) of those given IVIG and antibiotics. Survival was associated with IgG serum levels above 800 mg/dl; but numbers are still too small to prove efficacy and other well-designed and carefully-controlled studies are needed.

References

1. Baker, C. J. Intravenous immunoglobulin in low birthweight infants: Prevention. *In* "Intravenous Immunoglobulin", NIH Consensus Development Conference on Intravenous Immunoglobulin: Prevention and Treatment of Disease, pp. 61–67; 1990.
2. Fischer, G. W. Use of intravenous immunoglobulin during the treatment of infection in low birth weight infants. *op. cit.* pp. 79–83.

Intravenous immunoglobulin in neonates: a decade of experience

GERALD W. FISCHER and LEONARD E. WEISMAN

Uniformed Services University of The Health Sciences, F. Edward Hébert School of Medicine, Bethesda, Maryland, USA

Immunoglobulin has been used for many years to prevent and treat infections in children and adults. However, its potential usefulness had not been fully explored in neonates until the recent introduction of IVIG into our therapeutic armamentarium. In the late 1970s and early 1980s investigators began to analyze the effect of IVIG in animal models (1) and newborn babies with bacterial sepsis (2). This paper will review this decade of experience that we have now accumulated on the role of IVIG in neonates.

Prevention of neonatal sepsis with IVIG

Several authors have evaluated IVIG as a means of preventing neonatal sepsis (Table 1). Of the four published articles, three have shown some benefit and one showed no benefit. Three of the studies were not blinded and the total number of septic babies in each study was small.

The paper by Haque *et al.* (3) reports 100 preterm neonates (divided into two groups) who were treated with 120 mg/kg of IVIG (Intraglobulin®), either at birth or at birth and 8 days. A third group of 50

Immunotherapy with Intravenous Immunoglobulins
ISBN 0–12–370725–0

Table 1
Prevention of neonatal sepsis with IVIG

Author	Benefit	Blind	Gestation (weeks) or birth weight (kg)	Proven sepsis		P Value[a]	
				IVIG	No IVIG	1-tailed	2-tailed
1. Haque	Yes	No	30–37	4/100 (4%)	8/50 (16%)	0.015	0.02
2. Chirico	Yes	No	24–34	2/43 (5%)	8/40 (20%)	0.034	0.044
3. Clapp	Yes	Yes	< 2.0	0/56 (0%)	7/59 (8%)	0.008	0.013
					9/85[b]	0.008	0.012
4. Stabile	No	No	26–34	5/46 (13%)	3/48 (8%)	0.33	0.48

[a] Fisher's exact test.
[b] Patients that were not entered in study.

babies did not receive IVIG. All babies were observed for infection for 12 days. Patients were randomized and matched for gestational age, sex and birth weight. Proven sepsis developed in 2/50 (4%), 2/50 (4%), and 8/50 (16%) patients who received one dose, two doses, or no IVIG therapy respectively. Gram-negative rods accounted for all infections (*Escherichia coli* = 6, *Salmonella* = 3, *Klebsiella* = 2, *Serratia* = 1). There was no difference in the incidence of infection between either IVIG group and the no therapy group ($P = 0.09$ Fisher's exact test). Only by combining both IVIG groups together and comparing that group to the no therapy group was statistical significance achieved ($P = 0.02$ Fisher's exact test). Death occurred in two infected patients who received no IVIG, though this was not statistically significant ($P = 0.52$ Fisher's exact test) when compared to no deaths in the IVIG group. Both deaths were secondary to *Salmonella* infection.

In the report by Chirico *et al.* (4, 5) 83 preterm neonates were given either no therapy or 500 mg/kg of IVIG (Sandoglobulin®) every week for 4 weeks and observed for 100 days for infection. Patients were randomized but the clinicians were not blinded. Septicemia occurred in 2/43 (5%) treated patients and 8/40 (20%) controls resulting in a statistically significant difference ($P = 0.044$ Fisher's exact test). When statistics are recomputed with a limited observation period of 42 days (consistent with passive IgG effect) there are three less infected control patients and the therapy is not significant ($P = 0.25$ Fisher's exact test).

The third study to report benefit, Clapp *et al.* (6) gave 115 preterm infants 600 to < 2000 g in the first 48 h of life, either IVIG (Sandoglobulin®) at 0.5–1.3 g/kg every 2 weeks to maintain serum IgG at a set value of 700 mg/dl, or placebo. In this study the patients were randomized and the clinicians were blinded to therapy. Eighty-five patients whose parents declined entry into the study did not receive IVIG or placebo but were also followed for infections. Sepsis occurred in 0/56 (0%), 7/59 (12%) and 9/85, IVIG-treated, placebo-treated and non-randomized patients respectively. The incidence of infection between the three groups was significantly different ($P < 0.04$, using a 2×3 Fisher's exact test). When one compares the incidence of infection between the IVIG and placebo groups or the IVIG and non-randomized group, there was also a statistically significant difference ($P = 0.013$, 2×3 Fisher's exact test).

A paper by Stabile *et al.* (7) reported that IVIG was of no benefit, after treating 93 neonates at birth (≤ 34 weeks gestation or ≤ 1500 g) with either 500 mg/kg/day of IVIG (Venogamma®) on days 1, 2, 3, 7,

14, 21, 28, or nothing. The patients were randomized but clinicians were not blinded as to study assignment. Proven sepsis was observed in 5/46 (13%) and 3/48 (8%) of IVIG and control infants respectively ($P = 0.46$ Fisher's exact test). Meningitis occurred in 3 of the 5 infected IVIG-treated patients and 1 of 3 infected control patients.

Together these studies show some evidence of benefit when IVIG prophylaxis is used to prevent sepsis in neonates. However, the total number of sepsis cases is small and only one of the reported studies was blinded. Further complicating critical analysis is the use of different IVIG preparations and dosage regimens. In addition, the spectrum of bacterial pathogens was quite different between the studies. Larger, blinded and controlled studies may help clarify some of these confounding issues.

Treatment of neonatal sepsis with IVIG

Three groups have published reports on the use of IVIG in the treatment of neonatal sepsis and meningitis (Table 2).

Sidiropoulos and co-workers (2, 8, 9) were the first to report on the role of IVIG in treating neonates. Eighty-two neonates with suspected sepsis received antibiotics alone or antibiotic plus daily infusions of IVIG (Sandoglobulin®) for 6 days (preterm 15 ml/day, term 30 ml/

Table 2
Treatment of neonatal sepsis with IVIG

Author	Blind	Gestation (weeks)	Death 2° Infection		*P* value[a]	
			IVIG	No IVIG	1-tailed	2-tailed
1. Sidiropoulos	No	27–42	2/20 (10%)	4/15 (27%)	0.20	0.37
		27–37	1/13 (8%)	4/9 (44%)	0.07	0.12
		27–34	1/8 (13%)	4/9 (44%)	0.18	0.29
2. Haque	Yes	30–37	1/21 (5%)	4/23 (17%)	0.20	0.35
3. Friedman	No	26–42	2/12 (17%)	7/12 (58%)	0.045	0.09

[a] Fisher's exact test.

day). Term neonates therefore received a total dose of up to 3.9 g/kg while preterms (< 38 weeks) received 1.6–2.4 g/kg. Patients were randomized by alternating entry into treatment groups and clinicians were not blinded to therapy. Sepsis was proven in 20/41 (49%) and 15/41 (37%) of the immunoglobulin-treated and control patients respectively. Gram-negative rods accounted for 63% of bacterial infections. Death occurred in 2/20 (10%) and 4/15 (27%) of immunoglobulin and control groups respectively ($P = 0.37$ Fisher's exact test). Death in infected preterms (< 38 weeks) were analyzed separately, and because of small numbers, the mortality rate of 1/13 (8%) in the immunoglobulin group and 4/9 (44%) in the control group just approached significance using a 1-tailed test ($P = 0.07$ Fisher's exact test), but were not significantly different using a 2-tailed test ($P = 0.12$, Fisher's exact test).

Haque *et al.* (10) tested 60 neonates with suspected infection with antibiotics for 10 days plus four daily infusions of either 5 ml/kg/day of 10% dextrose or 5% IVIG (Pentaglobin®) for total dose of 1 g/kg. The babies were randomized using sealed envelopes and clinicians were blinded to patient therapy. This product was stated to be IgM-enriched and each 250 mg contained: 30 mg IgM, 30 mg IgA, and 190 mg IgG. That amoung of IgM would seem physiologically insignificant. While the published paper reports a statistical significance of $P < 0.001$, by the Student's *t*-test, by using a more appropriate analysis, no significant difference was found ($P = 0.35$, Fisher's exact test).

In the third treatment study Friedman *et al.* (11) treated 12 patients with neutropenia (< 3500 neutrophils) and high titers (≤ 1:10) of GBS antigen by latex agglutination with antibiotics and IVIG (Sandoglobulin®) 800 mg/kg/day. All patients were < 2 weeks old. This study was neither blinded or prospectively controlled, since the IVIG-treated patients were compared with 12 historical controls that had neutropenia and high GBS antigen titers and received only antibiotics and supportive care. Mortality in the IVIG-treated group was 2/12 (17%) while in historical controls it was 7/12 (50%). There was, however, not a statistically significant difference between the group ($P = 0.09$, 2-tailed Fisher's exact test).

Together these studies also show some evidence of benefit when IVIG is used in combination with antibiotics to treat neonatal sepsis. The total number of treated cases is small, however, and the spectrum of bacterial pathogens treated varied greatly from one study to another. It is difficult, therefore, to determine if therapy with IVIG is uniformly beneficial. In certain babies with infections due to encapsulated organisms, such as group B *Streptococcus* IVIG may be highly beneficial, while IVIG may have little or no effect on babies with other types of bacterial infections. Blinded, controlled studies that evaluate larger numbers of babies will be important to clarify the therapeutic role of IVIG in neonatal sepsis.

Discussion

While the efficacy of IVIG in neonates is not clearly established, IVIG has proven quite safe in neonates given prophylactic or therapeutic doses of IgG. Animal studies have shown that high-dose IVIG (> 2000 mg/dl) might impair microbial clearance (12, 13). Lower doses, however, should provide adequate elevation of serum antibody levels in neonates. Of critical importance is the requirement that the IVIG lot contains functional antibodies to the appropriate pathogens. Two critical factors in predicting efficacy for IVIG therapy or prophylaxis are (1) the infecting organism and (2) the composition of the IVIG preparation. The most common causes of early onset neonatal sepsis in the United States continue to be group B *Streptococcus* and *Escherichia coli*. Both of these pathogens are encapsulated and antibody plays an important role in effective phagocytosis and killing of these bacteria. In other parts of the world, different pathogens may be important and neonates may not require opsonic antibody for effective clearance. In addition, the role of antibody to other neonatal pathogens such as *Staphylococcus epidermidis*, *Candida albicans* and enterococci remains to be determined. Therefore, the role of IVIG therapy is less clear in settings where pathogens unresponsive to antibody therapy might predominate, such as late onset sepsis and infection. Further studies will be critical to clarify the role of IVIG in these settings.

Given the current data, two groups of babies may benefit from IVIG therapy. Small premature babies with low levels of IgG and recurrent infections may benefit from IVIG prophylaxis. In addition, infected neonates with overwhelming sepsis may be suitable for IVIG as adjunctive therapy to antibiotics, when other extraordinary treatments are under consideration (i.e. exchange blood transfusion, neutrophil transfusion, etc.). There is no evidence at this time that high-dose therapy provides any additional efficacy and large amounts of IVIG may cause harm. Therefore, current data suggests that 500–1000 mg/kg per dose would be appropriate for therapy. One dose of IVIG may be effective for therapy, however to prevent infection, repeat doses may need to be given every 2–3 weeks.

IVIG is currently not the standard of medical care in all neonates to prevent or treat neonatal infections. The published studies available for review are each relatively small, utilized different study designs, and IVIG preparations. Several large multicenter studies are either completed or nearing completion. Bussel and colleagues (14) have presented partial data on 240 babies given prophylactic Sandoglobulin® to prevent late onset infections. Preliminary data are only published on 125 patients. There was no significant decrease in infections in IVIG-treated patients (30/61, 49% IVIG vs. 23/65, 35% placebo). A recent abstract from another large multicenter study (15) suggested that IVIG provided some protection against late onset infection in premature infants when repeated doses were given (Gammagard®, 540 babies enrolled). A third large multicenter trial is now completed using Sandoglobulin® to prevent or treat neonatal sepsis (16, 17). In this study there were over 700 babies $\leqslant$ 12 h old and $\leqslant$ 2000 g enrolled and followed for 8 weeks. It will be important to analyze the final results of these large, well-controlled trials before we establish the role of IVIG in neonates.

References

1. Fischer, G. W., Hunter, K. W., Wilson, S. R. and Hensen, S. A. The role of antibody in group B streptococcal infections in immunoglobulins. *In* "Characteristics and Uses of Intravenous Preparations" (Eds Alving, B. M. and Ginlayson, J. S.) Vol. 1, p. 81. US Government Printing Office, Washington, DC; 1980.
2. Sidiropoulos, D., Boehme, U., von Muralt, G., Morell, A. and Barandun, S. Immunglobulinsubstitution bei der Behandlung der neonatalen Sepsis. *Schweiz med Wschr* 111: 1649–1655; 1981.
3. Haque, K. N., Zaidi, M. H., Haque, S. K., Bahakim, H., *et al.* Intravenous immunoglobulin for prevention of sepsis in preterm and low birth weight infants. *Pediatr. Infect. Dis.* 5: 622–625; 1986.
4. Chirico, G., Rondini, G., Plebani, A., Chiara, A., *et al.* Intravenous gammaglobulin therapy for prophylaxis of infection in high-risk neonates. *J. Pediatr.* 110: 437–442; 1987.
5. Chirico, G., Rodini, G., Regazzi, M. B. and Ugazio, A. G. Reply to editor: Pharmacokinetics and effectiveness of intravenous immunoglobulin in neonates. *J. Pediatr.* 112: 326–327; 1988.
6. Clapp, D. W., Baley, J. E., Kliegman, R. M., Baily, J. E., Shenker, N., *et al.* Use of intravenously administered immune globulin to prevent nosocomial sepsis in low birth weight infants. Report of a pilot study. *J. Pediatr.* 115: 973–978; 1989.
7. Stabile, A., Miceli Sopo, S., Romanelli, V., Pastore, M. and Pesaresi,

M. A. Intravenous immunoglobulin for prophylaxis of neonatal sepsis in premature infants. *Arch. Dis. Child.* 63: 441–443; 1988.
8. Sidiropoulos, D., Boehme, U., von Muralt, G., Morell, A. and Barandun, S. Immunoglobulin supplementation in prevention or treatment of neonatal sepsis. *Pediatr. Infect. Dis.* 5: S193–S194; 1986.
9. von Muralt, G. and Sidiropoulos, D. Experience with intravenous immunoglobulin treatment in neonates and pregnant women. *Vox Sang* 51 (Suppl. 2): 22–29; 1986.
10. Haque, K. N., Zaidi, M. H. and Bahakim, H. IgM-enriched intravenous immunoglobulin therapy in neonatal sepsis. *Am. J. Dis. Child.* 142: 1293–1296; 1988.
11. Friedman, C. A., Wender, D. F., Temple, D. M. and Rewson, J. E. Intravenous gamma globulin as adjunct therapy for severe group B streptococcal disease in the newborn. *Am. J. Perinatol.* 6: 453–456; 1989.
12. Kim, K. S. and Hong, J. K. High dose human intravenous immunoglobulin may impair therapeutic benefit of penicillin G against experimental group B streptococcal bacteremia and meningitis. *Pediatr. Res.* 21: 417a; 1987.
13. Weisman, L. E. and Lorenzetti, P. M. High dose of human intravenous immunoglobulin suppresses neonatal group B streptococcal immunity in rats. *J. Pediatr.* 115: 445–450; 1989.
14. Bussel, J. B., LaGamma, E. F. and Giuliano, M. Intravenous gammaglobulin prophylaxis of late sepsis in VLBW infants: A randomized placebo controlled trial. *Pediatr. Res.* 23: 471A (abstract 1614); 1988.
15. Baker, C. J. and the Neonatal IVIG Collaborative Study Group. Multicenter trial of intravenous immunoglobulin to prevent late-onset infection in preterm infants: preliminary results. *Pediatr. Res.* 25: 275A (abstract 1633); 1989.
16. Weisman, L. E., Stoll, B., Kueser, T., Rubio, T., Frank, G., Heiman, H., Subramanian, S., Hankins, C., Hemming, V. and Fischer, G. W. Intravenous immunoglobulin (IVIG) therapy of neonatal sepsis. *Pediatr. Res.* 27: 277A (abstract 1647); 1990.
17. Weisman, L. E., Stoll, B., Kueser, T., Rubio, T., Frank, G., Heiman, H., Subramanian, S., Hankins, C., Hemming, V. and Fischer G. W. Intravenous immunoglobulin (IVIG) prophylaxis of late-onset septicemia in neonates. *Pediatr. Res.* 27: 277A (abstract 1648); 1990.

Discussion

A. D. B. Webster

It is important to comment that the study of children and adults with antibody deficiency shows that antibodies are not of major importance in protection against group B *Streptococcus* and Gram-negative infections. This suggests that other factors are more critical, for instance mannan-binding proteins, neutrophil adhesins, etc. However, high-titer specific antibodies may be able to override defects in these persons.

G. W. Fischer
Since older children and adults do not commonly become infected with pathogens such as group B *Streptococcus* and *E. coli* (even when immunoglobulin deficiency is present), there are clearly factors other than antibody that are also important in immunity to these bacteria. While pathogen-specific antibody is necessary for efficient phagocytosis and killing of encapsulated organisms, we must continue to study the effect of IVIG on other immunologic factors that may be important in preventing these neonatal infections.

C. J. Baker
In the study of Weisman *et al.* was the mortality among IVIG recipients (1/14) significantly different from that in placebo recipients (5/17)? What was the distribution of etiologic agents in the 30 blood culture isolates from these septic neonates?

G. W. Fischer
The infections-related mortality in the IVIG plus antibiotics treatment group (1/14) was not significantly better than the infections-related mortality in the placebo plus antibiotics group (5/17). However, the number of patients with sepsis on entry is small despite entering over 750 neonates in the study.

T. Alsaker
Please comment on potential side effects of IVIG, especially the problem of hypertension in small babies.

G. W. Fischer
Side effects of IVIG have not been a problem in neonatal studies to date. Elevated blood pressure did not occur outside the normal range for premature infants in our study. Animal studies have suggested, however, that high doses of IVIG might cause Fc receptor blockade. Therefore doses of 500–1000 mg/kg would seem appropriate for neonates until this potential problem is resolved.

Passive immunization for the protection of infants and young children from respiratory infection by respiratory syncytial virus

VAL G. HEMMING[1] and GREGORY A. PRINCE[2]

[1]Department of Pediatrics, The Uniformed Services University of the Health Sciences, Bethesda, Maryland, USA
[2] National Institute of Allergy and Infectious Diseases, Bethesda, Maryland, USA

The respiratory syncytial virus (RSV) was first isolated and characterized about 30 years ago (1–3). Subsequently RSV proved to be a ubiquitous virus, or group of viruses, responsible for frequent human respiratory infections, especially in infants and young children. Wherever sought, annual epidemic or endemic RSV infections have been documented throughout the world (3–11). Most infections are mild, brief and limited mostly to the upper respiratory tract. However, RSV infections of the very young or elderly often involve the lower respiratory tract and may be sufficiently severe to require hospitalization (8–14). Respiratory RSV infections of immunocompromised patients are commonly severe and may disseminate resulting in the death of the patient (15–16). Children with chronic lung disease or congenital cyanotic heart disease also experience substantial morbidity and mortality when infected with RSV (17–18). Nosocomial spread of RSV among hospitalized patients is a common and serious problem (19–22). Not long after the discovery and characterization of RSV it

Immunotherapy with Intravenous Immunoglobulins
ISBN 0-12-370725-0

was clear that infection prevention by immunization would be extremely desirable. Efforts at RSV vaccine development were well underway by the early 1960s.

The formulation of an effective and safe RSV vaccine has proved to be difficult. In the early 1960s a killed (inactivated by exposure to dilute formalin) whole virus vaccine was developed and tested in children. The unexpected and unfortunate outcome of this vaccine trial is well known and will not be further discussed here (23–26). Subsequently, other vaccines were developed and tested including attenuated or temperature–sensitive mutant live viruses (27–32), "subunit" RSV antigen-specific vaccines utilizing monoclonal antibody technology and affinity chromatography to purify vaccine antigens, or by genetic engineering (cloning of RSV genes and insertion into virus vectors such as vaccinia) (35–39). To date, none of these immunization strategies has been successful for the protection of young patients at high risk of serious complications during RSV infection. The vaccine projects are further complicated by the observation that natural, primary RSV infection in the very young fails to induce fully protective immunity (9, 40). Fortunately, the inevitable recurrent RSV infections of children produce progressively less severe clinical disease with more upper and fewer lower respiratory tract signs and symptoms (40).

Our previous investigations in laboratory animals and children showed that passive immunization may preferentially protect the lower airways and lung during RSV infection (41–44). In contrast to active immunization with formalin-inactivated RSV vaccine (45), passive immunization of cotton rats, to reduce virus replication or prevent RSV infection, proved both safe and efficacious (42). A representative experiment is demonstrated in Table 1. Human IgG, containing sufficient titers of RSV neutralizing antibody, significantly reduced the amounts of RSV recovered from the lungs of infected animals. The lungs of passively immunized cotton rats did not exhibit histopathological changes similar to those of infected animals immunized with formalin-inactivated vaccine (45). Related therapeutic observations regarding safety were subsequently corroborated in RSV infections in owl monkeys (43) and in children hospitalized with RSV bronchiolitis and pneumonia (44).

In 1987, the data just cited were used by the National Institute of Allergy and Infectious Diseases (National Institutes of Health, NIH, Bethesda, Maryland, USA) to justify solicitation of applications for research proposals to examine whether passive immunization might reduce the incidence and severity of RSV infections in high-risk

Table 1
Prophylactic effect of Sandoglobulin® given intraperitoneal to cotton rats infected intranasally 24 h later with respiratory syncytial virus (RVS)

	Number of animals	Lung titer of RSV 4 days after challenge with 10^4 pfu of virus (geometric mean $\log_{10}$/g ± SE)
Sandoglobulin® 50 mg/10 g (titer ~ 1:3000 in 10% solution)	25	< 2.0[a]
Control (no Sandoglobulin®)	24	4.98 ± 0.12

[a] Significance compared to control values $P < 0.001$.

children. With NIH support we designed a multicenter collaborative project to test whether high-risk infants and young children (i.e. those with bronchopulmonary dysplasia or cyanotic congenital heart disease) would benefit from monthly infusions of human IgG containing sufficient amounts of RSV neutralizing antibody to maintain protective serum titers throughout the RSV infection season. It was presumed that screening commercially available IgG lots, prepared for intravenous infusion (IVIG) by the 60% plague-reduction RSV neutralization test (41, 46), should disclose high-titered lots for the proposed studies. However, screening of multiple IVIG lots from

Table 2
Respiratory syncytial virus neutralizing antibody titers[a] in different lots of human intravenous gammaglobulin[b]

Manufacturer			
Cutter	Sandoz	Hyland	MPHBL[C]
1100	680	520	1935
700	612	540	3200
330	500	575	
325	720	320	
420	910		
886	200		

[a] Reciprocal of geometric mean by 60% plaque reduction.
[b] 5% concentration—all kindly supplied by manufacturers.
[c] Massachusetts Public Health Biologic Laboratories.

three licensed manufacturers failed to identify any lots with titers sufficient (Table 2) to achieve the requisite antibody levels in the children (we predicted a requirement for a geometric mean titer of >1:2000 at a concentration of 5%)

The highest available titered lot of IVIG Gamimune N ® (Cutter Laboratories, Berkeley, California, titer 1:1100) was selected for the phase I of the passive immunization trial (safety and pharmacokinetics). Twenty-three infants with serious cardiac or pulmonary disease were enrolled and divided into three groups. The infants in each group received either 500 mg/kg, 600 mg/kg, or 750 mg/kg of immunoglobulin intravenously once monthly throughout the RSV season. The children tolerated the infusions with only minor difficulties. A number of these children experienced culture-proven RSV disease during the respiratory season but did not develop life-threatening illness (47). One small infant with very severe bronchopulmonary dysplasia and who had never left the hospital became infected with RSV and expired after a 2-week illness despite receiving 500 mg/kg of IVIG and treatment with ribavirin. RSV neutralizing titers were low in this child as they were in the other children. For example, trough titers (against the A2 RSV strain drawn about 30 days following the previous infusion) in the group receiving 500 mg/kg ranged from 25.0 ±5.9 to 33.0 ±20; the 600 mg/kg group 24.1 ±2.6 to 41.4 ±6.8; and in the 750 mg/kg group was 49.5 ±12.4 to 70.0 ±7.0 (SE). Despite the death of this child, the other results of the phase I trial resulted in approval from the Food and Drug Administration (FDA) to proceed to phase II of the RSV passive immunization trial.

Following an unsuccessful search for higher titered lots of IgG from the manufacturers licensed to sell IgG in the United States, a plan was devised to produce an RSV-enriched IVIG for use in the phase II trial. A collaborative RSV-IVIG development group was organized. Utilizing proprietary technology, an enriched human polyclonal RSV globulin for passive immunization was developed (MPHBL, Table 2). With NIH and FDA approval the RSV-enriched globulin was selected for use in the three-arm, blinded, controlled, phase II trial (group A, 750 mg/kg and group B, 150 mg/kg, both infused monthly, and group C, untreated controls). High-risk children similar to those studied in the phase I RSV trial were enrolled (prematurely born children with bronchopulmonary dysplasia, oxygen-dependent or recently oxygen-dependent, or children with cyanotic congenital heart disease and pulmonary hypertension) at three clinical centers (University of Colorado, University of Rochester and Children's National Medical Center of Washington, DC).

The first year of this 4-year prospective trial has just been completed without difficulty. Except for the ongoing review by the study's Data and Safety Monitoring Board, the data from the study will not be analyzed until the conclusion of the study. By that time there should be 100 children in each study arm. If the hypothesis of the study is valid, as predicted by our animal data, passive immunization with sufficient amounts of RSV-specific antibody should both reduce the incidence of RSV infections and decrease the severity of lower respiratory tract disease in these children.

In summary, RSV infection may be life-threatening to certain children. Present evidence suggests that active RSV immunization with live virus or subunit vaccines may not protect these children from primary or reinfection. Further, the epidemiologic properties of RSV makes it extremely difficult to protect children from virus exposure. We predict, therefore, that passive immunization with adequate amounts of RSV-enriched IVIG throughout the respiratory season will reduce hospitalization rates, morbidity and mortality in these very fragile children. At the next iteration of this conference we expect to report the successful completion of these IVIG trials and to demonstrate the efficacy of passive immunization to prevent or reduce the clinical severity of RSV infection in infants and young children.

Summary

The respiratory syncytial virus (RSV) is a common and serious cause of bronchiolitis and pneumonia in infancy, especially for infants with underlying diseases such as bronchopulmonary dysplasia or congenital heart disease. Prevention of RSV infection by primary immunization is yet not possible. We have shown that passive immunization, with human RSV-immune gammaglobulin (RSVIG), safely protects susceptible animals from lower respiratory tract RSV infection. These observations resulted in a multicenter, collaborative trial of RSVIG for prevention of serious RSV infections in high-risk infants and young children. The format of this ongoing study is presented and phase I safety data are discussed

References

1. Morris J. A. Jr. and Blount, R. E. Recovery of cytopathic agent from chimpanzees with coryza. *Proc. Soc. Exp. Biol. Med.* 92: 544–549; 1956.

2. Chanock, R., Roizman, B. and Myers, R. Recovery from infants with respiratory illness of a virus related to chimpanzee coryza agent (CCA). I. isolation, properties and characterization. *Am. J. Hyg.* **66**: 281–290; 1957.
3. Chanock, R. and Finberg, L. Recovery from infants with respiratory illness of a virus related to chimpanzee coryza agent (CCA). II. epidemiologic aspects of infection in infants and young children. *Am. J. Hyg.* **66**: 291–300; 1958.
4. Berkovich, S. and Taranko, L. Acute respiratory illness in the premature nursery associated with respiratory syncytial virus infections. *Pediatrics* **34**: 753–760; 1964.
5. Gardner, P. S., Elderkin, F. M. and Wall, A. H. Serological study of respiratory syncytial virus infections in infancy and childhood. *Br. Med. J.* **2**: 1570–1573; 1964.
6. Kim, H. W., Arrobio, J. O., Brandt, C. D., Jeffries, B. C., Pyles, G., Reid, J. L., Chanock, R. M. and Parrott, R. H. Epidemiology of respiratory syncytial virus infection in Washington D.C., I. importance of the virus in different respiratory tract disease syndromes and temporal distribution of infection. *Am. J. Epidemiol.* **98**: 216–225; 1973.
7. Parrott, R. H., Kim, H. W., Arrobio, J. O., Hodes, D. S., Murphy, B. R., Brandt, D. D., Camargo, E. and Chanock, R. M. Epidemiology of respiratory syncytial virus in Washington D. C., II. infection and disease with respect to age, immunologic status, race and sex. *Am. J. Epidemiol.* **98**: 289–300; 1973.
8. Martin, A. J., Gardner, P. S. and McQuillin, J. Epidemiology of respiratory syncytial viral infection among pediatric inpatients over a six year period in north-east England. *Lancet* **II**: 1035–1038; 1978.
9. Henderson, F. W., Collier, A. M., Clyde, W. A. Jr., and Denny, F. W. Respiratory syncytial virus infections, reinfections and immunity: a prospective, longitudinal study in young children. *N. Engl. J. Med.* **300**: 530–534; 1979.
10. Beem, M., Wright, F. H., Hamre, D., Egerer, R. and Oehme, M. Association of chimpanzee coryza agent with acute respiratory disease of children. *N. Engl. J. Med.* **263**: 523–530; 1960.
11. Tyrrell, D. A. J. A collaborative study of acute respiratory infections in Britain 1961–1964. *Br. Med. J.* **2**: 319–326; 1965.
12. Glezen, W. P., Paredes, A., Allison, J. E., Taber, L. H. and Frank, A. L. Risk of respiratory syncytial virus infection for infants from low-income families in relationship to age, sex, ethnic group, and maternal antibody level. *J. Pediatr.* **98**: 708–715; 1981.
13. Hall, W. J., Hall, C. B. and Speers, D. M. Respiratory syncytial virus infections in adults: clinical, virologic, and serial pulmonary function studies. *Ann. Intern. Med.* **88**: 203–205; 1978.
14. Garvie, D. G. and Gray, J. Outbreak of respiratory syncytial virus infection in the elderly. *Br. Med. J.* **281**: 1253–1254; 1980.

15. Hertz, M. I., Englund, J. A., Snover, D., Bitterman, P. B. and McGlave, P. B. Respiratory syncytial virus-induced acute lung injury in adult patients with bone marrow transplants: a clinical approach and review of the literature. *Medicine* **68**: 269–281; 1989.
16. Hall, C. B., Powell, K., MacDonald, M. E., Gala, C. L., Menegus, M. E., Suffin, S. C. and Cohen, H. J. Respiratory syncytial virus in children with compromised immune function. *N. Engl. J. Med.* **315**: 77–81; 1986.
17. Groothuis, J. R., Gutierrez, K. M. and Lauer, B. A. Respiratory syncytial virus in children with bronchopulmonary dysplasia. *Pediatrics* **82**: 199–203; 1988.
18. MacDonald, N. E., Hall, C. B., Suffin, S. C., Alexson, C., Harris, P. J. and Manning, J. A. Respiratory syncytial viral infection in infants with congenital heart disease. *N. Engl. J. Med.* **307**: 397–400; 1982.
19. Neligan, G. A. and Steiner, H. Respiratory syncytial virus infection of the newborn. *Br. Med. J.* **3**: 146–147; 1970.
20. Hall, C. B., Douglas, R. G. Jr., Geiman, J. M. and Messner, M. K. Nosocomial respiratory syncytial virus infections. *N. Engl. J. Med.* **293**: 1343–1346; 1975.
21. Mintz, L., Ballard, R. A., Sniderman, S. H., Roth, R. S. and Drew, W. L. Nosocomial respiratory syncytial virus in an intensive care nursery: rapid diagnosis by direct immunofluorescence. *Pediatrics* **64**: 149–153; 1979.
22. Hall, C. B. and Douglas R. G. Jr. Modes of transmission of respiratory syncytial virus. *J. Pediatr.* **99**: 100–103; 1981.
23. Kapikian, A. Z., Mitchell, R. H., Chanock, R. M., Shvedoff, R. A. and Stewart, C. E. An epidemiologic study of altered clinical reactivity to respiratory syncytial virus (RS) infection in children previously vaccinated with an inactivated RS virus vaccine. *Am. J. Epidemiol.* **89**: 405–421; 1969.
24. Kim, H. W., Canchola, J. G., Brandt, C. D., Pyles, G., Chanock, R. M., Jensen, K. and Parrott, R. H. Respiratory syncytial virus diseases in infants despite prior administration of antigenic inactivated vaccine. *Am. J. Epidemiol.* **89**: 422–434; 1969.
25. Fulginiti, V. A., Eller, J. J., Sieber, O. F., Joyner, J. W., Minamitani, M. and Meiklejohn G. Respiratory virus immunization I. A field trial of two inactivated respiratory virus vaccines; an aqueous trivalent para-influenza virus vaccine and an alum-precipitated respiratory syncytial virus vaccine. *Am. J. Epidemiol.* **89**: 435–448; 1969.
26. Chin, J., Magoffin, R. L., Shearer, L. A., Schieble, J. H. and Lennette, E. H. Field evaluation of a respiratory syncytial virus vaccine and a trivalent parainfluenza virus vaccine in a pediatric population. *Am. J. Epidemiol.* **89**: 449–463; 1969.
27. Friedenwald, W. T., Forsyth, B. R., Smith, C. B., Gharpure, M. S. and Chanock, R. M. Low-temperature grown RS virus in adult volunteers. *J. Am. Med. Assoc.* **204**: 690–694; 1968.

28. Kim, H. W., Arrobio, J. O., Brandt, C. D., Wright P., Hodes, D., Chanock, R. M. and Parrott, R. H. Safety and antigenicity of temperature sensitive (ts) mutants of respiratory syncytial virus in infants and children. *Pediatrics* 52: 56–63; 1973.
29. McIntosh, K., Arbeter, A. M., Stahl, M. K., Orr, I. A., Hodes, D. S. and Ellis, D. R. Attenuated respiratory syncytial virus vaccines in asthmatic children. *Pediatr. Res.* 8: 689–696; 1974.
30. Wright, P. F., Shinovaki, T., Fleet, W., Sell, S. H., Thompson, J. and Karzon, D. T. Evaluation of live attenuated respiratory syncytial virus vaccine in infants. *J. Pediatr.* 88: 931–939; 1976.
31. Belshe, R. B., Van Voris, L. P. and Mufson, M. A. Parenteral administration of live respiratory syncytial virus vaccine: results of a field trial. *J. Infect. Dis.* 145: 311–319; 1982.
32. Wright, P. F., Belshe, R. B., Kim, H. W., Van Voris, L. P. and Chanock, R. M. Administration of a highly attenuated, live respiratory syncytial virus vaccine to adults and children. *Infect. Immunol.* 37: 397–400; 1982.
33 Walsh, E. E., Hall, C. B., Briselli, M., Brandriss, M. W. and Schlesinger, J. J. Immunization with glycoprotein subunits of respiratory syncytial virus to protect cotton rats against viral infection. *J. Infect. Dis.* 155: 1198–1204; 1987.
34. Routledge, E. G., Wilcocks, M. M., Samson, A. C. R., Morgen, L., Scott, R., Anderson, J. J. and Toms, G. L. The purification of four respiratory syncytial virus proteins and their evaluation as protective agents against experimental infection in BALB/c mice. *J. Gen. Virol.* 69: 292–303; 1988.
35. Ball, L. A., Young, K. K-Y., Anderson, K., Collins, P. L. and Wertz, G. W. Expression of major glycoprotein G of human respiratory syncytial virus from recombinant vaccinia virus vectors. *Proc. Natl. Acad. Sci. USA* 83: 246–250; 1986.
36. Elango, N., Prince, G. A., Murphy, B. R., Venkatesan, S., Chanock, R. M. and Moss, B. R. Resistance to human respiratory syncytial virus (RSV) infection induced by immunization of cotton rats with a recombinant vaccinia virus expressing the RSV G Glycoprotein. *Proc. Natl. Acad. Sci. USA* 83: 1906–1910; 1986.
37. Olmstead, R. A., Elango, N., Prince, G. A., Murphy, B. R., Johnson, P. R., Moss, B., Chanock, R. M. and Collins P. L. Expression of the F glycoprotein of respiratory syncytial virus by a recombinant vaccinia virus: comparison of the individual contributions of F and G glycoproteins to host immunity. *Proc. Natl. Acad. Sci. USA* 83: 7462–7466; 1986.
38. Stott, E. J., Ball, L. A., Young, K. K, Furze, J. and Wertz, G. W. Human respiratory syncytial virus glycoprotein G expressed from a recombinant vaccinia virus vector protects mice against live virus challenge. *J. Virol.* 60: 607–613; 1986.
39. Wertz, G. W, Stott, E. J., Young, K. K-Y., Anderson, K. and Ball,

L. A. Expression of the fusion protein of human respiratory syncytial virus from recombinant vaccinia virus vectors and protection of vaccinated mice. *J. Virol.* 61: 293–301; 1987.

40. Glezen, W. P., Taber, L. H., Frank, A. L. and Kasel, J. A. Risk of primary infection and reinfection with respiratory syncytial virus (1986). *Am. J. Dis. Child.* 140: 543–546; 1986.
41. Prince, G. A., Horswood, R. L. and Chanock, R. M. Quantitative aspects of passive immunity to respiratory syncytial virus infection in infant cotton rats. *J. Virol.* 55: 517–520; 1985.
42. Prince, G. A., Hemming, V. G., Horswood, R. L. and Chanock, R. M. Immunoprophylaxis and immunotherapy of respiratory syncytial virus infection in the cotton rat. *Vir. Res.* 3: 193–206; 1985.
43. Hemming, V. G., Prince, G. A., Horswood, R. L., London, W. T., Murphy, B. R., Walsh, E. E., Fischer, G. W., Weisman, L. E., Baron, P. A. and Chanock, R. M. Studies of passive immunotherapy of respiratory syncytial virus in the respiratory tract of a primate model. *J. Infect. Dis.* 152: 1083–1987; 1985.
44. Hemming, V. G., Rodriguez, W., Kim, H. W., Brandt, C. D., Parrott, R. H., Burch, B., Prince, G. A., Baron, P. A., Fink, R. J. and Reaman, G. Intravenous immunoglobulin treatment of respiratory syncytial virus infections in infants and young children. *Antimicrob. Agents Chemother.* 31: 1882–1886; 1987.
45. Prince, G. A., Jenson, A. B., Hemming, V. G., Murphy, B. R., Walsh, E. E., Horswood, R. L. and Chanock, R. M. Enhancement of respiratory syncytial virus pulmonary pathology in cotton rats by prior intramuscular inoculation of formalin-inactivated virus. *J. Virol.* 57: 721–728; 1986.
46. Hemming, V. G., Prince, G. A., London, W. T., Murphy, B. R., Baron, P. A., Horswood, R. L., Fischer, G. W. and Chanock, R. M. Immunoglobulins in respiratory syncytial virus infections. In "Clinical Use of Intravenous Immunoglobulins" (Eds Morell, A. and Nydegger, U. E.), pp. 285–294. Academic Press, London; 1986.
47. Groothuis, J., Rodriguez, W., Hall, C. and Hemming, B. Intravenous gammaglobulin for prevention of respiratory syncytial virus disease in high-risk infants. *Pediatr. Res.* 27: abstract 1012 (APS-SPR, Anaheim, CA); 1990.

Discussion

R. van Furth

Is it correct that there is a safe vaccine that can be given in adults and that it is protective? If so, would it then be more appropriate to vaccinate adults, and prepare a hyperimmune serum from those individuals? Why is this not done?

V. G. Hemming

At least three live virus RSV vaccines have been given to adult humans. Each gives a secondary immune response. As all adults have been previously infected with RSV it is difficult to know the "quality" of this response in terms of protection. I believe such vaccines might be used to boost neutralizing antibody titers to RSV in donors. Hyperimmune plasma might be used to prepare anti-RSV-enriched IVIG.

M. Xanthou

What is the earliest post-natal age at which you start passive immunization?

V. G. Hemming

Once it has been established that RSV-Ig will prevent or reduce RSV disease in infants and children, I believe there will be no lower age limit for passive immunization. Prematures and infants residing in nurseries are at risk for nosocomial RSV infections. If proven safe and efficacious, I believe that use of RSV passive immunization will ultimately be possible in nursery patients including small prematures.

Part III
Secondary immunodeficiencies and infections

Use of immunoglobulin therapy in secondary antibody deficiencies

E. RICHARD STIEHM

Division of Immunology, UCLA Department of Pediatrics, Los Angeles, California, USA

The secondary immunodeficiencies

Patients with secondary immunodeficiency have had (or will have if they survive the neonatal period) a normal immune system some time in their life, but as a result of their age or some other primary condition, one or more limbs of their immune system is abnormal, making them unusually susceptible to infections. Usually the immune system recovers when the primary illness is reversed (e.g. feeding a malnourished child) but in some instances (e.g. removing the spleen) permanent defects or progressive immunodeficiency (e.g. HIV infection) occurs, resulting in a patient with life-long susceptibility to infection.

A treatise on the secondary immunodeficiencies will read like a junior Merck Manual because of the extensive scope of the topic (1, 2). These disorders are much more common than the primary immunodeficiencies, and may effect as many as 50% of hospitalized individuals. Further, they are increasing in numbers as care of tiny prematures improves, as the population ages, as new treatments for underlying diseases are developed, as diagnostic methods to recognize

Immunotherapy with Intravenous Immunoglobulins
ISBN 0–12–370725–0

subtle immunodeficiency improves, and the use of transplantation and immunosuppressive drugs increases. Needless to say, the worldwide occurrence of HIV infection, the secondary immunodeficiency *sine qua non*, has greatly expanded the scope and interest in this problem.

Secondary immunodeficiency can involve one or more limbs of the immune system (Fig. 1). The T-cell system is the limb of the immune system most frequently involved, since it is the most metabolically active and most susceptible to acute endocrine and metabolic events. The antibody system, primarily because of the long half-life of IgG and the ample pool of precursor B cells, is far less susceptible to acute stress and illness. Nevertheless, secondary antibody defects are not unusual, particularly in certain chronic illnesses. Less common are secondary deficiencies of phagocytic and complement systems. In general, factors affecting T-cell immunity may also affect phagocytic cells, and factors inhibiting synthesis or increasing the loss of serum immunoglobulins may have a similar although less clinically apparent effect on serum complement proteins.

Table 1 presents a long list of secondary disorders affecting the immune system, categorized into eight main categories and several minor categories. Each of these disorders has been shown to have

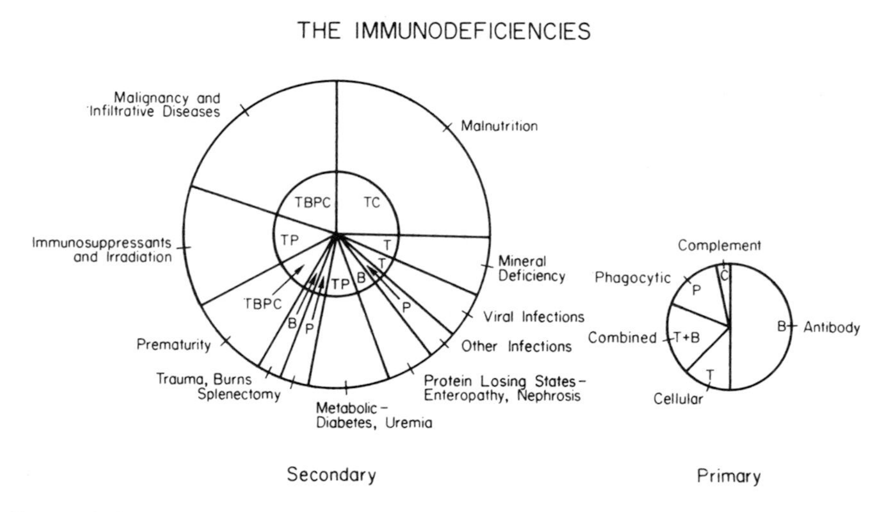

Figure 1. Immunologic defects in primary and secondary immunodeficiencies. The relative sizes of the circles emphasize the dominance of secondary immunodeficiencies in human disease. In the secondary immunodeficiency figure, the arrows indicate which limb of the immune system is primarily involved: B, antibody system; T, cellular immune system; P, phagocytic system; C, complement systems.

Table 1
The secondary immunodeficiencies

I. Age extremes
- (a) Premature infants
- (b) Newborn infants
- (c) Infants in first year of life
- (d) Aged individuals

II. Hereditary and metabolic disorders
1. Chromosomal disorders
   - (a) Down's syndrome
   - (b) Turner's syndrome
   - (c) Chromosome 18 abnormalities
2. Diabetes mellitus
3. Protein losing enteropathies
4. Nephrotic syndrome
5. Inherited enzyme defects
6. Myotonic dystrophy
7. Sickle cell anemia
8. Nutritional disturbances
   - (a) Protein calorie malnutrition
   - (b) Obesity
   - (c) Iron deficiency
   - (d) Mineral deficiency
   - (e) Vitamin deficiency
9. Uremia
10. Cirrhosis

III. Immunosuppressive drugs and agents
1. Radiation
2. ATG, ALG, OK-T3
3. Corticosteroids
4. Cyclosporin
5. Cytotoxic drugs
6. Anticonvulsants

IV. Infectious diseases
1. HIV infection
2. Congenital infection
   - (a) Rubella
   - (b) CMV
3. Acute viral infection
   EBV
4. Chronic viral infection
5. Acute bacterial infection

Table 1 continued

6. Parasitic diseases
   (a) Malaria
   (b) Trypanosomiasis

V. Hematologic disorders
1. Histiocytosis
2. Sarcoidosis
3. Acute leukemia
4. Chronic leukemia
5. Multiple myeloma
6. Hodgkin's disease and lymphoma
7. Invasive cancer

VI. Autoimmune diseases
1. Lupus erythematosus
2. Chronic active hepatitis

VII. Trauma and surgery
1. Anaesthesia
2. Shock
3. Burns
4. Surgery
5. Splenectomy

VIII. Post-transplantation period
1. Bone marrow transplants
2. Solid organ transplants

significant defects of the immune system in most but not all affected patients. Despite its length it is probably incomplete, particularly the list of infectious agents that may adversely affect the immune system.

Table 2 details the disorders which have significant antibody deficiencies. I have divided them into those in which immunoglobulin therapy (either intravenous or intramuscular) is of probable or proven benefit, and those in which immunoglobulin therapy is of possible benefit. References are given in the table for those in which immunoglobulin has been proven to be efficacious.

Mechanisms of secondary antibody deficiency

Several mechanisms may be responsible for secondary antibody deficiencies (Table 3). Excessive loss of immunoglobulin may result

Table 2
Secondary antibody deficiencies in which immunoglobulin therapy may be beneficial

Proven or probable benefit
Pediatric AIDS (3)
Multiple myeloma (4)
Chronic lymphocytic leukemia (5)
Hypogammaglobulinemia of prematurity (6)
Transient hypogammaglobulinemia of infancy in high-risk groups (7)
Post-bone marrow transplantation (7a)
Possible benefit
Nephrotic syndrome
Protein losing enteropathy with severe diarrhea
Severe burns
Severe viral diseases[a]
Severe bacterial diseases[a]
Severe malnutrition with kwashiorkor
Exfoliative dermatitis
Post-solid organ transplantation

[a] With specific antibody depletion.

Table 3
Causes of secondary antibody deficiency

1. Excess immunoglobulin loss
2. Immunoglobulin hypercatabolism
3. Polyclonal B-cell activation
4. Hematopoietic malignancy
5. B-cell malignancy
6. Immunodysregulation with excess T-suppressor function
7. T-cell deficiency with decreased T-helper function
8. Failure of antigen processing
9. Excess consumption of specific antibody
10. Inhibition of Ig class or subclass synthesis
11. Immaturity of the B-cell system

in immunoglobulin deficiency; for clinically significant antibody deficiency to occur, the loss must be massive and/or accompanied by a defect in Ig synthesis. Nevertheless in severe protein-losing enteropathy, severe renal disease (e.g. nephrosis) or severe skin disease (e.g. burns) sufficient loss may occur to result in profound immunoglobulin deficiency. IgG may also be lost in the lungs in some tiny prematures in the first days of life, thus accentuating their physiologic hypogammaglobulinemia. Often patients with immunoglobulin loss have less trouble with infection than patients with immunoglobulin synthetic defects, despite similarly low Ig levels; in the former antibody synthesis is often increased or accelerated, so that circulating antibodies are present but short-lived. In nephrosis and possibly in burns, there may be simultaneous inhibition of antibody synthesis (8). Patients with gastrointestinal loss often have concomitant lymphopenia due to lymphocyte loss in the gastrointestinal tract. These patients tend to lose other serum proteins including complement proteins. An albumin level less than 3.0 g/dl should alert the clinician to the occurrence of possible hypogammaglobulinemia and lymphopenia.

Hypercatabolism of IgG may occur in a few disorders, notably myotonica dystrophica (mean IgG half-life of 11.6 days vs. normal IgG half-life of 20–25 days). This may lead to hypogammaglobulinemia (9). Patients with Wiskott-Aldrich syndrome also have rapid IgG catabolism, but significant hypogammaglobulinemia rarely occurs in this disorder (10).

A temporary or permanent shut-down of both primary and secondary antibody synthesis may occur in a number of disorders, rendering the patients very susceptible to infection. Such is the case in pediatric AIDS, chronic lymphocytic leukemia and multiple myeloma. Such patients have a broad defect in antibody production for both new antigens and for secondary responses and/or resting antibody levels. Many of those disorders have decreased numbers of B cells, often with lymphopenia and/or bone marrow infiltration. Patients with non-specific B-cell activation may have many B cells and hypergammaglobulinemia but lack specific antibody responses.

In other secondary antibody-deficiency disorders the principal defect may be one in which pre-existing antibody levels are normal but the primary responses to a neoantigen are defective. Defective T-cell responses or excessive T suppression may be occurring. Examples may include adults with HIV, Hodgkin disease, lupus erythematosus and other hypergammaglobulinemic states. Often the repertoire of pre-existing antibody keeps these patients clinically well until a new agent not previously encountered emerges and then the patient develops severe or persistent infection.

Another cause of secondary antibody immunodeficiency is excess consumption of a specific antibody because of persistent or acute infection but with normal immunoglobulin levels and antibody titers to most other agents. This may be the case in patients with shock or abdominal trauma with Gram-negative sepsis who have depleted their antibody to Gram-negative endotoxins. In acute viral infection such as cytomegalovirus infection (CMV) or chronic viral infection such as human immunodeficiency virus (HIV) or bacterial infection such as subacute bacterial endocarditis (SBE) a large antigen load may deplete antibody early in the course of the disease. In these conditions additional specific antibody may be of considerable therapeutic benefit to help clear the bloodstream of the offending agent and promote antibody-dependent cellular cytotoxicity (ADCC) of infected cells. Treatment of CMV pneumonia with combined ganciclovir and IVIG (11, 12) and treatment of far advanced HIV with hyperimmune plasma are examples (13).

Finally certain illnesses may shift the immunoglobulin balance by inhibiting synthesis of one or more IgG subclasses or Ig classes. Pediatric HIV can result in subclass deficiency (14) while phenytoin and other anticonvulsants may result in IgA deficiency, with a propensity to recurrent infection (15). Other drugs have been implicated too (16).

Indications for IVIG in secondary immunodeficiency

When should immunoglobulin be used in secondary immunodeficiency? Table 4 outlines some guidelines for such therapy. Of particular importance is to judge the severity of the clinical or laboratory abnormality. In primary immunodeficiency one always gives IVIG to a child with an IgG < 100 mg/dl; but if the IgG is $>$ 400 mg/dl and there is some antibody synthesis, immunoglobulin may not be necessary. The same criteria are applicable to asymptomatic patients with secondary hypogammaglobulinemia. A reasonable general rule is that if the IgG is less than 200 mg/dl or if the total Ig (IgG + IgM + IgA) is less than 400 mg/dl the patient is a good candidate for IVIG. Patients with IgG levels between 200 and 400 mg/dl and total Ig levels between 400 and 600 mg/dl should also be

Table 4
Laboratory guidelines for use of IVIG in secondary antibody deficiencies

1. Hypogammaglobulinemia
   (IgG $<$ 200 mg/dl; IgG + IgM + IgA $<$ 400 mg/dl)
2. Low resting antibody titers to natural antigens
3. Poor antibody response to vaccine antigens
4. Rapid loss of antibody titers to vaccine antigens
5. Low antibody titers to infecting organisms

considered for immunoglobulin therapy, particularly if they have decreased antibody levels and/or multiple infections.

Low resting specific antibody titers to certain antigens can also be used as an indicator of B-cell function. These natural antibodies—antibodies to ubiquitous antigens present in all normal subjects including isohemagglutinins *E. coli* antibodies (17), streptococcal A antibodies (18), and cardiolipin antibodies (4), are low in patients with primary and secondary antibody deficiencies. A standard battery of such tests to define antibody deficiency would be desirable.

Poor antibody responses to vaccine antigen challenge, even in the face of normal or elevated IgG levels, is also an indication for IVIG therapy, particularly if accompanied by recurrent infection. Some patients with partial antibody deficiency have short-lived antibody responses (often limited to an IgM response) but after 2–3 months the antibody falls to preimmunization levels. Thus it is important to assess antibody titers serially after immunization if antibody deficiency is suspected.

Finally, a selective antibody defect (or continued consumption) to an infecting organism may occur, leading to continued chronic infection. The half-life of specific antibody may be considerably less than the IgG half-life (19). Under these circumstances, it will be important to select an immunoglobulin that has adequate levels of specific antibody and monitor the rapidity of its disappearance from the circulation (18).

Certain clinical observations can be used as a guideline for immunoglobulin therapy (Table 5) in the presence of infection and the absence of hypogammaglobulinemia. Patients with recurrent or persistent infections despite adequate antibiotic treatment are good candidates for a trial of IVIG therapy. Patients with continuous diarrhea, particularly associated with weight loss or failure to gain weight, or those that have malabsorption or demonstrate hypogammaglobulinemia may be considered for a trial of immunoglobulin therapy. Other tests to identify a specific microbial cause of the diarrhea or identify the cause of the failure to thrive must be done. Infection with an organism that cannot be eradicated with antibiotics alone should be considered for a trial of immunoglobulin therapy, particularly if there is demonstrable deficiency of antibody to the infecting organism.

A final use of immunoglobulin is in patients with infection and an autoimmune disease that may be responsive to immunoglobulin such as thrombocytopenic purpura or immune neutropenia. In such cases IVIG in conjunction with antibiotics may be preferable to steroids or other immunosuppressive drugs.

Table 5
Clinical guidelines for use of IVIG in infection in the absence of hypogammaglobulinemia

1. Recurrent or persistent infection despite continuous use of high-dose antibiotics for 6–12 weeks
2. Continuous diarrhea or weight loss
3. Gastroenteritis with persistent diarrhea and failure to thrive
4. Infection and coexistent autoimmune illness

Guidelines for IVIG in secondary immunodeficiency

When IVIG is used in secondary immunodeficiency, the following guidelines are suggested. Give a large initial dose (400–800 mg/kg), usually double the maintenance dose at onset of therapy. Measure the IgG level after each infusion and do trough levels before subsequent infusions. A trough IgG level of 600–800 mg/dl is highly desirable. Consider increasing the dose if localized infection is present and high dose of immunoglobulin is needed in the central nervous system, gastrointestinal tract, or respiratory tract. When IVIG is given to patients without hypogammaglobulinemia a clinical goal and a time to reach the goal must be established. If the goal is not achieved, consider adding or substituting other forms of therapy.

Summary

Secondary antibody deficiencies occur frequently in newborns, children and adults in a wide variety of illnesses. Several different mechanisms cause these antibody deficiencies including immunoglobulin loss, accelerated catabolism, T-cell abnormalities, polyclonal B-cell activation with failure of primary antibody synthesis, infiltration of the marrow, malignant B-cell proliferation, and immaturity of the B-cell system. In some secondary antibody deficiencies, immunoglobulin therapy is of proven or probable benefit, e.g. in prematurity and infancy, multiple myeloma, chronic lymphocytic leukemia, and pediatric AIDS. In other secondary immunodeficiencies immunoglobulin therapy may be of possible benefit e.g. in nephrotic syndrome, protein-losing enteropathy, burns, severe infections, severe malnutrition, severe dermatitis and post-bone marrow transplantation. Guidelines for the treatment of secondary antibody deficiency with intravenous immunoglobulin are presented.

Acknowledgement

Supported in part by NIH grants AI-15332 and HD-09008 from the US Public Health Service.

References

1. Shearer, W. T. and Anderson, D. C. The secondary immunodeficiencies. In "Immunologic Disorders in Infants and Children" (Ed. Stiehm, E. R.), pp. 400–425. W. B. Saunders, Philadelphia; 1989.
2. Waldmann, T. A. Primary and acquired immunological diseases. In "Immunodeficiency Diseases", 4th edn (Eds Samter, M., Talmage, D. W., Frank, M. M., Austen, K. F. and Claman, H. N.) pp. 411–465. Little Brown, Boston; 1988.
3. Stiehm, E. R. Human immune serum globulin for IV use could prevent infection in children. *AIDS Med. Rep.* 2: 129–134; 1989.
4. Schedel, I. Application of immunoglobulin preparations in multiple myeloma. *In* "Clinical Use of Intravenous Immunoglobulins" (Eds Morell, A. and Nydegger, U. E.) pp. 123–132. Academic Press, London; 1986.
5. Cooperative Group for the Study of Immunoglobulin in Chronic Lymphocytic Leukemia. Intravenous immunoglobulin for the prevention of infection in chronic lymphocytic leukemia: A randomized, controlled clinical trial. *N. Eng. J. Med.* 319: 902–907; 1988.
6. Clapp, D. W., Kliegman, R. M., Baley, J. E., Shenker, N., Kyllonen, K., Fanaroff, A. A. and Berger, M. Use of intravenously administered immune globulin to prevent nosocomial sepsis in low birth weight infants: Report of a pilot study. *J. Pediatr.* 115: 973–978; 1989.

7a. Sullivan, K. M., Kopecky, K. J., Jocom, J. *et al.* Immunodeficiency and antimicrobial efficacy of intravenous immunoglobulin in bone marrow transplantation. *N. Eng. J. Med.* 323: 705–712; 1990.

7. Santosham, M., Reid, R., Ambrosino, D. M., Wolff, M. C., Almeido-Hill, J., Priehs, C., Aspery, K. M., Garrett, S., Croll, L., Foster, S., Burge, G., Page, P., Zacher, B., Moxon, R., Chir, B. and Siber, G. R. Prevention of *Haemophilus influenzae type B* infections in high-risk infants treated with bacterial polysaccharide immune globulin. *N. Engl. J. Med.* 317: 923–929; 1987.
8. Schapner, H. W. The immune system in minimal change nephrotic syndrome. *Pediatr. Nephrol.* 3: 101–120; 1989.
9. Wochner, R. D., Drews, G., Strober, W. and Waldmann, T. A. IgG metabolism in myotonic dystrophy. *In* "Progress in Neurogenetics", pp. 219–266. Excerpta Medica Foundation, Amsterdam; 1969.
10. Blaese, R. M., Strober, W., Levy, A. L. and Waldmann, T. A.

Hypercatabolism of IgG, IgA, IgM and albumin in the Wiskott-Aldrich syndrome. *J. Clin. Invest.* **50**: 2331–2338; 1971.
11. Reed, E. C., Bowden, R. A., Dandliker, P. S., Lilleby, K. E. and Meyers, J. D. Treatment of cytomegalovirus pneumonia with ganciclovir and intravenous cytomegalovirus immunoglobulin in patients with bone marrow transplants. *Ann. Intern. Med.* **109**: 783–788; 1988.
12. Emanuel, D., Cunningham, I., Jules-Elysee, K., Brochstein, J. A., Kernan, N. A., Laver, J., Stover, D., White, D. A., Fels, A., Polsky, B., Castro-Malaspina, H., Peppard, J. R., Bartus, P., Hammerling, U. and O'Reilly, R. J. Cytomegalovirus pneumonia after bone marrow transplantation successfully treated with the combination of ganciclovir and high-dose intravenous immune globulin. *Ann. Intern. Med.* **109**: 777–782; 1988.
13. Karpas, A., Hill, F., Youle, M., Vivienne, C., Gray, J., Byron, N., Hayhoe, F., Tenant-Flowers, M., Howard, L., Gilgen, D., Oates, J. K., Hawkins, D. and Gazzard, B. Effects of passive immunization in patients with the acquired immunodeficiency syndrome-related complex and acquired immunodeficiency syndrome. *Proc. Natl. Acad. Sci. USA* **85**: 9234–9237; 1988.
14. Church, J. A., Lewis, J. and Spotkov, J. M. IgG subclass deficiencies in children with suspected AIDS. *Lancet* **1**: 279; 1984.
15. Bardana, E. J., Gabourel, J. D., Davies, G. H. and Craig, S. Effects of phenytoin on man's immunity. Evaluation of changes in serum immunoglobulins, complement, and antinuclear antibody. *Am. J. Med.* **74**: 289–296; 1983.
16. Ochs, H. D. and Wedgwood, R. J. Disorders of the B-cell system. *In* "Immunologic Disorders in Infants and Children", 3rd edn (Ed. Stiehm, E. R.), pp. 226–256. W. B. Saunders, Philadelphia; 1989.
17. Webster, A. D. B., Efter, T. and Asherson, G. L. *Escherichia coli* antibody: A screening test for immunodeficiency. *Br. Med. J.* **3**: 16–18; 1974.
18. Ayoub, E. M., Dudding, B. A., and Cooper, M. D. Dichotomy of antibody response to group A streptococcal antigens in Wiskott-Aldrich syndrome. *J. Lab. Clin. Med.* **72**: 971–979; 1968.
19. Rand, K. H., Houck, H., Ganju, A., Babington, R. G. and Elfenbein, G. J. Pharmacokinetics of cytomegalovirus specific IgG antibody following intravenous immunoglobulin in bone marrow transplant patients. *Bone Marrow Transpl.* **4**: 679–683; 1989.

Discussion

F. Kanakoudi-Tsakalidou
You mentioned that one of the criteria for giving IVIG treatment to patients with secondary ID is an IgG level of < 2 g/l or IgG + IgM + IgA of < 4 g/l.

Do you believe that IgG level *per se* could be a satisfactory criteria or would we better say "a low level of IgG in co-estimation with patient's clinical condition"? We have the example of the "normal" or even the "transient" hypogammaglobulinemia of infancy. We may find IgG levels of less than 2 g/l in a number of infants who remain completely healthy for months.

E. R. Stiehm

In general, I agree. Many patients can have low levels of IgG for months without clinical illness. They are still *susceptible* to infection. I do not advocate use of gammaglobulin for most cases of transient or physiologic hypogammaglobulinemia but I do use it if the patient is having coexistent infection.

T. Gardner

You suggest that: (a) poor response to vaccine, (b) rapid loss of antibody titer post-vaccine, and (c) poor antibody titer response to infection may help identify patients suitable for IVIG. Presumably you are referring to AIDS patients. Is there any evidence that these parameters may be used to identify chronic lymphocytic leukemia or multiple myeloma patients that are susceptible to infection?

E. R. Stiehm

Patients with partial antibody deficiencies of all types may have these immunologic defects. Specific examples include nephrotic syndrome patients, myeloma patients, and CMV patients. These criteria are useful in all situations.

G. Gaedicke

I disagree in declaring healthy newborns and children in the first year of life as being immunodeficient. Immunodeficiency is defined as being a pathological state, but the impaired immune functions in early life are transient and related to the normal development of the immune system. Would you be so kind as to comment on that?

E. R. Stiehm

Perhaps I should have used "immunologically immature". The net effect is the same; the immune system cannot fight infection as well as normal adults, with the result that there is increased morbidity and mortality. The history of medicine is to help nature, and such measures can decrease infant mortality and morbidity.

Immunoprophylaxis in "septic-risk" patients undergoing surgery for gastrointestinal cancer. Preliminary results of a randomized, controlled, multicenter clinical trial

FERDINANDO CAFIERO and MARCO GIPPONI

Divisione di Oncologia Chirurgica, Istituto Nazionale per la Ricerca sul Cancro, Genoa, Italy

Introduction

Post-operative infections still represent a major cause of morbidity, mostly in neoplastic patients undergoing surgery for gastrointestinal cancer (1, 2). Multiple risk factors, such as pathogens (3), impairment of host defense mechanisms (3), environment (3), disease site and staging (4, 5), previous anti-neoplastic treatment (6, 7), anaesthesia (8), operative stress (9), advanced age associated with compromised performance status (10), and nutritional deficiency (11–13) deeply affect a patient's predisposition to septic complications. In this view, pathogens have certainly attracted the greatest attention, especially when clean-contaminated or contaminated surgical procedures are being performed; this has prompted the need to define which kind of intervention requires an antibiotic prophylaxis. In the field of

Immunotherapy with Intravenous Immunoglobulins
ISBN 0–12–370725–0

gastro-intestinal surgery, there is general consensus on short-term parenteral antibiotic prophylaxis in colo-rectal surgery and, according to recent reports, in surgery for gastric or biliary tract obstructing neoplasms as well (14, 15).

However, despite antibiotic prophylaxis, post-operative infections are not definitely prevented in any circumstance; an outlook to other risk factors, such as host defense, might contribute to improve the outcome for these patients. Host defense effector mechanism deficits certainly play a major role in the onset of infections, even though pre-operative host defense abnormalities have hardly ever been documented; this fact has prevented the adoption of any timely and selective immunoprophylaxis. Remarkably, only in the post-operative period do patients who develop infections often show a concomitant significant reduction of some humoral markers such as CH50, C3, C4 and IgG (16).

Therefore, a rational approach to selective immunoprophylaxis might consist in the pre-operative identification of "septic-risk" patients who, by definition, are likely to develop septic complications and, consequently, such an impairment of humoral response. The adoption, in this subset of patients, of an immunoglobulin prophylaxis could counterbalance the specific and transient post-operative humoral effector mechanism deficit, thus contributing to the reduction of post-operative infections.

On these grounds, a randomized clinical trial to evaluate the effectiveness and tolerability of peri-operative prophylaxis with intravenous immunoglobulins (IVIG) in "septic-risk" patients undergoing surgical treatment for gastrointestinal cancer was undertaken.

Materials and methods

From July 1986 to May 1989, 298 patients undergoing surgical treatment for gastrointestinal cancer were pre-operatively evaluated to select "septic-risk" patients who would have been recruited in the randomized clinical trial. The following centers participated in this trial: Division of Surgical Oncology, Istituto Nazionale per la Ricerca sul Cancro, Genoa; Istituto di Patologia Chirurgica, University of Genoa, School of Medicine, and I Division of General Surgery, Sampierdarena Hospital, Genoa. The pre-operative selection is carried out by means of an original screening test based on a discriminant equation where absolute values of total serum proteins, serum albumins, $\alpha 1-$, $\beta-$, $\gamma-$ globulins, and the score of Multitest skin testing are weighed: results of this equation above the optimal discriminant threshold allow the detection of "septic-risk" patients (17).

Prophylaxis in patients undergoing colo-rectal surgery (COLON group) includes mechanical bowel preparation and parenteral short-term cefoxitin (2 g at 1 h prior to operation, 2 g at the end of the operation, and 2 g every 6 h for 24 h) (18) randomly associated with IVIG (15 g on the day prior to operation, on the 1st and 5th post-operative day); in NON-COLON group (abdominal oesophagus, stomach, small intestine, extra-hepatic biliary tract, liver and pancreas) prophylaxis is based on random administration of IVIG following the same dosage.

Post-operative septic complications are analyzed both to assess the predictivity of the screening test used to select "septic-risk" patients, and to evaluate the efficacy of immunoprophylactic measures. Septic complications include wound infections and extra-operative site infections, such as lung and genito-urinary tract infections. Secondary sepsis, i.e. anastomotic dehiscence with clinical and radiologic confirmation, is considered separately for the evaluation of screening test predictivity, since such infections are mainly related to operative technique, insufficient blood supply of gastrointestinal stumps and less than optimal bowel preparation, and, consequently, can hardly be predicted pre-operatively (19).

Tolerability is carefully evaluated during and soon after IVIG infusion, looking for possible side effects, such as nausea, vomiting, fever, tachycardia, dyspnea, precordial and back pain, or flushing, that could be related to phlogistic or anaphylaxis reactions (20).

Statistical analysis of pre-and post-operative monitoring of serum IgG, IgA, and IgM included Student's t-test for paired data, in order to detect significant differences ($P < 0.05$) between pre- and post-operative serum immunoglobulin levels within a specific group of patients (i.e within patients who developed post-operative infections or with a regular outcome): Student's t-test for unpaired data was used to compare serum immunoglobulins levels in septic versus patients with a regular post-operative outcome.

Results

At the present time, 298 patients have been pre-operatively screened; there were 120 "septic-risk" patients (40%) who were recruited in the randomized clinical trial, with 77 patients included in the COLON and 43 in the NON-COLON group (Table 1). The remaining 178 "non-septic risk" patients underwent routine prophylaxis, with a careful follow-up of post-operative infections. The percentage of patients with different types of post-operative infections are illustrated in Figure 1.

The predictivity of the screening method used to detect "septic-risk" patients was assessed in 213 out of 298 patients. The other 85

Table 1
"Septic-risk" patients who were recruited in the randomized clinical trial, stratified by type of surgery (COLON, NON-COLON)

	COLON		NON-COLON	
	IG+A	A	IG	C
Patients (n)	41	36	22	21
Age (years)	67±1.4	66±1.3	64±1.7	66±1.7
Sex (M/F)	15/26	16/20	8/14	10/11
Septic-risk score				
Males	0.85±0.03	0.83±0.03	0.85±0.03	0.86±0.04
Females	11.1±0.8	13.4±0.7	12.5±0.7	10.3±1.4
Multitest score				
Males	0.47±0.13	0.25±0.11	1.25±0.84	0.60±0.22
Females	2.3±0.41	2.4±0.39	2.7±0.55	4.2±0.71
Length of anesthesia (h)	2.9±0.1	3.1±0.1	3.1±0.2	2.9±0.2

Mean values ± SEM.

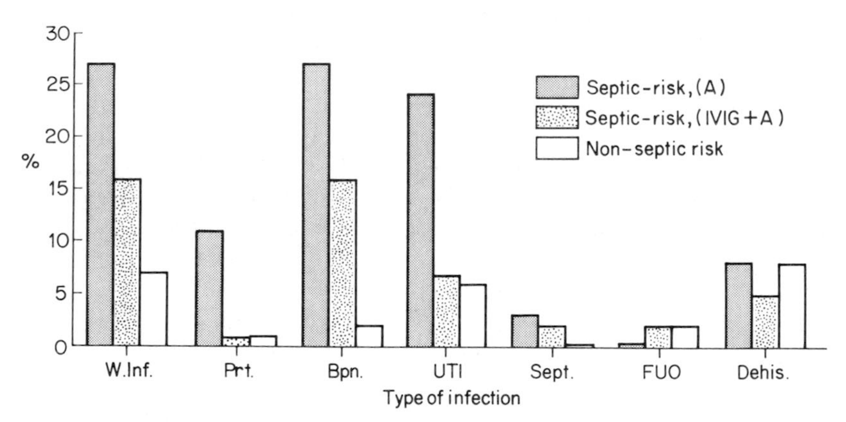

Figure 1. Percentage of patients with different types of post-operative infections. W. Inf., wound infection; Prt., peritonitis; Bpn; bronchopneumonia; UTI, urinary tract infection; Sept; septicemia; FUO, fever of unknown origin; Dehis; anastomotic dehiscence.

patients were not comparable as 63 "septic-risk" were randomized in the immunoprophylaxis arm, while 4 "septic-risk" patients of the control group and 18 "non-septic-risk" patients developed secondary infections (i.e. secondary to anastomotic dehiscence). Thus, the evaluation group included 53 "septic-risk" patients, belonging to the control subset, and 160 "non-septic-risk" patients, neither of which developed secondary infections.

Sensitivity and specificity have not been calculated because of their artificial variation due to the exclusion of "septic-risk" patients, randomized for IVIG prophylaxis; the outcome of these latter might have been improved by immunoprophylactic procedures. Positive predictivity was 73.5%, negative predictivity 82.5%, and global predictivity 80.2% (Table 2).

Table 2
Assessment of predictivity of the screening test used to detect "septic-risk" patients

	Test		
Infection	Positive	Negative	Total
Present	39	28	67
Absent	14	132	146
Total	53	160	213

Positive predictivity: (39/53) = 73.5%
Negative predictivity: (132/160) = 82.5%
Global predictivity: (171/213) = 80.2%

As regards post-operative septic complications in "septic-risk" patients, both COLON and NON-COLON groups showed a significant reduction of infections in patients who were randomized for immunoprophylaxis (Table 3). In the COLON group there were 20 infections in 19 patients treated with IVIG plus antibiotic prophylaxis versus 35 infections in 28 control patients who had only antibiotic prophylaxis ($P < 0.005$). In the NON-COLON group there were 10 infections in 10 patients of the IVIG prophylaxis subset versus 21 infections in 15 control patients ($P < 0.04$). No matter what the kind of prophylaxis regimen was, post-operative infections were constantly lower in "non-septic-risk" as compared to "septic risk" patients (Table 4).

Table 3

Post-operative infective events in "septic-risk" patients COLON (n = 77) and NON-COLON (n = 43), related with the prophylaxis schedule: noteworthy, some patients developed more than one type of infection

Surgery		Type of post-operative infections									Regular outcome	P
		Wound inf.	Prt	Extra-op Bpn	Extra-op UTI	Sept	FUO	D	Total (i)	Total (*)		
COLON												
A+Ig	(41)	6	—	7	3	1	1	2	20	19	22	0.005
A	(36)	11	3	9	9	—	—	3	35	28	8	
NON-COLON												
Ig	(22)	4	1	3	1	—	—	1	10	10	12	0.04
C	(21)	5	4	7	3	—	1	1	21	15	6	
Total	(120)											
Ig	(63)	10	1	10	4	1	1	3	30	29	34	
No-Ig	(57)	16	7	16	12	—	1	4	56	43	14	

Legend: Prt, peritonitis; Bpn, broncopneumonia; UTI, urinary tract infection; Sept., septicemia; FUO, fever unknown origin; D, anastomotic dehiscence.
Total: (i), overall infective events; (*), number of patients with post-operative infections

Table 4

Distribution of post-operative infections in "non-septic-risk" patients, by type of surgery (COLON, NON-COLON)

Surgery	Type of post-operative infections								Regular outcome
	Wound inf.	Prt	Extra-op. Bpn	Extra-op. UTI	Sept	FUO	D	Total	
COLON (n= 114)	9	1	3	5	—	1	11	30 26.3%	84 73.6%
NON-COLON (n= 64)	3	—	5	1	—	—	7	16 25%	48 75%
Total (n= 178)	12	1	8	6	—	1	18	46	132

Legend: Prt, peritonitis; Bpn, broncopneumonia; UTI, urinary tract infection; Sept, septicemia; FUO, fever unknown origin; D, Anastomotic dehiscence

Table 5
Pre- and post-operative mean values (± SEM) of serum IgG, IgA, and IgM (mg %) in COLON patients (N = 77) in two arms of prophylaxis schedule [(IG + A) or (A)], considering significant differences separately within septic and non-septic patients (*), and between the two subgroups of patients (**).

	(IG + A) (*n*=41)				(A) (*n*=36)			
	Infection (*n*=19)		No-infection (*n*=22)		Infection (*n*=28)		No-infection (*n*=8)	
	Mean	(±SEM)	Mean	(±SEM)	Mean	(±SEM)	Mean	(±SEM)
	┌──── 0.01 ────┐				┌──── n.s. ────┐			
IgG pre	767	(142)	1036	(148)	1035	(193)	1186	(226)
	n.s.		0.01		0.01		n.s.	
	┌──── 0.01 ────┐				┌──── 0.01 ────┐			
IgG post	886	(178)	1315	(129)	819	(140)	1057	(169)
IgA	157	(54)	202	(71)	182	(84)	155	(35)
IgA	172	(66)	240	(118)	172	(86)	164	(65)
IgM	105	(54)	110	(44)	114	(44)	107	(54)
IgM	140	(100)	137	(52)	124	(73)	109	(49)

(*) Student's *t*-test for paired data.
(**) Student's *t*-test for unpaired data.

Interesting results were supplied by statistical analysis of pre- and post-treatment monitoring of serum immunoglobulins in the COLON group (Table 5). In IVIG-treated patients, a regular post-operative outcome was correlated with a significant increase of serum IgG ($P < 0.01$), while only a slight— but not significant—increase of IgG was detected in septic patients. In the control group, a significant reduction of serum IgG ($P < 0.01$) was evidenced in septic as opposed to non-septic patients. Considering serum IgG levels in septic versus non-septic subjects, within the specific group of prophylaxis schedule (IVIG plus antibiotic or antibiotic), significant differences ($P < 0.01$) of basal and final IgG values in IVIG-treated patients and of final IgG levels only in control patients were observed, respectively.

As regards side effects following IVIG treatment, the infusion had to be stopped in two patients because of the onset of increasing dyspnea, tachycardia, flushing, and precordial feeling of oppression related to drug administration.

Discussion

The rationale of this randomized, controlled, multicenter, clinical trial is based on the assumption that "septic-risk" patients undergoing surgery for gastrointestinal cancer are more likely to develop an impairment of humoral effector mechanisms. Consequently, these "septic-risk" patients represent a suitable sample for evaluating the efficacy of a passive humoral immunoprophylaxis of post-operative septic complications.

In this view, the pre-operative selection of "septic-risk" patients takes on a primary relevance, especially when the unpredictive value of the pre-operative assessment of immunity parameters in such patients is considered (21, 22). The predictivity of the screening test used to detect "septic-risk" patients seemed to work rather well and allowed a high prevalence of post-operative infections (73.5%) in the target population of control patients recruited in the randomized trial to be discerned.

As anticipated, pre-operative IgG serum level assay in the control group did not reveal significant differences in patients who would or would not have developed post-operative infections; a significant serum IgG decrease, limited only to post-operative assays, was evidenced in patients who developed septic complications. Thus, as suggested by Shinagawa and co-workers (16), patients with post-operative infections do have a concomitant post-operative deficit of humoral effector mechanisms which is not evidenced pre-operatively.

These preliminary results seem to indicate a significant advantage for the immunoprophylaxis group (IVIG-treated patients), with a reduction of post-operative infections both in COLON ($P < 0.005$) and in NON-COLON ($P < 0.04$) subsets. This crude evaluation of the effectiveness of immunoprophylaxis as compared to standard prophylaxis is further supported by the significant trends towards serum IgG reduction in control patients who developed post-operative septic complications, and serum IgG increase in IVIG-treated patients who had a regular outcome.

Remarkably, a threshold value of post-operative serum IgG, approximately 1000 mg%, seems to discriminate patients who will develop septic complications from those with a normal post-operative course. In fact, in the IVIG-treated group, patients with final serum IgG levels above 1000 mg% hardly ever develop septic complications, while patients with lower values have a higher rate of infections, notwithstanding immunoprophylactic measures. This suggests that there is a subset of "septic-risk" patients who present a less than optimal increase of serum IgG following IVIG infusion. On the other hand, in the control group, patients who develop post-operative septic complications, as compared to those with a normal outcome, show a clear-cut reduction of serum IgG levels in the post-operative period, far below the threshold of 1000 mg%.

A limited immunoprotein synthesis might thus explain the different behavior of patients defined as "septic-risk" who actually develop post-operative infections, but a definitive confirmation is required following the conclusion of the trial.

As regards post-operative infections despite passive IVIG reintegration in the immunoprophylaxis group, an insufficient dose, a high consumption, or a deficit of other than humoral effector mechanisms might justify the occurrence, although significantly lower, of post-operative septic complications.

Summary

This chapter describes the preliminary results of an ongoing randomized, controlled, multicenter, clinical trial of immunoprophylaxis of post-operative infections with intravenous immunoglobulins (IVIG) in "septic-risk" patients undergoing surgery for gastrointestinal cancer. Immunoprophylaxis is randomly associated with antibiotic prophylaxis in patients undergoing colo-rectal (COLON) surgery while, in the other types of gastrointestinal (NON-COLON) surgery, prophylaxis is based only on random administration of IVIG.

Up to now, 120 patients have been included (COLON $n = 77$. NON-COLON $n = 43$); this preliminary assessment shows a reduction of septic complications in IVIG prophylaxis versus control subset both in COLON (20 and 35 infections, respectively; $P < .005$) and in NON-COLON group (10 and 21 infections, respectively; $P < .04$), with a significant trend of serum IgG levels correlated with post-operative infection outcome.

Acknowledgement

This work has been partly supported by grant from the CNR, no. 88.0553.44.

References

1. Pietsch, J. B. and Meakins, J. L. Predicting infection in surgical patients. *Surg. Clin. North Am.* **59**: 185–197; 1979.
2. Bozzetti, F., Baticci, F. and Terno, G. Impact of cancer site and treatment on the nutritional status of the patients. "Proc. II ESPEN Congress", Newcastle, p. 46. 7–10 September 1980.
3. Meakins, J. L., Pietsch, J. B., Christou, N. V. and Maclean, L. D. Predicting surgical infection before operation. *World J. Surg.* **4**: 439–450; 1980.
4. Dionigi, R., Dominioni, L. and Campani, M. Infections in cancer patients. *Surg. Clin. North Am.* **60**: 145–158; 1980.
5. Orita, K., Miwa, H. and Fukuda, H. Preoperative cell-mediated immune status of gastric cancer patients. *Cancer* **38**: 2343–2347; 1976.
6. Brambilla, G., Parodi, S., Cavanna, M. and Baldini, L. The immunodepressive activity of N-diazoacetylglycine in some transplantation system. *Transplantation* **10**: 100–104; 1979.
7. Campbell, A. C., Hersey, P. and Hardling, B. Effects of anticancer agents on immunological status. *Br. J. Cancer* **28** (s): 254–259; 1973.
8. Slade, M. S. Immunodepression after major surgery in normal patients. *Surgery* **78**: 363–369; 1975.
9. Park, S. K., Wallacc, H. A., Brody, J. I., Blakemore, W. S. Immunodepressive effect of surgery. *Lancet* i: 53–56; 1971.
10. Weksler, M. E. and Hutteroth, T. H. Impaired lymphocyte function in the aged human. *J. Clin. Invest.* **53**: 99–105; 1974.
11. Vint, F. W., Post-mortem findings in the natives of Kenya. *East Africa Med. J.* **15**: 155–161; 1969.
12. Neuman, C. G. Non-specific host factors and infection in malnutrition—A review. *In* "Malnutrition and the Immune Response" (Ed. Suskind, R. M.), pp. 355–378. New York, Raven Press; 1977.
13. Kniker W. T., Anderson, C. T. and Roumiantzeff, M. The Multitest System: a standardized approach to evaluation of delayed hypersensitivity and cell mediated immunity. *Ann. Allergy* **43**: 73–80; 1979.
14. Baum, M. L., Anish, D. S., Chalmers, T. C., Sacks, H. S., Smith, Jr, H. and Fagerstrom, R. M. A survey of clinical trial of antibiotic prophylaxis in colon surgery: evidence against further use of no-treatment controls. *N. Engl. J. Med.* **305**: 795–799; 1981.
15. Kaiser, A. B. Antimicrobial prophylaxis in surgery. *N. Engl. J. Med.* **315**: 1129–1138; 1986.
16. Shinagawa, N., Takaoka, T. and Yura, J. A sequential, prospective analysis of humoral immunodepression and infection following biliary tract surgery. *In* II International Symposium on "Infections in the Immunocompromised Host" (Eds Easmon, F. and Gaya, H.), pp. 119–123. Academic Press, London; 1983.
17. Cafiero, F., Gipponi, M., Bonalumi, U. *et al.* Identificazione preoperatoria

del paziente "a rischio" di complicanze settiche dopo chirurgia per neoplasia dell'apparato digerente. Studio policentrico multifasico. *Min. Chir* 44: 2169–2180; 1989.
18. Sertoli, M. R., Cafiero, F., Campora, E., Parodi, E., Rosso, R. and Berti Riboli, E. A randomized trial of systemic versus oral prophylactic antibiotic treatment in colo-rectal surgery. *Chemotherapy* 1: 375–378; 1982.
19. Killingback, M. J. Infection and surgical technique in colo-rectal surgery. *In* "Infection in Surgery: Basic and Clinical Aspects" (Eds Watts, J. M. and Finlay-Jones, J. J.) Churchill Livingstone, Edinburgh; 1981.
20. Barandun, S. and Morell, A. "Adverse Reactions to Immunoglobulin Preparations". Institute for Clinical and Experimental Cancer Research, University of Bern, Tiefenau-Hospital CH-3004 Bern, Switzerland. Academic Press, London; 1981.
21. Cafiero, F., Gipponi, M., Moresco, L. *et al.* Selection of preoperative haematobiochemical parameters for the identification of patients "at risk of infection" undergoing surgery for gastrointestinal cancer. *Eur. J. Surg. Onc.* 15: 247–252; 1989.
22. Cafiero, F., Gipponi, M., Roncella, S., Bonalumi, U., Bonassi, S. and Stabilini, L. Surface marker analysis of peripheral blood mononuclear cells from patients with gastrointestinal tumors. *J. Exp. Clin. Cancer Res.* 6: 91–96; 1987.

Discussion

G. W. Fischer

It is interesting that several patients that became infected did not have a post-IVIG infusion rise in serum IgG. What were the infections and infecting pathogens in these patients?

M. Gipponi (F. Cafiero)

They were mostly wound infection (with mixed pathogens) and bronchopneumonia (we have no data on microbiology in these cases, only Rx chest). Wound infections were commonly sustained by Gram-negative aerobic and anaerobic pathogens (*B. fragilis/E. coli, Enterococcus* (G+), *Pseudomonas*), while *S. aureus* was not so frequent.

A. M. Munster

1. What happens to your statistics if you take out the urinary tract infections?
2. The levels of IgG in all patients seem to be normal or near-normal. Should we try to reach supernormal levels?

M. Gipponi (F. Cafiero)

1. First, the aim was to reduce overall infection rate and the study was sized for that purpose; therefore any statistical comparison of subsets of patients might not have enough power to select a significant difference—with the number of patients presently recruited. Secondly, our results simply reflect the common epidemiologic situation by type of infection that is characteristic of surgical patients. As you know, in fact, UTI is the most frequent cause of infective morbidity, followed by wound infections and bronchopneumonia.
2. Post-op infection are associated with a decrease of serum IgG, as it was confirmed in our antibiotic prophylaxis (A) group and in non-specific risk patients who developed infections. This decrease occurs in the immediate post-operative days (transient humoral deficit? specific antibody consumption?). The key point is that IVIG prophylaxis may counter-balance this transient deficit, mostly by supplying specific antibody for more likely pathogens of post-operative infections.

Non-specific immunotherapy and intravenous gammaglobulin administration in surgical sepsis

L. DOMINIONI, A. BENEVENTO, M., ZANELLO[1], R. GENNARI, M. C. BESOZZI, M. HOURCADE and R. DIONIGI

Department of Surgery, University of Pavia, Ospedale Multizonale di Varese, Italy
[1] Istituto di Anestesia e Rianimazione, Universita di Bologna, Italy

Introduction

During the last two decades a decrease in the overall incidence of post-operative infections has been observed as a result of improved prophylactic measures, including: (1) accurate pre-operative preparation (nutritional support, physiotherapy, correction of metabolic imbalances); (2) rational use of antibiotic prophylaxis; (3) improved anesthesiologic techniques; (4) improved post-operative care.

Extensive studies on the immunologic status of surgical patients have shown that the susceptibility to post-operative infections and the risk of developing fatal sepsis are influenced not only by operative field contamination, but also by the condition of peri-operative immunologic impairment and by defective acute-phase responses (1). The importance of immunologic defenses and of acute-phase responses for control of surgical infections is well known (1, 2). The immunologic mechanisms of defense that have been found to be essential for

Immunotherapy with Intravenous Immunoglobulins
ISBN 0-12-370725-0

resistance to bacterial pathogens include humoral and cell-mediated immunity, neutrophil functions, the reticuloendothelial system, macrophages and a large number of endogenous mediators of immune and inflammatory responses which are released into the plasma in response to infection (3–5).

Severe surgical infections, due either to extensive bacterial contamination or to a deficit of immune competence, are characterized by a complex septic response, which may progress to septic shock or toward multiple organ failure (MOF) and death (6).

The septic state is a complex clinical syndrome which may develop in response to infection (bacterial, fungal or viral) (7). The purpose of the septic response is to create optimal conditions for microbial elimination, by modifying the internal environment by means of hemodynamic, hormonal, metabolic and immunological reactive changes.

During the last two decades extensive clinical and experimental studies have elucidated the most relevant changes which take place during the septic response to surgical infection. The pathophysiological alterations caused by severe bacterial invasion can be classified as: (a) local effects on the infected tissues; (b) acute-phase reactions; (c) secondary effects on target organ-systems.

The condition of severe sepsis is frequently encountered in multiple trauma and in patients undergoing dirty surgical procedures or who are markedly immunocompromised; mortality among severely septic surgical patients remains very high (1).

Immunocompromise during sepsis

From the immunological viewpoint, the septic state is characterized by a severe compromise of immunoreactivity, which may be documented by appropriate tests of immunologic functions. In fact the following immunologic derangements are documented during sepsis: (1) decrease in peripheral blood total lymphocyte count; (2) decreased circulating T cells; (3) low response of T cells to mitogenic stimulation. Immunoglobulin levels during severe sepsis are within normal levels, however, they are higher in survivors than in non-survivors from sepsis (8).

Other factors contributing to the compromise of defense mechanisms during infection and sepsis are the following: (1) broken or defective anatomic barriers as a result of surgery, trauma, burns or invasive maneuvers; (2) extensive consumption of specific (antibody) or non-specific (complement or fibronectin) opsonic factors, resulting in impaired phagocytosis; (3) compromised oxidative metabolism of phagocytes, which have a reduction of bactericidal capacity; (4) depressed cell-mediated immunity.

Non-specific immunotherapy in sepsis

Numerous therapeutic strategies have been tried in an attempt to strengthen defense mechanisms in septic patients; they can be divided conceptually into two types: (1) stimulation of the non-specific defense mechanisms; (2) specific immunotherapy. In the first group, non-specific immunity has been stimulated by BCG and by *Corynebacterium parvum*; however, only modest results have been obtained (9).

Another substance utilized as a non-specific immunostimulator is muramyldipeptide a well-characterized component of the mycobacterium cell wall. This substance was shown to be effective when given in association with antibiotics (10).

Recent studies have shown that gamma-interferon has the capacity to stimulate *in vitro* macrophages and monocytes (10).

Studies have been conducted in multiple trauma to test whether the administration of fibronectin in patients with documented fribronectin deficit could reduce the incidence of infectious complications (11, 12). The results of that study indicated that exogenous fibronectin did not influence the clinical course of multiple trauma and did not prevent sepsis or septic shock.

Use of polyvalent IgG in sepsis

Non-specific immunotherapy has also been attempted by using polyvalent immunoglobulins for prophylaxis of bacterial infections. Studies *in vitro* have shown that intact IgG favors opsonization and phagocytosis (13, 14). Moreover, intact Fc gammaglobulins have shown efficacy in decreasing mortality in septic animals models (15, 16).

In a double-blind clinical study carried out in 1985 in 150 severely traumatized patients undergoing long-term artificial ventilation, the administration of intravenous immunoglobulins (IVIG) for prophylaxis of nosocomial infections has been tested. Patients given IVIG prophylactically received a total amount of 36 g of polyvalent intact Fc gammaglobulins, in three doses (12 g on day 0, + 5 and + 12). In these traumatized patients IVIG prophylaxis was shown to decrease the incidence of pneumonia, and the therapeutic use of antibiotics; however, no difference in the incidence of other infections was observed as compared to placebo controls (17). In that study serum levels of IgG significantly increased in the group treated with IVIG only on day 5. In the serum samples drawn later in the study, no difference in IgG levels was found when comparing the group treated vs. control groups. Theoretically, it might seem preferable to administer the whole high dose of IVIG immediately after trauma; however, in the study on multiple trauma patients referred to above, IVIG were given in three separate doses. The reason for the delayed and refracted administration of IVIG was to prevent initial loss of the drug due to hemorrhage and through the wounds, and to give optimal protection not only against early infections but also against late sepsis.

Another study was carried out recently in a surgical intensive care unit to assess the effect of early administration of IVIG in the prevention of surgical and post-traumatic sepsis.

Patients randomized in this study were severely traumatized or had undergone major surgical operations; none of these patients, however, was septic at the beginning of randomization with the following protocol: polyvalent IVIG 10 g prophylactically on post-operative days 1, 3, 5 and 10. Patients in the control group received four infusions of placebo DW 5%. The results of that study were the following (18): (1) after 2 weeks from operation, patients in the placebo group were still febrile, whereas patients receiving IVIG were non-febrile; (2) serum C3 and C4 levels were significantly higher in IVIG-treated patients; (3) blood cultures, performed on a routine basis post-operatively, were always negative in IVIG-treated patients, whereas six bacteremic episodes were found in control patients; (4) clinically relevant sepsis was diagnosed in six patients of the placebo group vs. three patients in the IVIG group; (5) mortality was lower (although not significantly) in the IVIG-treated patients (6.7% vs. 23.5%). Altogether the data of that study suggest that IVIG contributes to reduce the incidence of sepsis in severely traumatized patients.

To conclude the review of clinical investigations carried out to test the effect of IVIG in septic patients we report the results of a study carried out at our institution.

High-dose polyvalent immunoglobulins in severely septic surgical patients

The purpose of our investigation was to verify if high-dose IVIG in severely septic patients could reduce mortality. A randomized double-blind study was thus carried out comparing the administration of IVIG (Sandoglobulin®) vs. placebo (human albumin) in severely septic surgical patients. Only patients with sepsis score ≥ 20 (meaning a mortality risk ≥ 70% (19)) were accepted into this protocol. The schedule of administration of IVIG and placebo is given in Table 1.

Table 1
Schedule of treatment in the intravenous gammaglobulin (IVIG) patients

Randomization	Day 0	Day 1	Day 5
Body weight ≥ 50 kg	4 × 6 g vials	4 × 6 g vials	2 × 6 g vials
Body weight < 50 kg	3 × 6 g vials	3 × 6 g vials	2 × 6 g vials

At the beginning of ICU treatment, the two groups of patients were similar for severity of sepsis, age, concomitant disease, type of surgical procedure, intra and peri-operative procedures, antibiotic administration.

The results of the study indicated a significantly reduced mortality in patients with severe surgical sepsis treated with polyvalent IVIG as compared to placebo control patients (mortality: 38% vs. 67% respectively ($P < 0.05$)).

In conclusion, the results of our study in patients with severe surgical sepsis were the following: (1) IVIG plus multimodal treatment of sepsis, including antibiotics, reduce mortality significantly; (2) the reduction of mortality seems to be due to a decreased incidence of lethal septic shock.

Summary

Surgical patients with severe septic complications have a high incidence of mortality due to septic shock and multiple organ failure. The septic state is characterized by several organ systems alterations, including a marked compromise of immunoreactivity. Non-specific immunotherapy trials for treatment of sepsis are reviewed. High dose immunoglobulin administration to severely septic surgical patients resulted in a significantly improved survival rate.

Acknowledgement

This work was supported by funds from Ministero Pubblica Istruzione (40%, 1988), and by CNR Grant Contract No. 8702818.52.

References

1. Dominioni, L., Dionigi, R., Zanello, M. *et al.* Sepsis score and acute-phase protein response as predictors of outcome in septic surgical patients. *Arch. Surg.* 122: 141–146; 1987.
2. Alexander, J. W., Stinnett, J. D., Ogle, C. *et al.* A comparison of immunological profiles and their influence on bacteremia in surgical patients with a high risk of infection. *Surgery* 86: 94–104; 1979.
3. Michie, H. R., Guillou, P. S. and Wilmore, D. V. Tumor necrosis factor and bacterial sepsis. *Br. J. Surg.* 76: 670–671; 1989.
4. Schirmer, W. J., Schirmer, J. M. and Fry, D. E. Recombinant human tumor necrosis factor produces hemodynamic changes characteristic of sepsis and endotoxemia. *Arch. Surg.* 124: 445–448; 1989.
5. Border, J. R. Hypothesis: sepsis, multiple systems organ failure, and the macrophage. *Arch. Surg.* 123: 285–286; 1988.
6. Fry, D. E., Pearlstein, L., Fulton, R. L. *et al.* Multiple system organ failure. *Arch. Surg.* 115: 136–140; 1980.
7. Deutschmann, C. S., Konstantinides, F. N., Tsai, M. *et al.* Physiology and metabolism in isolated viral septicemia: further evidence of an organism-independent, host-dependent response. *Arch. Surg.* 122: 21–25; 1987.
8. Nishijima, M. K., Takezawa, J., Hosotsubo, K. K. *et al.* Serial changes in cellular immunity of septic patients with multiple organ-system failure. *Critic Care Med.* 14: 87–91; 1989.
9. Polck, H. C. Jr. Non-specific host defence stimulation in the reduction of surgical infection in man. *Br. J. Surg.* 74: 969–970; 1987.
10. Polk, H. C. Jr., Galland, R. B. and Ausobosky, J. R. Non-specific enhancement of resistance to bacterial infection. Evidence of an effect supplemental to antibiotics. *Ann. Surg.* 196: 436–441; 1982.
11. Grossman, J. E., Plasma fibronectin and fibronectin therapy in sepsis and critical illness. *Rev. Infect. Dis.* 9: S420–S430; 1987.
12. Mansberger, A. R., Doran, J. E., Trat, R. *et al.* The influence of fibronectin administration on the incidence of sepsis and septic mortality in severely injured patients. *Ann. Surg.* 210: 297–307; 1989.
13. Fisher, G. *et al.* Functional antibacterial activity of a human intravenous immunoglobulin preparation: *in vitro* and *in vivo* studies. *Vox Sang* 44: 269–299; 1983.
14. Van Furth, R., Leigh, P. C. J. and Klein, F. Correlation between opsonic activity for various microorganisms and composition of Gammaglobulin preparation for intravenous use. *Rev. Infect. Dis.* 149: 511–517; 1984.
15. Pollack, M. Antibody activity against pseudomonas aeruginosa in immune globulins prepared for intravenous use in humans. *Rev. Infect. Dis.* 147: 1090–1098; 1983.

16. Barandum, S. *et al.* Applicazioni cliniche della immunoglobulina (Gammaglobulina). "Rassegna dello Stato Attuale" (Ed. Lattman, P.), pp. 35–39. Sandoz S. A., Basilea; 1982.
17. Glinz, W., Grob, P. J., Nydegger, U. E. *et al.* Polyvalent immunoglobulins for prophylaxis of bacterial infections in patients following multiple trauma. *Intensive Care Med.* 11: 288–294; 1985.
18. Mao, P., Enrichens, F., Olivero, G. *et al.* Early administration of intravenous immunoglobulins in the prevention of surgical and post-traumatic sepsis: a double blind randomized clinical trial. *Surg. Res. Commun.* 5: 93–98; 1989.
19. Dominioni, L. and Dionigi, R. The grading of sepsis and the assessment of its prognosis in the surgical patient: a review. *Surg. Res. Commun.* 1: 1–11; 1987.

Control of infection following major burns: the immunological approach

ANDREW M. MUNSTER

Baltimore Regional Burn Center and the Department of Surgery, Johns Hopkins University, Baltimore, Maryland, USA

The phenomenon of post-traumatic immunosuppression in general, and post-burn immunosuppression in particular, has been recognized for 25 years (1, 2). The burn wound itself makes a substantial contribution to the phenomenon by providing a portal of entry for massive loads of endotoxin (3) and possibly other immunosuppressive/toxic substances (4); otherwise, thermal injury, traumatic injury and elective surgical intervention share common systemic immunosuppressive effects, depending on the "dose" of the injury (5).

What makes post-traumatic immunosuppression important to the clinician is that, with the conquest of transportation problems and improvements in the management of post-burn shock, most of the mortality now due to thermal injury is attributable to sepsis and to pulmonary complications which accompany sepsis (6). Further, the risk of death and septic complications has been directly related to immunosuppression as measured by a number of different *in vivo* and *in vitro* parameters. For example, skin test responsiveness is related to burn size (7). Lymphocyte responsiveness to mitogens and antigens is suppressed in proportion to the size of the injury (8), including burns, and longitudinal analysis permits separation of septic from non-septic

Immunotherapy with Intravenous Immunoglobulins
ISBN 0–12–370725–0

patients at about the time of onset of sepsis (5, 9). Neutrophil function is altered in several aspects, and such perturbations can also be related to the onset of sepsis in burn patients (10). Of great interest, the depletion of serum immunoglobulin G level can also be prognostically tied to burn survival and the development of sepsis (11).

In other aspects of immune changes following thermal injury, the picture is somewhat less clear cut. There are changes in peripheral lymphocyte populations, with changes in compartmentalization (12, 13). There is no agreement as to whether phenotypic changes (generally resulting in lower total T-cell numbers, drastic lowering of helper T cells, variable changes in suppressor T cells, and the appearance of immature markers) is of functional significance, due to a change in traffic between the circulating blood and nodes/spleen, and whether these changes are a cause or result of infection. Of importance are recent findings that although, as previously mentioned, IgG and to a lesser degree IgA levels are depressed following major thermal injury, B-cell function and IgG production is normal or supernormal quite soon after injury (14). The suppression of early IgM synthesis following trauma can be partially modulated by lymphokine administration, particularly by IL-2 (15). The neutrophil dysfunction following thermal injury (16) has been most recently attributed to altered leukotriene generation (17).

In brief, almost every aspect of the immune mechanism which has been investigated following major burns has been found to be depressed in proportion to the size of the burn.

Until quite recently, investigators felt that although post-burn immunosuppression was multifaceted, immunomodulation, perhaps combined with appropriate replacement therapy, would, in time, restore immune function. This optimism has not been borne out by most approaches. In a typical experiment, mortality rate of experimental animals could be improved early, or slightly, but the eventual end result was rarely a significant improvement. Our early work in the area was typical: *Pseudomonas*-infected, burned rats were treated by super-natants from spleen cell cultures from immunized animals. The immunized animals died more slowly, but eventually there was no difference from controls (18). This experience was reproduced by many investigators.

Is post-burn immunosuppression due to a defect?

Questions began to be raised about the *mechanism* of immunosuppression with the hypothesis that suppressor T-cell proliferation, in order to prevent autoimmune disease, was somehow instrumental in the phenomena observed (19). This theory has been challenged since the advent of phenotypic markers (13, 20) and on theoretical grounds, since the appearance of soluble free IL-2 receptor, evidence of immune activity, is much increased in burn patients' lymphocyte cultures (21, 22), even as IL-2 receptor expression is depressed (24). Nevertheless, suppressor T cells clearly appear following thermal injury (23). Further, prostaglandins and endotoxin, both inducers of suppressor T cells, have been documented to be increased following thermal injury (24–27). The significance of suppressor cell activity is still not clear.

By the mid-1980s, it became clear that the inflammatory response following thermal injury had a critical role in post-burn immunosuppression, and that the macrophage-monocyte axis was a key component of these alterations. Interleukin-1 was an early candidate for a suppressive monokine, being released in conjunction with PGE2 from endotoxin-stimulated macrophages (28). Very recently, tumor necrosis factor (TNF) has been found to be correlated with infection and mortality in burn patients (29). Furthermore, the presence of endotoxin which originates from the burn wound (3, 30) or from the gastrointestinal tract by translocation (31) induces interleukin-6 production; the height of IL-6 can be strongly correlated both with serum endotoxin concentration and with clinical complications (32); both can be controlled by the administration of the endotoxin antagonist, polymyxin B. Adding to the maze of interlocking reactions is the role of the neuroendocrine axis: opioid peptides are known to modulate both neutrophil and lymphocyte function, and alterations in plasma opioid levels do indeed occur after burns (33).

In summary, the immunosuppression following trauma, particularly burns, is an important component of septic morbidity and mortality in patients. Initially thought to be principally an "acquired immunodeficiency", the syndrome is now known to be a complex array of biochemical and immunological change, involving the secretion of many cytokines and other mediators, the teleological reason for whose appearance is still incompletely understood. Intervention in this difficult situation can be classified as being in one of several directions: replacement therapy, mediator administration, mediator blockage, endotoxin blockage, immunomodulation (biological response modifiers), and other measures including general and nutritional support, mechanical removal of toxic substances, and early closure of the burn wound. These will now be each considered in turn.

Replacement therapy: classic active and passive vaccination

Gammaglobulin replacement in burn patients was attempted as early as 1964 (34). Active immunization has been used in many trials, employing polyvalent, monovalent or serotype and even strain-specific vaccines (35). Active vaccination is undoubtedly successful; its failure as a universal prophylactic against sepsis in burns is more due to the constantly changing flora and specificity of the colonizing organisms than to any inherent problem in the process of vaccination. Passive vaccination, or immunoglobulin replacement, emerged as a desirable objective with early observations that immunoglobulin depletion was common after major burns, and the extent of depletion could be correlated with the incidence of sepsis and septic death (11, 36, 37).

Unfortunately, the advent of the highly purified and concentrated immunoglobulins available for intravenous use has not, so far, been reported to reduce the occurrence of sepsis and septic mortality in patients. Initial trials from several centers (38–40) universally report immediate correction of serum immunoglobulin concentration, including subclasses, but with little effect on outcome. Our group looked in detail at T-cell function, neutrophil phagocytosis and intracellular kill, and found no substantial differences between treated and untreated patients. Burleson *et al.* (41) found no changes in the proportion of total, helper or suppressor T cells between IgG-treated and untreated patients, but a slight increase in *in vitro* secretion of IgM by Pokeweed mitogen (PMW)-stimulated B cells, in the treated patients.

Clearly, immunoglobulin replacement alone will not solve the problem of sepsis in the burn patients, because of several other key perturbations in addition to Ig depletion. To address this problem, combination therapy has been attempted by some investigators. Combination of thyroxin replacement with IgG (42), immunoglobulin and antibiotic (43) or immunoglobulin together with polymyxin B to reduce the endotoxin load (44) have been attempted with promising results. This type of approach will have to be explored further.

Perhaps the most promising work recently has been that of Holder (45). Arguing that pathogenicity is a combined effect of bacterial load, protease activity, and exotoxin A, he demonstrated that a combination of therapies directed at these three factors in burned infected mice was superior to any treatment alone. Immunoglobulin replacement will undoubtedly continue to be a valuable therapeutic modality in the treatment of burned patients, but not alone; other host-directed or germ-directed treatments will have to be used in combination.

Fibronectin is a major opsonizing protein in man. As other proteins, it is severely depleted after burn and trauma and the extent of depletion can be correlated with sepsis (46). Even though the depletion can be reversed by the administration of fibronectin (47), a recent very tightly controlled trial in a large series of trauma patients failed to yield clinically significant improvement in outcome (48).

Thus it would seem that replacement therapy of catabolized/leaking plasma protein components alone is unlikely to eliminate the susceptibility of burn patients to sepsis.

Biological response modifiers

Ever since Lemperle (49) attempted to use restim and glucan to stimulate the reticuloendothelial system of burned rats and mice in 1970, there have been dozens of immunomodulatory agents used to stimulate the depressed host response following burn injury. These have included, recently, CP-46665, CP-20961, Levamisol, MDP, TP-5 and lithium (50), thymopentin and isoprinosine (51), Biostim or RU 41 740 (52), cimetidine and cyclophoshamide (53), Methysoprinol (54), Thymopentin TP-5 (55), as well as nutritional agents such as vitamin E and arginine (56, 57). Recently, glucan made a reappearance in the treatment of trauma patients (58). In this latter study, improvement in sepsis and mortality was accomplished by an improvement in skin test reactivity and increased serum levels of IL-1 beta. The theoretical and practical difficulties inherent in the use of biological response modifiers (BRMs), however, include phase variations in response and some fairly critical species differences (59); as well, most BRMs appear to require pretreatment, which is clearly not clinically practical for the burn patient. In a well-controlled double-blind study Waymack *et al.* (60) were unable to demonstrate any improvements in patient mortality, infectious complications or the need for antibiotic use with the use of thymopentin.

Mediator therapy

I am defining mediator, in contrast to a biological response modifier, as a monokine or cytokine occurring in man during normal immunological or inflammatory responses. As mentioned before, our laboratory made an extensive attempt at what was then called "thymocyte reconstituting factor" or TRF therapy in the burned, *Pseudomonas*-challenged rat (18). This material was probably mainly interleukin-2, unidentified at that time.

Transfer factor was recently used to treat 57 patients in an intensive care unit with improvements in immune parameters, but this series was not randomized (61). The addition of IL-2 was ineffective in restoring the reduction of PWM-induced IgG and IgM synthesis in a large group of trauma patients' B cells (62). However, the addition of normal T cells or supernatants from isoantigen-stimulated cell cultures did provide effective stimulation. The same group of investigators successfully reversed the impaired expression of IL-2R in burn patients with exogenous IL-2; the clinical results of this intervention, however, could not be evaluated (63).

Suppression of IL-2 production and of IL-2R expression on lymphocytes is clearly a central phenomenon in post-burn immunosuppression; but convincing clinical evidence that passive replacement with IL-2 or other mediators will result in substantial clinical improvement has not, to date, been forthcoming.

Mediator and endotoxin blockade

These two approaches are bracketed together, because there is strong evidence that most of the biological effects of endotoxin are mediated by monokines and cytokines, and that endotoxemia is a universal phenomenon following burn injury. That mediator administration and mediator blockade could both be beneficial is theoretically possible, given the existence of a multitude of feed-back loops, and the different experimental conditions with regard to timing and dosage; but from the pragmatic clinical point of view, this proposition is extremely difficult.

Prostaglandins, particularly E2 have been extensively investigated post-burn, since PGE2 is released early post-burn, its release is stimulated by injury as well as endotoxin, and it is known to induce suppressor cell proliferation. Inhibition of prostanoids and other cyclooxygenases has been attempted by antibody in an animal study (64), and by systemic or topical ibuprofen (65, 66). Prostaglandin inhibition, however, while abolishing some components of the inflammatory response, appears to have little effect on the immune response itself (67). Ibuprofen also inhibits some of the clinical effects of tumor necrosis factor, supporting the hypothesis that some of the effects of TNF may be mediated through the cyclooxygenase pathway (68). The antifungal agent ketokonazole is a potent inhibitor of thromboxane synthetase, and has been reported to reduce the incidence of the adult respiratory distress syndrome in a series of surgical intensive care patients (69). By reducing the effect of thromboxane B2 synthesis and secretion as an initiating factor, this therapy could potentially be valuable in burn patients as well.

Indomethacin is a prostaglandin synthetase inhibitor and available for clinical intravenous use. In 43 patients undergoing major surgical procedures, Faist and colleagues (70) demonstrated an improvement in parameters of cell-mediated immunity, particularly IL-2R expression; statistically significant reduction in septic complications or mortality was not, however, obtained.

Combination therapy with mediator blockade and biologic response modification is promising; thymopentin and indomethacin together accomplished remarkable immunorestoration in a series of animal burn experiments (71). Such "blockade" can be accomplished at the effector cell membrane level also, since T cells are known to have both slow and rapid calcium channels; presumably, rapidly increasing intracellular Ca^2 concentration can lead to cell damage, and calcium-channel blockade is a theoretically sound approach to this problem. Our laboratory has attempted to do this with Verapamil, but doses sufficient to kill animals were inadequate in producing any improvement in the post-burn suppression of antibody synthesis (72). Recently, the Michigan group (73) reported success with the Ca^2-blocking agent diltiazem in improving post-hemorrhagic macrophage antigen presentation in mice. The problem with this approach is, of course, that cells critical to resuscitation and recovery (e.g. the cardiac cell) also depend on calcium entry for activation, and calcium blockage could be, in this instance, a very two-edged sword.

Because endotoxemia is universal in large burns both early and late, and it appears to be related to injury size (3): because endotoxin induces this secretion of many mediators of the inflammatory response such as TNF and IL-1, our laboratory has concentrated over the last 5 years on control of endotoxemia as one approach to immunorestoration.

Endotoxin in animals and man can be neutralized in several ways: by monoclonal antibody, charcoal hemofiltration, antiendotoxin $F(ab')_2$ fragments, competitive inhibition or analogs, and polymyxin B. To a lesser extent, commercially available IgG preparations also carry anti-endotoxin activity (74–77).

We have had extensive laboratory and clinical experience with the administration of polymyxin B to burned animals and patients. Polymyxin B therapy improves *in vitro* immunological parameters, particularly the helper/suppressor T-cell ratio, natural killer cell function, and IL-2 responsiveness, while lowering the measured level of plasma endotoxin. Improvements in septic morbidity and mortality as a result of polymyxin therapy are suggestive but not, at this point, statistically significant (78). The most exciting recent finding is that endotoxin-regulated induction of interleukin-6, an excellent marker of severity of diseases and injury, can be down-regulated with polymyxin B (32).

It is likely that in combination with immunomodulation, the reduction of endotoxemia, by down-regulating mediator induction, may be of clinical benefit.

General measures

In addition to good nursing care, adequate nutritional support, maintenance of good oxygenation and blood haemoglobin levels, the early excision and closure of the burn wound has definite beneficial immunologic effects. Stratta and colleagues (79) measured immunologic profiles in 26 patients undergoing excisional surgery and found improvement in several parameters, although all of these were humoral; no improvement in cell-mediated immunity was demonstrated. For patients with pulmonary dysfunction, excisional surgery may actually produce a transient deterioration due to release of thromboxane from wound manipulation (80). Possibly the immunologic improvement from wound closure is related to a lowered endotoxin load (30).

Finally, the maintenance of a cheerful, supportive atmosphere resulting in diminished stress for the patient is of definite immunologic benefit, and in this respect, laughter may be the best medicine of all (81).

Conclusion

The discovery of the complexities of the immune response to injury have tempered the optimism with which the potential for immunotherapy of trauma and burns was viewed 10 years ago; this potential, nevertheless, still exists. Needed now are large prospective, randomized trials of combination therapy, in which control of endotoxemia, stimulation of cell-mediated immunity, and inhibition of excess cyclooxygenase production are combined with the administration of immunoglobulin. The data from isolated therapies are promising enough to spur combined therapy to achieve immunological control of septic complications in burn and trauma patients.

Summary

Immunosuppression is a common consequence of major burns, and it becomes more severe with increasing burn size. Almost every facet of the immune response which has been investigated has been found to be suppressed, but the precise etiology of the exchanges is still incompletely understood. Current thinking favors the concept of downregulation of the immune response by mediators of the inflammatory reaction rather than an intrinsic failure of immune competent cells. Therapies which have been attempted, including replacement of immunoglobulins and fibronectin, the use of biological response modifiers, the administration of cytokines and the blockage of inflammatory mediators, as well as intervention in the endotoxemia manifested by burn patients, has, to date, met with only limited success. It is likely that to accomplish upregulation of the response, so that clinical complications and septic mortality can be reduced in these patients, will require combination therapy.

References

1. Riddle, F. R. and Berenbaum, M. C. Postoperative depression of the lymphocyte response to phytohemagglutinin. *Lancet* 1: 747; 1967.
2. Alexander, J. W. and Moncrief, J. A. Alterations of the immune response following severe thermal injury. *Arch. Surg.* 93: 75; 1966.
3. Winchurch, R. A., Thupari, J. N. and Munster, A. M. Endotoxemia in burn patients: Levels of circulating endotoxin are related to burn size. *Surgery* 102: 808; 1987.
4. Schonenberger, G. A., Burkhardt, F., Kahlberger, F. *et al.* Experimental evidence for a significant impairment of host defense for gram negative organisms by a specific cutaneous toxin produced by severe burn injuries. *Surg. Gynae. Obstet.* 141: 222; 1975.
5. Keane, R. M., Munster, A. M., Birmingham, W. *et al.* Prediction of sepsis in the multitrauma patient by assays of lymphocyte responsiveness. *Surg. Gynae. Obstet.* 156: 163; 1987.
6. Pruitt, B. A., Jr. Infection: Cause or effect? *In* 'Lipid Mediators in the Immunology of Shock" (Ed. Paubert-Braquet, M.). Plenum, New York; 1987.
7. Munster, A. M., Eurenius, K., Katz, R. M. *et al.* Cell mediated immunity after thermal injury. *Ann. Surg.* 177: 139; 1973.
8. Munster, A. M., Eurenius, K., Mortensen, R. F. *et al.* Ability of splenic lymphocytes from traumatised animals to induce a GvH reaction. *Transplantation* 14: 106; 1972.
9. Munster, A. M., Winchurch, R. A., Keane, R. *et al.* The *in vitro* skin

test: A reliable and repeatable assay of immunologic competence in the surgical patient. *Ann. Surg.* **194**: 345; 1981.
10. Alexander, J. W. and Wixon, D. Neutrophil dysfunction and sepsis in burn injury. *Surg. Gynae. Obstet.* **130**: 431; 1967.
11. Munster, A. M., Hoagland, H. C. and Pruitt, B. A., Jr. The effect of thermal injury on serum immunoglobulins. *Ann. Surg.* **172**: 965; 1970.
12. Organ, B. C., Antonacci, A. C., Chiao, J. *et al.* Changes in lymphocyte number and phenotype in seven lymphoid compartments after thermal injury. *Ann. Surg.* **210**: 780; 1989.
13. Burleson, D. G., Mason, A. D. and Pruitt, B. A., Jr. Lymphocyte subpopulation changes after thermal injury with infection in an experimental model. *Ann. Surg.* **207**: 208; 1988.
14. Faist, E., Ertel, W., Baker, C. C. and Heberer, G. Terminal B-cell maturation and immunoglobulin (Ig) synthesis *in vitro* in patients with major injury. *J. Trauma* **29**: 2; 1989.
15. Ertel, W., Faist, E., Nestle, C. *et al.* Dynamics of immunoglobulin synthesis after major trauma. Influence of recombinant lymphokines. *Arch. Surg.* **124**: 1437; 1989.
16. Moran, K. and Munster, A. M. Alterations of the host defense mechanism in burned patients. *Surg. Clin. North Am.* **67**: 47; 1987.
17. Koller, M., Konig, W., Brom, J. *et al.* Studies on the mechanisms of granulocyte dysfunction in severely burned patients—evidence for altered leukotriene generation. *J. Trauma* **29**: 435; 1989.
18. Munster, A. M., Leary, A. G., Spicer, S. S. *et al.* The effect of lymphocytotherapy on the course of experimental pseudomonas sepsis. *Ann. Surg.* **179**: 482; 1974.
19. Munster, A. M. Posttraumatic immunodepression is due to activation of suppressor T-cells. *Lancet* **1**: 1329; 1976.
20. Xu, D., Deitch, E. A., Sittig, K. *et al. In vitro* cell mediated immunity after thermal injury is not impaired. *Ann. Surg.* **208**: 768; 1988.
21. Xiao, G. X., Chopra, R. K., Adler, W. H. *et al.* Altered expression of IL-2 receptors in burn patients. *J. Trauma* **28**: 1669; 1988.
22. Sparkes, B. G., Teodorczyk-Injeyan, J. A., Peters, W. J. *et al. In* "Lipid Mediators in the Immunology of Shock" (Ed. Paubert-Braquet, M.). Plenum, New York; 1987.
23. Kupper, T. S. and Green, D. R. Immunoregulation after thermal injury: Sequential appearance of I-J+, LY-1 T-suppressor inducer cells and LY-2 T-suppressor effector cells following thermal trauma in mice. *J. Immunol.* **133**: 3047; 1984.
24. Teodorczyk-Injeyan, J. A., Sparkes, B. G., Peters, W. J. *et al.* Prostaglandin E related impaired expression of Interleukin-2 receptor in the burn patient. *In* "Advances in Prostaglandin, Thromboxane and Leukotriene Research" (Eds Samuelsson, B., Pauletti, R. and Raniwell, P. W.) Vol. 17. Raven Press, New York; 1987.
25. Ninneman, J. L. and Stockland, A. E. Participation of prostaglandin E

in immunosuppression following thermal injury. *J. Trauma* **24**: 201; 1984.
26. Miller, C. L. and Clandy, B. J. Suppressor T-cell activity induced as a result of thermal injury. *Cell Immunol.* **44**: 201; 1979.
27. Munster, A. M., Winchurch, R. A., Thupari, J. N. *et al.* Reversal of postburn immunosuppression with low-dose polymyxin. *Br. J. Trauma* **26**: 995; 1986.
28. Chouaib, S., Chatenoud, D., Klatzmann, D. and Fradelizi, D. The mechanism of inhibition of human IL-2 production. II. Prostaglandin E2 induction of suppressor T lymphocytes. *J. Immunol.* **132**: 1851; 1984.
29. Ma-ano, M. A., Fong, Y., Moldawer, L. L. *et al.* Serum cachectin/TNF in critically ill patients with burns correlates with infection and mortality. *Surg. Gynae. Obstet.* **170**: 32; 1990.
30. Dobke, M. K., Simoni, J. and Ninneman, J. L. Endotoxemia after burn injury: Effect of early excision on circulating endotoxin levels. *J. Burn Care Rehab.* **10**: 107; 1989.
31. Deitch, E. A. and Berg, R. Bacterial translocation from the gut: A mechanism of infection. *J. Burn Care Rehab.* **8**: 475; 1987.
32. Guo, Y., Dickerson, C., Chrest, F. *et al.* Increased levels of circulating Interleukin-6 (IL-6) in burn patients. *Clin. Immunol. Immunopath.* **54**: 361; 1990.
33. Deitch, E. A., Xu, D. and Bridges, R. M. Opiods modulate human neutrophil and lymphocyte function: Thermal injury alters plasma beta-endorphin levels. *Surgery* **104**: 41; 1988.
34. Kefalides, N. A., Aranaja, B. *et al.* Evaluation of antibiotic prophylaxis and gamma-globulin, plasma, albumin and saline soaks in severe burns. *Ann. Surg.* **159**: 496; 1964.
35. Munster, A. M. Immunization therapy in burn patients. *In* "The Art and Science of Burn Care" (Ed. Boswick, J. A. Jr.,). Aspen Publications, Rockville, MD; 1987.
36. Daniels, J. C., Larson, D. L., Abston, S. *et al.* Serum protein profiles in thermal burns. *J. Trauma* **14**: 137; 1974.
37. Arturson, G., Hogman, C. F., Johansson, S. G. *et al.* Changes in immunoglobulin levels in severely burned patients. *Lancet* **1**: 546: 1969.
38. Waymack, J. P., Jenkins, M. E. and Alexander, J. W. A prospective trial of prophylactic intravenous immune globulin for the prevention of infections in severely burned patients. *Burns* **15**: 71; 1989.
39. Munster, A. M., Moran, K. T., Thupari, J. *et al.* Prophylactic intravenous immunoglobulin replacement in high risk burn patients. *J. Burn Care Rehab.* **8**: 376; 1987.
40. Hansborough, J. F., Miller, L. M., Field, T. O., Jr. *et al.* High dose intravenous immunoglobulin therapy in burn patients: Pharmacokinetics and effects on microbial opsomization and phagocytosis. *Pediatr. Infect. Dis. J.* **7**: 549; 1988.

41. Burleson, D. G., Mason, A. D., McManus, A. T. and Pruitt, B. A., Jr. Lymphocyte phenotype and function changes in burn patients after intravenous IgG therapy. *Arch. Surg.* 123: 1379; 1988.
42 Annual Report Institute of Surgical Research, US Army R. D. Command, 1986, p. 269.
43. Minukhin, V. V. *et al.* Effectiveness of tobramycin and immunologic preparations in experimental Pseudomonas infection. *Antibio. Khimioter.* 34: 286; 1989.
44. Munster, A. M. Unpublished data.
45. Holder, I. A. and Neely, A. N. Combined host and specific Anti-*Pseudomonas* therapy for *Pseudomonas aeruginosa* infections in burned patients. *J. Burn Care Rehab.* 10: 131; 1989.
46. Lanser, M. E., Saba, T. M. and Scovill, W. A. Opsonic glycoprotein (fibronectin) levels after burn injury: Relationship to extent of burn and development of sepsis. *Ann. Surg.* 192: 782; 1980.
47. Saba, T. M., Blumenstock, F. A., Shah, D. M. *et al.* Reversal of opsonic deficiency in surgical, trauma and burn patients by infusion of purified plasma fibronectin. Correlation with experimental observations. *Am. J. Med.* 80: 229; 1986.
48. Mansberger, A. R., Doran, J. E., Treat, R. *et al.* The influence of fibronectin administration on the incidence of sepsis and septic mortality in severely injured patients. *Ann. Surg.* 210: 297; 1989.
49. Lemperle, G. Depression and stimulation of host defense mechanisms after severe burns. *Plastic. Recon. Surg.* 45 435; 1970.
50. Stinnett, J. D., Loose, L. D., Mishell, P. *et al.* Synthetic immunomodulators for prevention of fatal infections in a burned guinea pig model. *Ann. Surg.* 198: 53; 1983.
51. Faist, E. D. Immune enhancing effects of thymopentin, indomethacin and isoprinosine in patients with major trauma. *In* "Immune Consequences of Trauma, Shock and Sepsis" (Eds Faist, E. D. and Ninneman, J.). Springer-Verlag, Berlin; 1989.
52. Christou, N. V., Zakaluzny, I., Marshall, J. C. *et al.* The effect of the immunomodulator RU 41740 on the specific and nonspecific immunosuppression induced by thermal injury or protein deprivation. *Arch. Surg.* 1213: 297; 1988.
53. Waymack, J. P. and Alexander, J. W. Immunomodulators for the prevention of infections in the burned guinea pig. *J. Burn Care Rehab.* 5: 363; 1987.
54. Donati, L., Lazzarin, A., Signorini, M. *et al.* Preliminary clinical experience with the use of immunomodulators in burns. *J. Trauma* 23: 816; 1983.
55. Hamilton, G., Zoch, G. and Meissl, G. Effects of thymopentin treatment in severely burned patients. *In* "Immune Consequences of Trauma, Shock and Sepsis" (Eds Faist, E. D. and Ninneman, J.). Springer-Verlag, Berlin; 1989.
56. Haberal, M., Hamaloglu, E., Bora, S. *et al.* The effects of vitamin

E on immune regulation after thermal injury. *Burns* **14**: 388; 1988.
57. Daly, J. M., Reynolds, Thom, *et al.* Immune and metabolic effects of arginine in the surgical patient. *Ann. Surg.* **208**: 512; 1988.
58. Browder, W., Williams, D., Pretus, H. *et al.* Beneficial effect of enhanced macrophage function in the trauma patient. Material presented to the 101st meeting of the Southern Surgical Association, Hot Springs, VA, December 1989.
59. Davies, M. Phase variations in the modulation of the immune response. *Immunol. Today* **4**: 103; 1983.
60. Waymack, J. P., Jenkins, M., Warden, G. D. *et al.* A prospective study of thymopentin in severely burned patients. *Surg. Gynae. Obstet.* **164**: 423; 1987.
61. Lokai, J., Kuklined, P., Taborska, D. *et al.* Dialysable leukocyte extract in the therapy of sepsis. *In* "Immune Consequences of Trauma, Shock and Sepsis" (Eds Faist, E. D. and Ninneman J.) Springer-Verlag, Berlin; 1989.
62. McRitchie, D. I., Girotti, M. J., Rotstein, O. D. *et al.* Impaired antibody production in blunt trauma. *Arch. Surg.* **125**: 91; 1990.
63. Teodorczyk-Injeyan, J. A., Sparkles, B. G., Mills, G. B. *et al.* Impaired expression of Interleukin-2 receptor (IL-2R) in the immunosuppressed burn patient: Reversal by exogenous IL-2. *J. Trauma* **27**: 180; 1987.
64. Freeman, T. R. and Shelby, J. Effect of anti-PGE antibody on cell-mediated immune response in thermally injured mice. *J. Trauma* **28**: 190; 1988.
65. Katz, A., Ryan, P., Lalonde, C. *et al.* Topical ibuprofen decreases thromboxane release from the endotoxin-stimulated burn wound. *J. Trauma* **26**: 157; 1986.
66. Rockwell, W. B. and Ehrlich, H. P. Ibuprofen in acute-care therapy. *Ann. Surg.* **211**: 78: 1990.
67. Gadd, M. and Hansborough, J. F. Postburn suppression of lymphocyte and neutrophil functions is not reversed by prostaglandin blockade. *J. Surg. Res.* **48**: 84; 1990.
68. Evans, D. A., Jacobs, D. O., Revhaug, A. *et al.* The effects of tumor necrosis factor and their selective inhibition by ibuprofen. *Ann. Surg.* **209**: 320; 1989.
69. Slotman, G. J., Burchard, K. W., D'Arezzo, A. S. *et al.* Ketokonazole prevents acute respiratory failure in critically ill surgical patients. *J. Trauma* **28**: 654; 1988.
70. Faist, E., Ertel, W., Cohnert, T. *et al.* Immunoprotective effects of cyclooxygenase inhibition in patients with major surgical trauma. *J. Trauma* **30**: 8; 1990.
71. Magshudi, M. and Miller, C. L. The immunomodulating effect of TP5 and indomethacin in burn acquired hypoimmunity. *J. Surg. Res.* **37**: 133; 1984.

72. Winchurch, R. A. and Munster, A. M. Unpublished data, 1987.
73. Ertel, W., Morrison, M., Ayala, A. *et al.* Immunoprotective effect of a calcium channel blocker on macrophage antigen presentation, function, la expression and Interleukin-1 (IL-1) synthesis following hemorrhage. Material presented to the 51st meeting of the Soriety of University Surgeons, Los Angeles, 8–10 February, 1990.
74. Bende, S. and Bertok, L. Elimination of endotoxin from the blood by extracorporeal activated charcoal hemoperfusion in experimental canine endotoxing shock. *Circ. Shock* **19**: 239; 1986.
75. Bertok, L. and Szeberenyi, S. Effects of radio-detoxified endotoxin on the liver microsomal drug metabolizing enzyme system in rats. *Immunopharmacology* **6**: 1; 1983.
76. Harkonen, S. and Mischak, R. Clinical studies of monoclonal antiendotoxin antibody—XMMEN-OE5. *Clin. Res.* **35**: 143A; 1987.
77. Dunn, D. L., Mach, P. A. *et al.* Anticore endotoxin F(ab′)2 fragments protect against lethal effects of gram negative bacterial sepsis. *Surgery* **96**: 440; 1984.
78. Munster, A. M., Xiao, G. X. *et al.* Control of endotoxemia in burn patients by use of polymyxin B. *J. Burn Care Rehab.* **10**: 327; 1989.
79. Stratta, R. J., Warden, G. D., Ninneman, J. L. *et al.* Immunologic parameters in burned patients: Effect of therapeutic interventions. *J. Trauma* **26**: 7; 1986.
80. Demling, R. H., Katz, A., Lalonde, C. *et al.* The immediate effect of burn wound excition on pulmonary function in sheep: The role of prostanouds, oxygen radicals and chemoattractants. *Surgery* **101**: 44; 1987.
81. Berk, L. S., Tan, S. A. and Fry, W. F. Neuroendocrine and stress hormone changes during mirthful laughter. *Am. J. Med. Sci.* **298**: 390; 1989.

Discussion

J. M. Dwyer
Are there data to suggest that a T-cell toxin is released from burnt skin?

A. M. Munster
A great deal has been written about intravenous immunotoxin, mostly by Schönenberger and Allgöwer, right here in Switzerland. The problem is that anti-endotoxic therapy, for example passage over Sephadex coated with polymyxin B, abolishes the activity of the "toxin". No one is totally convinced that it exists.

T. Jungi
You highlighted the pathophysiological similarities between burns and endotoxin effects. As endotoxin activates macrophages, as many of the immunomodulations you mentioned seem to be beneficial. I wonder to what extent macrophage activation is harmful or beneficial. I also would like to know whether you measured cytokines other than IL-6, which have a proven immunosuppressive activity, such as transforming-growth-factor-B and interleukin-1-antagonist.

A. M. Munster
We have measured IL-1, which is elevated, and TNF, which is very erratically and inconsistently elevated. One must remember that this is a "chronic" model of endotoxemia and levels of monokines with short half-lives are quite difficult to measure. I believe that modest monophage activation is beneficial, but that strong induction is harmful.

J. E. Doran
Could the changes in IL-6 seen in your patients be used as a prognostic indicator? Did increases in IL-6 occur *before* clinical changes or only concomitantly?

A. M. Munster
The IL-6 increases seemed to occur just prior to the clinical appearance of major, life-threatening complications. I think it could indeed be used as a prognostic marker.

H. M. Chapel
Frank Whitehead reported increased catabolism of IgG to $F(ab')_2$ some 20 years ago. Do you think this could be a reason for the failure of replacement IgG to work in these patients. It might account for the reduced endotoxin levels but no clinical efficacy.

A. M. Munster
This is a distinct possibility. I don't believe that $F(ab')_2$ measurements have been repeated since that report of Whitehouse and Hardy.

IVIG indication in patients with low-grade B-cell tumors

HELEN CHAPEL[1], HELEN GRIFFITHS[1] and MARTIN LEE[2]

[1] *Department of Immunology, John Radcliffe Hospital, Oxford, UK*
[2] *Baxter Healthcare Corporation, California, USA*

Introduction

The fact that many patients with low-grade B-cell tumors have secondary hypogammaglobulinemia has been known for many years (1), but the clinical significance of these low serum IgG levels has not been clear. First reports of hypogammaglobulinemia secondary to chronic lymphocytic leukemia (CLL) were published in the 1950s, when the use of total protein measurements and electrophoresis resulted in underestimation of the proportion of patients with CLL who were hypogammaglobulinemic. Despite this, correlations were shown by Fairley and Scott (2) between gammaglobulin levels and both disease duration and recurrence of infections.

The increased incidence of infections in patients with CLL was formally demonstrated by Twomey. He compared CLL patients with aged matched controls who were followed up for myocardial infection and found a fivefold increase in the risk of infection (3). The infections suffered by CLL patients were predominantly bacterial (3, 4), similar to the infections seen in patients with primary hypogammaglobulinemia. Furthermore, the respiratory tract was a common site for such

Immunotherapy with Intravenous Immunoglobulins
ISBN 0–12–370725–0

infections though bacterial infections were also seen in the skin, urinary tract and blood; it is of interest that there are few reports of gastrointestinal infections. We have looked more recently for a correlation between infections and serum IgG. In 29 patients with secondary hypogammaglobulinemia, 15 suffered from multiple or life-threatening infections in the 2-year period preceding the serum IgG measurement, compared with only 2 out of 27 with normal IgG levels (J. North, personal communication). Correlation with serum IgA levels was poor in these patients and this may account for the paucity of gastrointestinal infections (5).

We have studied the effect of intravenous immunoglobulin replacement therapy on the incidence of infection in patients with chronic lymphocytic leukemia and low-grade non-Hodgkin's lymphoma in an attempt to provide both better clinical management of these patients and to validate the clinical significance of the hypogammaglobulinemia in relation to infections.

IVIG replacement studies

Two studies were performed in patients with low-grade B-cell tumors who were at risk of infection. Patients received infusions of either 400 mg/kg of IVIG or an equivalent volume of normal saline at 3-weekly intervals. The patients were randomized and neither the patients nor their attendants knew the nature of the treatment. The data were analyzed blind. Patients were eligible if they had a serum IgG level less than 50% below the local limit of normal or had had a recent major infection. For the multicenter study, stratification was done by center and by IgG level (above or below 4 g/l). No exclusions were made for age or stage of disease. Eight-one patients were analyzed at the end of the study. Patients in the two treatment groups were found to be comparable for age, sex, disease duration, disease stage, previous therapy, previous infection history and immunological and hematological laboratory parameters (6). Bacterial infections occurred less frequently in the 41 patients receiving immunoglobulin; there were 23 bacterial infections in this group compared with 42 in the 40 control patients ($P = 0.01$, one-tailed). Not surprisingly there was seasonal variation in the bacterial infections in the patients in the placebo group (Fig. 1) although this was not statistically significant. When the analysis was conducted on only those 57 patients who had completed a full year (to counteract this variation), there were 14 bacterial infections in the 28 patients receiving IVIG compared with 36

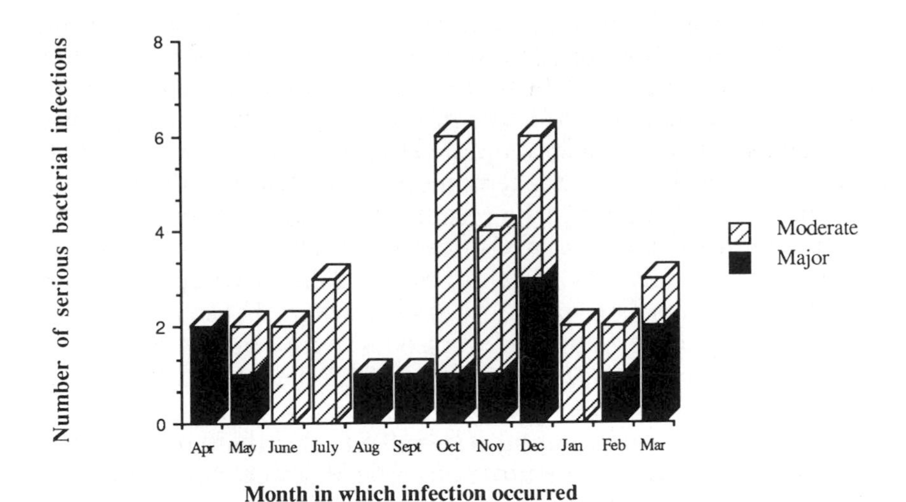

Figure 1. Seasonal variation of serious bacterial infections in 29 placebo patients who completed a full year of infusions.

in the 29 patients in the placebo group ($P = 0.001$, one-tailed). Not only was the overall number of bacterial infections reduced but there was trend to a reduction in the frequency of bacterial infections in individual patients (Table 1); only those who completed a full year were included in this analysis also. The incidence of significant fungal and viral infection was low and was similar in the two groups, with 8 viral and 3 fungal infections in the immunoglobulin group and 10 viral and 2 fungal in the placebo group. Trivial infections were also equal between the two groups (6).

Table 1
Frequency of bacterial infections in 57 patients who completed a full year of study

Number of infections	Number of patients	
	IVIG	Saline
0	18	13
1	7	6
2	2	4
3	1	3
4	0	2
5	0	1
Total	28	29

The incidence of adverse reactions was low, with minor adverse reactions in only 23 out of 1235 infusions (2%). It was of interest that adverse reactions occurred in some patients whilst receiving placebo (saline), though the rate was lower in this group (Table 2). There was some concern that administration of relatively large doses of IVIG to patients who had received chemotherapy (and might therefore be neutropenic) might result in Fc receptor blockade of phagocytic cells and thus increase the risk of septicemia. Analysis of all septicemic episodes in the study was therefore undertaken. Such episodes only occurred in patients with stage C disease, of whom 32 had entered into the study. The eight septicemic episodes were equally distributed between the two groups; namely 5 out of 19 stage C patients in the IVIG group suffered from septicemia compared with 3 out of 13 stage C patients in the placebo group ($P = 0.84$). Furthermore, the IgG levels in these patients at the times of septicemia were not particularly high (2.5–12.5 g/l).

Table 2
Adverse reactions in all patients receiving either IVIG or saline infusions

Nature of reactions	Treatment group	
	IVIG	Saline
Chills ± fever	6	1
Sleepiness	7	2
Low backache	1	0
Leg cramps	1	0
Nausea	1	0
Flushing	0	2
Transient weakness and anxiety	0	2
Total	16	7
Number of infusions	610	625

At the end of 12 months the 12 patients entered in Oxford were crossed over to receive the alternative therapy for a further 12 months. Patients continued to be followed with completion of daily diaries and history and examination at every visit, along with measurements of C-reactive protein, immunoglobulin measurements and liver function tests. (The IgG measurements were withheld from the physicians to preserve blinding.) A 2-year study in this group of patients is difficult to complete due to their underlying, albeit their low-grade malignancy, but 191 IVIG and 162 saline infusions were given (7). Six patients remained free of serious infections while receiving IVIG compared with only one whilst receiving saline. As in the multicenter study, the reduction in infections was predominantly in the bacterial infections (Table 3). When analyzed by the crossover method of Mainland (8), this reduction was shown to be statistically significant ($P = 0.001$).

Table 3
Number of infections by severity and etiology, in patients whilst receiving IVIG or saline infusions

Infections	Etiology	IVIG	Saline
Major	Bacterial	0	9
	Viral	1	1
	Fungal	1	0
Moderate	Bacterial	3	11
	Viral	3	0
	Fungal	0	1
	Unknown	1	1
Trivial		23	22

Further analysis of the serum IgG level at the time of infection showed that 18 of the serious bacterial infections in these patients occurred whilst the serum IgG level was below the lower limit of normal (IgG< 6.4 g/l) compared with only 5 whilst the IgG level was within the normal range (Table 4). Since this was a crossover study, a significant carryover effect from one period of therapy to the next had to be excluded. In terms of overall infection rate, there was no difference between those patients who received IVIG first compared with those who received placebo first ($P = 1.00$, Fisher's exact test). This conclusion is supported by an initial rapid decrease in IgG levels when patients were switched from IgG to placebo (Fig. 2), though measurements of the half-lives of the infused IgG in these patients showed that they were not reduced.

We also took the opportunity to analyze the rate of loss of IgG following infusions at intervals throughout the year in 15 patients receiving IVIG in the multicenter study. Total serum IgG measurements were made, pre-, 30 min post- and on days 7 and 21 after the 1st, 5th, 8th, 13th and 17th infusions. The differences between these IgG measurements at these time points in individual patients were analyzed by one-way repeated measures analysis of variance; there

Table 4
Serum IgG levels at the time of serious infection in patients in crossover study

Type of infection		Serum IgG level at time of infection	
		> 6.4 g/l	< 6.4 g/l
Major	Bacterial	0	9
	Viral	0	2
	Fungal	1	0
Moderate	Bacterial	5	9
	Viral	3	0
	Fungal	0	1
	Unknown	1	1

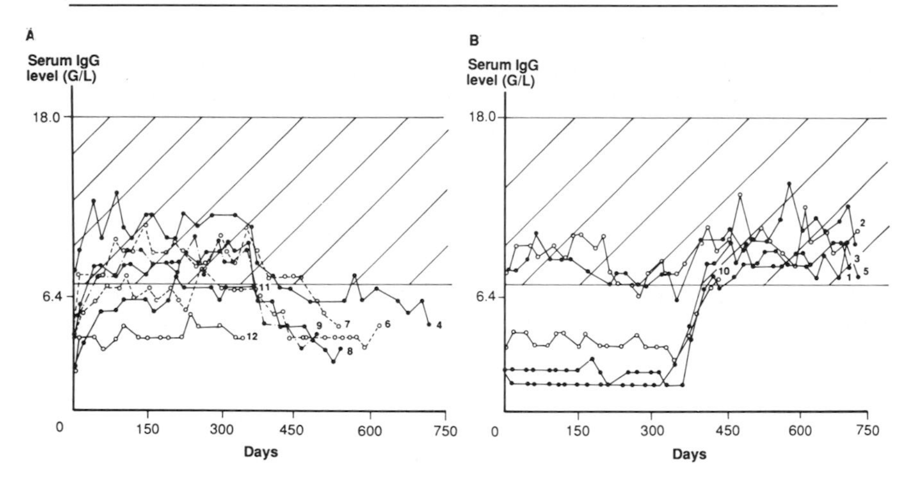

Figure 2. Serum IgG levels (pre-infusion) over the 2-year period. Hatched areas indicate the normal ranges. (A) Patients receiving immunoglobulin in the first year and saline in the second year. (B) Patients receiving saline in the first year and immunoglobulin in the second year.

were no significant differences. Furthermore, the mean levels at days 7 and 21 after the 5th, 8th, 13th and 17th infusions were unchanged, suggesting that catabolism of IgG was not altered during the year.

Conclusion

The incidence of major and moderate bacterial infections was significantly reduced by the administration of 400 mg/kg of IVIG every 3 weeks. The maintenance of the serum IgG levels within the normal range was associated with fewer infections, particularly serious bacterial infections. Analysis of the patients in the multicenter study who received only placebo infusions showed that the overall rate of serious bacterial infection was approximately 60%, suggesting that total IgG measurements or a history of infection is insufficient to predict those at particular risk with any precision.

Summary

Infection is a cause of significant morbidity and mortality in patients with low-grade B-cell tumors. This is associated with the high incidence of secondary hypogammaglobulinemia in these patients. Clinical trials of prophylactic intravenous immunoglobulin (IVIG) replacement therapy have been successful in preventing serious bacterial infections, confirming that hypogammaglobulinemia is a major factor in the immune pathogenesis of these infections.

Acknowledgements

These studies were supported by Baxter Healthcare Corporation, Hyland Division who also provided Gammagard, the IVIG preparation used in both clinical trials.

References

1. Chapel, H. M. Hypogammaglobulinaemia and chronic lymphocytic leukaemia. *In* "Chronic Lymphocytic Leukaemia: Recent Progress and Future Direction" (Eds Gale, R. P., and Rai, K. R.) pp. 383–389. Alan R. Liss, New York; 1987.
2. Fairley, G. H. and Scott, B. G. Hypogammaglobulinaemia in CLL. *Br. Med. J.* 4: 920–924; 1961.
3. Twomey, J. J. Infections complicating multiple myeloma and CLL. *Arch. Intern. Med.* 132: 562–565; 1973.
4. Shaw, R. K., Szwek, C., Bogg, D. R. *et al.* Infection and immunity in chronic lymphocytic leukaemia. *Arch. Intern. Med.* 106: 467–478; 1960.
5. Chapel, H. M., and Bunch, C. B. Mechanisms of infection in chronic lymphocytic leukaemia. *Seminars Haemat.* 24: 291–296; 1987.
6. Co-operative group for the study of immunoglobulin in CLL. Intravenous

immunoglobulin for the preventation of infection in CLL, a randomized, control clinical trial. *N. Engl. J. Med.* 319: 902–907; 1988.
7. Griffiths, H., Brennan, V., Lea, J. *et al.* Crossover study of immunoglobulin replacement therapy in patients with low grade B-cell tumors. *Blood* 73: 633–638; 1989.
8. Mainland, D. "Elementary Medical Statistics" 2nd Edn, Saunders, Phil. pp. 236, 1963.

Discussion

A. Morell
Were the infections observed in the IVIG and in the placebo group caused by different microorganisms?

H. Chapel
S. pneumoniae and *H. influenzae* were the predominant organisms identified in both treatment groups, and there were no differences between the groups in the range of organisms detected.

J. Herrera
A few years ago, Dr Besa in Philadelphia treated some patients with chronic lymphocytic leukemia with IVIG. He observed diminished infections, but he could also show an antiproliferative effect of IVIG infusions, i.e. diminished lymphadenopathy and a decrease in total lymphocyte counts. Can you confirm these findings and what would be the mechanism for these effects?

H. Chapel
We looked in the multicenter study for changes in platelet counts and hemoglobulin levels as well as circulating lymphocyte counts. We could find no significant changes, either after each cycle or long term over the study year. We did not look at changes in life expectancy.

Frequency and pathogenic implication of reactivated lymphotropic herpesviruses in autoimmune and immune deficiency disorders

GERHARD R. F. KRUEGER,[1,2] DHARAM V. ABLASHI,[1,3,4] ALBERT RAMON[1,5] and UWE LEMBKE[1]

[1] *International Institute of Immunopathology eV, Cologne–Washington, Cologne, FRG;* [2] *Immunopathology Laboratory, Institute of Pathology, University of Cologne, Cologne, FRG;* [3] *Laboratory of Tumor Cell Biology, National Cancer Institute, NIH, Bethesda, Maryland, USA;* [4] *Department of Microbiology, Georgetown University Medical School, Washington, DC, USA;* [5] *Department of Microbiology and Clinical Chemistry, Hospital of the Belgian Armed Forces, Cologne, FRG*

Preface

Primary infections by human herpesviruses in the healthy individual usually remain latent or induce acute diseases of limited duration. Diseases include fever blisters or herpes genitalis, varicella, infectious mononucleosis and exanthem subitum. Specific treatment is usually not necessary. Coinciding with the progress in transplant surgery and more recently with the occurrence of acquired immune deficiency syndrome (AIDS), reactivated herpesvirus infections have caught the attention of the medical community. They are diagnosed with increasing frequency, can complicate significantly the course of the patient's

Immunotherapy with Intravenous Immunoglobulins
ISBN 0–12–370725–0

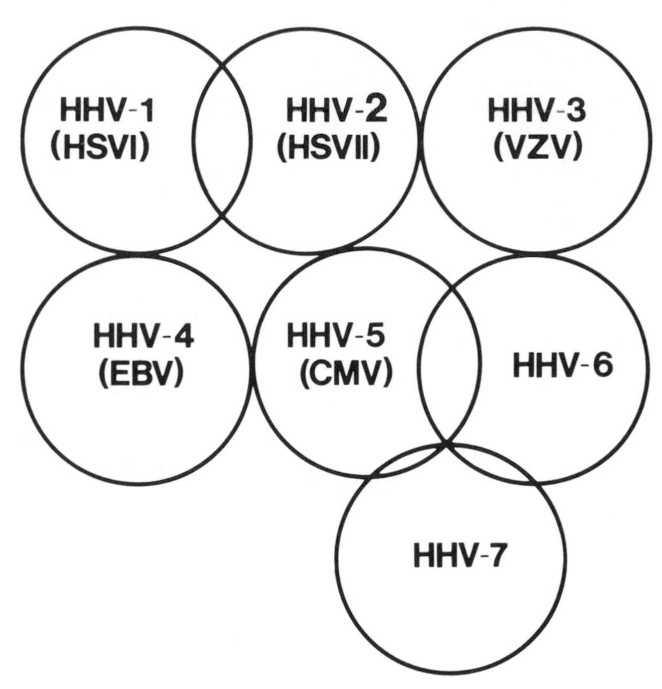

Figure 1. Currently identified human herpesviruses. The genetic relationship is indicated by overlapping circles. (The lymphotropic HHV–8 is not yet included.)

primary disease and thus require specific treatment. This applies especially to herpesviruses with pronounced lymphotropism. The present review will summarize current knowledge of this problem and its implications.

Herpesviruses and lymphotropism

Currently identified human herpesviruses are shown in Fig. 1. Overlapping circles in the figure refer to genetic relationships between individual members. Pathological sequelae of infection with these viruses depend on the target cell for infection and on the state of activity of the host's immune system at the time of infection (1–4). Primary infection by all members of the herpesvirus family and of normoreactive individuals usually remain clinically inapparent, leading to lifelong latency. HHV–1, HHV–2 and HHV–3 (HSVI and II, VZV) infect primarily non-lymphoid cells and cause acute disease secondary to an effective host defense and lysis of infected cells (e.g. of

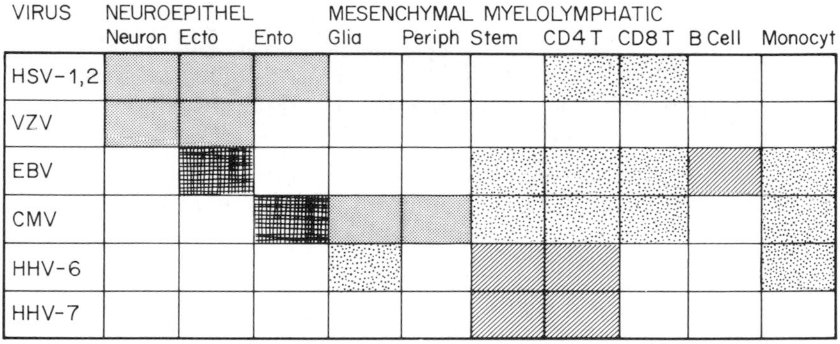

VIRUS NEUROEPITHEL MESENCHYMAL MYELOLYMPHATIC
Neuron Ecto Ento Glia Periph Stem CD4 T CD8 T B Cell Monocyt
HSV-1,2
VZV
EBV
CMV
HHV-6
HHV-7

Figure 2. Prevalent cellular tropism of human herpesviruses (see text).

neuroepithelial cells; Fig. 2). Again, lifelong latency follows. HSV was also shown in T helper and suppressor lymphocytes (CD4 and CD8 cells), yet specific diseases related to such infections are not yet known. HHV–4 (EBV), HHV–6 (formerly human B-lymphotropic virus, HBLV) and probably HHV–7 (RK virus of Frenkel *et al.*) (8) possess a pronounced lymphotropism and are able to infect B or T lymphocytes and their immature precursors (5–8). In addition, T lymphocytes from malignant lymphomas and dendritic reticular cells can carry EBV genomes. The CD21 (CR2, C3d complement receptor) serves as receptor for EBV infection of B lymphocytes. A receptor for HHV–6 is not yet known, the prime target cell for infection is the CD38/CD4 positive lymphoid cell. No receptor is yet known for HHV–7, which grows in CD4 cells and in cord blood cells. Upon primary infection in certain individuals the lymphotropic HHV–4 (EBV), HHV–6 and probably HHV–7 cause self-limited lesions in immunocompetent tissues such as infectious mononucleosis (IM) or Kikuchi's syndrome (4, 9–11). There is, however, some indication that HHV–4 (EBV) and HHV–6 also possess certain tropism for epithelial cells as seen from the association of EBV with nasopharyngeal and thymic carcinomas and hairy leukoplakia (12–14) and HHV–6 with exanthem subitum (4, 15). HHV–5 (CMV) can be shown in epithelial cells, mesenchymal cells and to a lesser extent in T or B lymphocytes. A cell receptor has not yet been identified. Acute primary infection with CMV rarely causes a disease: CMV mononucleosis was described only occasionally (3, 10, 16). Thus similar to certain genetic relationships among the individual herpesviruses, their cell tropism shows certain common features.

Frequency of latent infection and of reactivation

All herpesviruses, except for HHV–2 (HSV–2) and HHV–7, are present as latent infection in at least 50% of the general population, with EBV in over 90% (2, 4) (Table 1). HHV–2 is less frequent. Prevalence data for HHV–7 are not yet known. This means that a considerable percentage of the healthy population carries a significant load of inactive herpesvirus genomes which may become reactivated with adequate stimulation. As long as the human defense system (NK cells, K cells, cytotoxic T cells, interferons, etc.) is intact, virus reactivation will remain asymptomatic. Consequently, virus shedding is documented regularly in healthy individuals (Table 1) (2).

Table 1
Herpesvirus antibody prevalence and virus shedding in the healthy human population

Virus		Prevalence[a] %	Shedding[b] %
HHV–1	(HSV–1)	60–90	2–20
HHV–2	(HSV–2)	10–60	?
HHV–3	(VZV)	80	20
HHV–4	(EBV)	95	20
HHV–5	(CMV)	40–60	5–20
HHV–6	(HBLV)	60–80	?

[a] Rates depend upon population density and socio-economic class.
[b] Less frequent above age of 15 years.

Clinical implications of herpesvirus reactivation

Since herpesvirus shedding occurs in healthy individuals, reactivation as such is apparently not pathological. If disease follows reactivation, it appears rather as a consequence of an unusual degree and persistence of virus replication. This is well documented by the number of antigen- or genome-positive cells in various EBV or HHV–6 infections (Table 2). When reviewing conditions under which excessive herpes-virus reactivation and persistence may occur, two pathogenic mechanisms appear to prevail: continued abnormal stimulation of virus genome-carrying cells and defective host control of virus replication and spread (virus replication referring to intracellular reproduction of virus, spread to the sequential infection of new cells). Mechanisms

Table 2
Frequencies of herpesvirus-positive cells in various diseases[a]

EBV nuclear antigen (EBNA) in blood lymphocytes		total
Acute infectious mononucleosis	6–20%	$6\text{–}20 \times 10^8$
Latency in adults	$1/10^7\text{–}1/10^8$	$1\text{–}10 \times 10^2$
Virus reactivation: up to 50% of B lymphocytes		$10\text{–}20 \times 10^8$
HHV–6: ZVH14 genome in tissue lymphocytes		
Non-specific lymph node hyperplasia		$1/10^6$
Atypical polyclonal lymphoproliferation		$17.5/10^6$
Follicular center cell lymphoma		$5\text{–}20/10^6$
Sinusoidal B cell lymphoma		$230/10^6$
Hodgkin's disease		$760/10^6$

[a] Calculated for 70 kg young adult with 470×10^9 total lymphocytes; 2.2% blood lymphocytes = 10×10^9 and 20% B lymphocytes = 2×10^9

of stimulation causing virus reactivation are inadequately known yet (Table 3). Host control mechanisms include intracellular (e.g. interferons) activities and immune surveillance. Reactivated non-lymphotropic herpesviruses may cause excessive inflammatory necrotic and hemorrhagic lesions (17). Lymphotropic herpesviruses similarly cause upon reactivation necrotizing lymphadenitis, atrophy and/or hematopoietic hypoplasia (1), lesions like Kikuchi's syndrome, Rosai-Dorfman's syndrome or Kawasaki's disease (11, 18, 19) (Fig. 3). These lesions can cause severe damage to the lymphoid tissue, yet are usually still self-limited.

Table 3
Some suggested stimulants of herpesvirus reactivation

HSV1, 2; VZV	Excessive UV light exposure Other infections (cell stimulation/coinfection) Direct trauma to neurons carrying viral genomes Endocrine stimulation (stress, trauma, menses)
EBV, HHV–6, HHV–7	Endotoxin and plant agglutinin-type substances Other infections (cell stimulation/coinfection) Endocrine stimulation (e.g. steroids, stress) Increased cytokine production (e.g. interleukins) "Cocarcinogens" (plant and food components, e.g. phorbolesters, aflatoxin) Autoantibodies (e.g. anti-IgM for B cells)

Figure 3. Overview of subacute necrotizing lymphadenitis: Kikuchi's syndrome following HHV–6 reactivation. Note extensive tumor-like lympho-histiocytic proliferation. (Characteristic regions of cell necrosis are not evident at this magnification of 150×; H. & E. stain.)

Table 4 summarizes diseases which are associated with reactivation and persistent activity of lymphotropic herpesviruses. Atypical polyclonal lymphoproliferation (APL) as induced by EBV and/or HHV–6 mimics clinically systemic lymphoma and may even progress to overt malignant lymphoma (1, 20–25) (Fig. 4). The pathogenesis of this proliferative response is not yet completely understood. Both EBV and HHV–6 induce polyclonal lymphoproliferation as reactive response to surface glycoproteins of the virus and of virus-infected cells, a reaction that probably compares to the polyclonal B-cell stimulation by bacterial endotoxins. EBV-infected lymphoblastoid cells (LCLs) and HHV–6-stimulated macrophages may produce B-cell growth factors (BCGF, interleukin-6) causing rapid expansion of receptor-carrying B lymphocytes as well as enhancing the response of T lymphocytes to interleukin-2 (26–30). EBV-infected LCLs express BCGF receptors besides producing BCGF and thus stimulate their own expansion according to an autocrine mechanism. They also express highly immunogenic EBNA–2(–6) and late membrane protein (LMP), and

Table 4
Diseases frequently associated with reactivated lymphotropic human herpesviruses

Autoimmune Disorders		
Systemic lupus erythematosus and UCVD	HHV–6	(4, 42, 49)
Rheumatoid arthritis	EBV	(40)
Sjoegren's syndrome	HHV–6	(41, 42)
Sarcoidosis	HHV–6	(74)
Atypical polyclonal lymphoproliferation (APL)		
Castleman's disease	EBV, HHV–6	(20, 79)
Kikuchi's syndrome	HHV–6	(4, 11)
Kawasaki's disease	EBV	(19)
Lymphomatoid granulomatosis	EBV	(25)
Rosai–Dorfman's disease	HHV–6	(18)
Canale–Smith's syndrome	HHV–6	(21)
Chronic infectious mononucleosis	EBV, HHV–6	(77, 78)
APL, not otherwise specified	HHV–6, EBV	(20, 31, 75)
Malignant diseases		
Hodgkin's disease	HHV–6, EBV	(20, 31, 80)
Burkitt's lymphoma	EBV	(76)
Follicular center cell lymphomas	HHV–6	(20, 22–24, 31)
Sinusoidal B cell lymphoma	HHV–6	(20)
Peripheral T cell lymphoma	EBV, HHV–6	(20, 81)
Immune deficiency disorders		
Transplant recipients	EBV, HHV–6	(1, 43, 44)
Acquired immune deficiency syndrome	EBV, HHV–6	(34–39, 48)
Inherited immune deficiency syndromes	EBV (HHV–6?)	(1)
"Chronic fatigue syndrome"	HHV–6, EBV	(60, 61, 73)

probably survive and proliferate only in immunodeficient individuals (30).

Sustained lymphoproliferation may at least lower the threshold for incidental cell transformation and thus increase the risk of lymphoma development (20, 31). While EBV is known to be oncogenic (32), similar activities of HHV–6 are at best suggestive (33). In EBV-induced Burkitt's lymphoma (BL), transposition of the *c-myc* gene into the neighborhood of immunoglobulin heavy chain genes (e.g. 8; 14 translocations) with subsequent constitutive activation of the *c-myc* gene appears essential for malignant transformation. Current thoughts of EBV-induced lymphoma development were recently summarized by George Klein (30). Even if HHV–6 may not finally prove to be

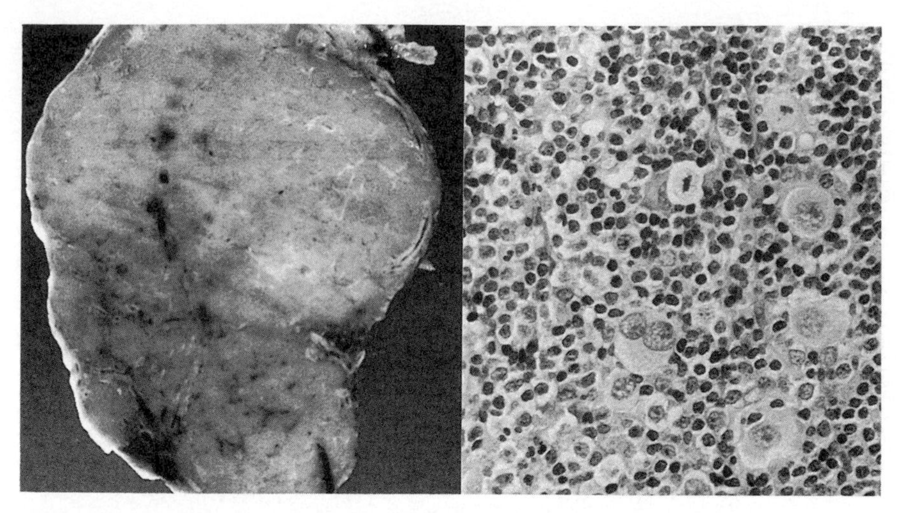

Figure 4. Lymph node changes in persistent active EBV infection simulating malignant lymphoma. (a) Gross features show complete effacement of structure with marked enlargement of the lymph node (longitudinal diameter 6.5 cm); (b) the histology shows a diffuse lympho-histiocytic population with giant cells. (375×; H. & E. stain.)

oncogenic, induction of polyclonal lymphoproliferation with reactivation of latent EBV and/or facilitation of double infections of cells by HHV–6 and oncogenic viruses can still facilitate the development of malignancies. In addition, herpesviruses exert distinct immunosuppressive activities (2). Their persistence and replication thus might favor the survival and proliferation of immortal (virally transformed) cells.

Suggestive viral interactions in herpesvirus infection

Evidence is accumulating in recent years that double viral infection of cells may contribute to the progress of diseases. Reactivation of latent herpesviruses such as EBV and HHV–6 during the course of HIV–1-induced ARC and AIDS has been repeatedly shown (34–39). Similar reactivations are documented as well in non-AIDS-related autoimmune and immune deficiency disorders as summarized in Tables 4 and 5 (40–44). Single cells can become infected by two different viruses such as by HHV–6 and HIV–1, HHV–6 and EBV, HHV–6 and measles virus, EBV and HIV–1 (45–49). This phenomenon appeared puzzling

Table 5
Reported HHV–6 isolates (as of March 1990)

Malignant lymphomas	Salahuddin *et al.*
Atypical polyclonal lymphoproliferation	Krueger *et al.*
Hairy cell leukemia/HIV+	Becker *et al.*
HIV+ patients	Tedder *et al.*
	Downing *et al.*
	Feorino *et al.*
	Lopez *et al.*
	Kaplan *et al.*
	Agut *et al.*
Exanthem subitum	Yamanishi *et al.*
	Kikuta *et al.*
Systemic lupus erythematosus and unclassified collagen-vascular disease	Krueger *et al.*
Rheumatoid arthritis	Krueger *et al.*
Chronic fatigue syndrome	Ablashi *et al.*
	Krueger *et al.*
Allograft recipients	Ward *et al.*
Chronic lymphopenia and Legionnaires' disease	Carrigan *et al.*
Healthy persons (saliva, blood)	Pietroboni *et al.*
	Krueger *et al.*

Reference D. V. Ablashi *et al.* (73).

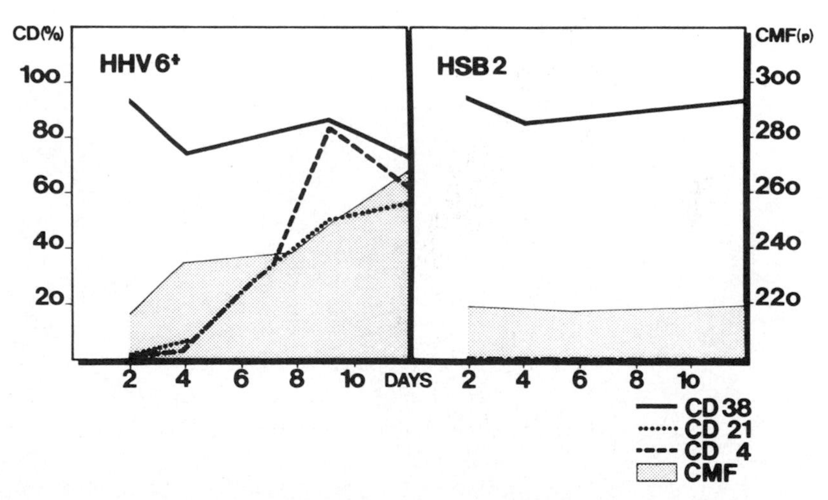

Figure 5. Cell membrane fluidity (CMF in poise [p]) and receptor expression (CD [%]) in HHV–6 infected (left) and in uninfected (right) CD38 positive stem cells. While no spontaneous changes are seen in uninfected cells, HHV–6 infection causes significant rigidification of the cell membrane (increase in poise) and expression of receptors such as CD21 (EBV receptor) and CD4 (HIV receptor). (See references 7, 50, 51.)

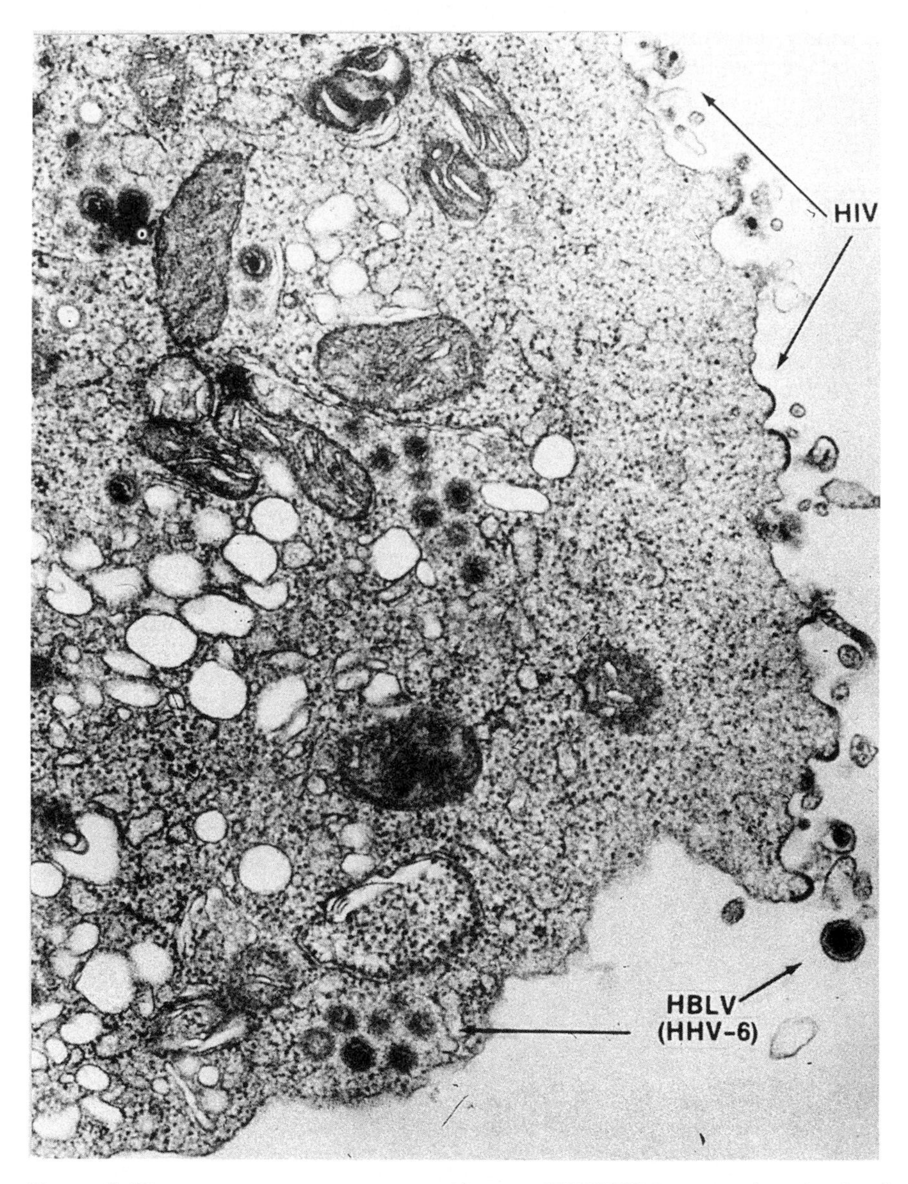

Figure 6. Electron microscopic picture of human CD38/CD4 positive lymphoid cell with double infection by HHV–6 and HIV–1. (From reference 55.)

since originally susceptible receptor-carrying cells for the individual viruses differed such as CD38/CD4 cells for HHV–6, CD4 cells for HIV–1 and CD21 cells for EBV (5–7). We were able to show, however, that stem cells carrying only the CD38 epitope expressed also CD4 and CD21 after infection with HHV–6 and thus became susceptible for HIV–1 and EBV infection (50, 51) (Figs 5 and 6). HHV–6 positive CD4 cells superinfected with HIV–1 show enhanced HIV gene expression, more pronounced reverse transcriptase activity and accelerated cell death (45, 52) (Figs 7 and 8). Within the doubly infected cells certain viral proteins are capable of post-transcriptional activation of promoters for different viruses (45, 52). HHV–6 infection activates the expression of a heterologous gene linked to the HIV–1 promoter. HIV–1 RNA expression in doubly infected cells is higher than in HIV–1 infection alone and parallels CAT enzymatic activity, suggesting that HHV–6 transactivation occurs at transcriptional and/ or post-transcriptional level (53). Similar interactions are suggested in EBV/HTLV1, 2 and HIV–1 coinfections (54, 55). Although HIV–1 is essentially T lymphotropic (and "monocytotropic"), it may also coinfect EBV-positive B lymphocytes (48, 55, 56). The two viruses then might interact at a molecular level by activation of a HIV transcriptional/

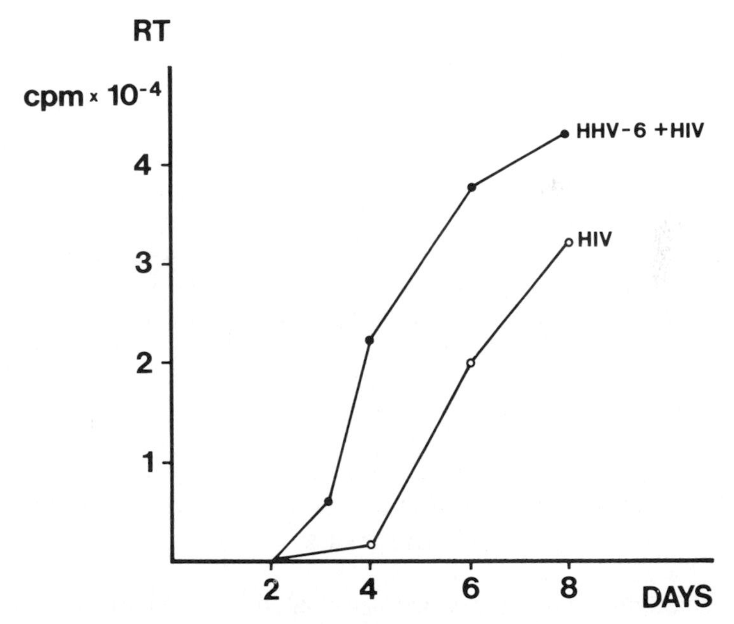

Figure 7. Reverse transcriptase (RT) activity in human CD38/CD4-positive lymphoid cells infected with HIV–1 alone or with HHV–6 and HIV–1.

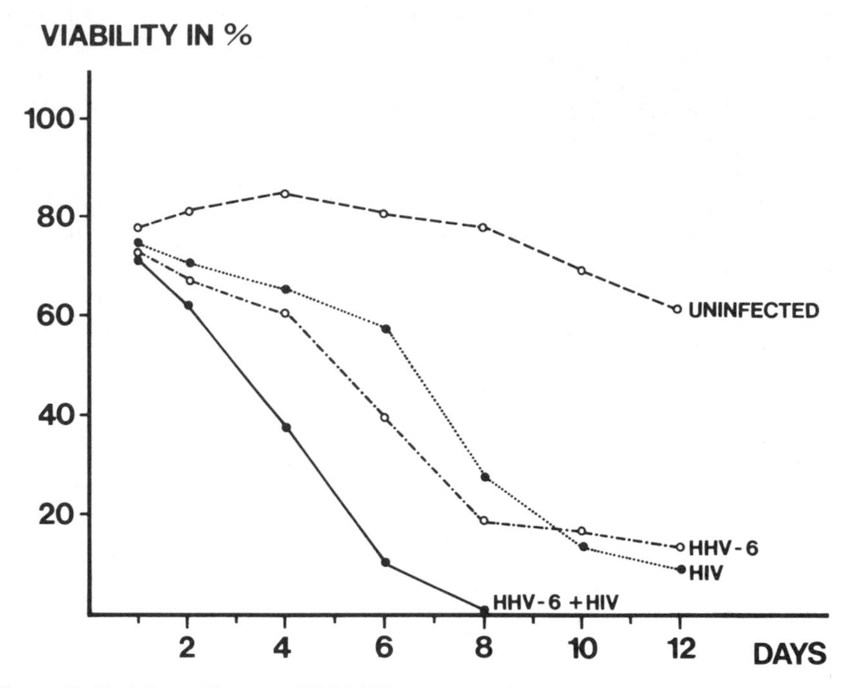

Figure 8. Viability of human CD38/CD4-positive lymphoid cells in single or double infections with HHV–6 and HIV–1.

post-transcriptional promoter through an EBV gene product (57). The EBV protein that transactivates HIV LTR also appears to transactivate its own EBV promoter BMLF–1. These findings further support earlier assumptions that HHV–6 and EBV infections may contribute to disease progression in AIDS (35). EBV and HHV–6 cooperation need to be investigated similarly at the molecular level in HIV-negative diseases since double infections by both viruses such as in infectious mononucleosis and in malignant lymphoproliferative diseases appear not a rare event (10, 20, 31).

Current therapeutic considerations in reactivated herpesvirus infections

Therapeutic endeavors in diseases associated with reactivated (herpes) virus infections should focus on two targets: (a) to correct immune dysfunction, and (b) to inhibit virus replication. Attempts to correct immune dysregulation were essentially less successful, partly because immune defects were quite variable, frequently delicate and only diagnostic by sophisticated methodology, or they are a symptom of another underlying disease. The matter is further complicated since reactivated lymphotropic herpesvirus themselves contribute to immune disturbances (1, 2). Among substances used for treatment of immune deficiency were non-specific stimulants (isoprinosine, amantadine, echinacin), thymic hormones, transfer factor, interleukins, interferons and immunoglobulins (58–60). In patients with persistent active EBV or HHV–6 infections and lymphoproliferative syndromes, interferon-alpha 2a with or without intravenous immunoglobulin showed significant improvement of the disease (61, 62). Intravenous immunoglobulin therapy is discussed by various authors during this symposium (63–69) and will not be repeated here. We have tested, however, commercially available immunoglobulin preparations from different sources for IgG antibody titers against EBV and HHV–6 and documented levels between 1:320 and 1:2580 (unpublished data). It may thus be worthwhile in future therapeutic planning to use immunoglobulin preparations with proven high antiviral titers in combination with antiviral drugs. This may possibly permit reduction of the load of extracellular virus, correct for some of the immune disturbances, and inhibit intracellular virus replication.

For treatment of viral infection, the currently available substances were administered, although they were usually less effective than in acute herpesvirus infections (70–72). In HSV–1 and 2, VZV and EBV intravenous acyclovir (ACV) may be helpful (58), not, however, in CMV and in HHV–6 infections. These viruses do not adequately activate a thymidine kinase necessary for activation of ACV through phosphorylation. Gancyclovir, phosphonoformate or other substances are tentatively administered in CMV or HHV–6 infections (3, 58). The use of gancyclovir yet is limited by its considerable toxicity.

Summary and conclusions

Reactivated infections with lymphotropic herpesviruses EBV and HHV–6 contribute to the pathology of a number of immune deficiency diseases and autoimmune disorders. They may also stimulate progressive lymphoproliferation with the risk of transition to malignant lymphoma. In addition, these viruses may enhance the effects of non-herpesvirus infections by coinfection of cells and transcriptional post-transcriptional transactivation. With additional new herpesvirus members isolated recently (suggestively HHV–7 and HHV–8 by Niza Frenkel, NIAID, and Zwi Berneman, NCI, National Institutes of Health, Bethesda, USA, respectively), the overall participation of herpesvirus infections in chronic diseases may be even more widespread than anticipated. Systematic patient studies are urgently needed to identify such relationships, thus providing the basis for adequate therapeutic intervention.

References

1. Purtilo, D. T., Tatsumi, E., Manolov G. *et al.* Epstein-Barr virus as an etiological agent in the pathogenesis of lymphoproliferative and aproliferative diseases in immune deficient patients. *Int. Rev. Exp. Pathol.* 27: 113; 1985.
2. Krueger, G. R. F. and Ramon, A. Overview of immunopathology of chronic active herpesvirus infection. *J. Virol. Methods* 21: 11; 1988.
3. Krueger, G. R. F. and Roewert, J. Klinische Immunpathologie der Cytomegalievirusinfektion. *AIDS Forsch (AIFO)* 3: 243; 1988.
4. Krueger, G. R. F. and Sander, C. What's new in human herpesvirus-6? Clinical immunopathology of the HHV–6 infection. *Path. Res. Pract.* 185: 915; 1989.
5. Fingeroth, J. D., Weiss, J. J., Tedder, T. F. *et al.* Epstein-Barr virus receptor of human B lymphocytes is the C3d receptor CR2. *Proc. Natl. Acad. Sci. USA* 81: 4510; 1984.
6. Lusso, P., Markham, P. D., Tschachler, E. *et al.* In vitro cellular tropism of human B-lymphotropic virus (human herpesvirus-6). *J. Exp. Med.* 167: 1659; 1988.
7. Krueger, G. R. F., Schonnebeck, M., Braun, M. *et al.* Enhanced cell membrane receptor expression following infection with human herpesvirus-6. *FASEB J.* 4: A343; 1990.
8. Frenkel, N., Schirmer, E. C., Wyatt, L. S. *et al.* Isolation of a new herpesvirus from human CD4+ T cells. *Proc. Natl. Acad. Sci. USA* 87: 748; 1990.
9. Henle, G. and Henle, W. The virus as an etiological agent of infectious mononucleosis. *In* "The Epstein–Barr virus" (Eds Epstein, M. and Achong, B. G.). Springer, Berlin; 1979.
10. Krueger, G. R. F., Ramon, A., Bertram, G. *et al.* Frequent double active infection with Epstein–Barr virus and human herpesvirus-6 in patients with acute infectious mononucleosis. *In Vivo.* (In press); 1991.
11. Eizuru, Y., Minematsu, T., Minamishima, Y. *et al.* Human herpesvirus 6 in lymph nodes. *Lancet* 1: 40; 1989.
12. Krueger, G. R. F. Nasopharyngeal carcinoma. *In* "Immune Deficiency and Cancer" (Ed. Purtilo, D. T.) Plenum, New York: 1984.

13. Dimery, I. W., Lee, J. S., Blick, M. *et al.* Association of the Epstein–Barr virus with lymphoepithelioma of the thymus. *Cancer* **61**: 2475; 1988.
14. Becker, J., Leser, U., Marschall, M. *et al.* EB-viral expression depends on the differentiated status of epithelial cells in oral hairy leukoplakia. *In* "Epstein–Barr virus and human disease 1988" (Eds Ablashi, D. V., Faggioni, A., Krueger, G. R. F. *et al.*). Humana Press, Clifton, NJ: 1989.
15. Yamanishi, K., Okuno, T., Shiraki, K. *et al.* Identification of human herpesvirus-6 as a causal agent for exanthem subitum. *Lancet* **2**: 1065; 1988.
16. Klemola, E., Kaariainen, R., von Essen, R. *et al.* Further studies on cytomegalovirus mononucleosis in previously healthy individuals. *Acta Med. Scand.* **182**: 311; 1967.
17. Krueger, G. R. F. Pathologie des immundefizienten erwachsenen Patienten. *Forschr. Antimikrob. Chemother.* **3–6**: 863; 1984.
18. Manak, M. Increased numbers of HHV–6 genome carrying cells in lymph nodes from patients with Rosai–Dorfman syndrome. *Personal communication.* (In preparation for publication.)
19. Kikuta, H., Taguchi, Y., Tomizawa, K. *et al.* Epstein–Barr virus genome positive T lymphocytes in a boy with chronic active EBV infection associated with Kawasaki-like disease. *Nature* **333**: 455; 1988.
20. Krueger, G. R. F., Manak, M., Bourgeois, N. *et al.* Persistent active herpesvirus infection associated with atypical polyclonal lymphoproliferation and malignant lymphoma. *Anticancer Res.* **9**: 1457; 1989.
21. Berthold, F., Krueger, G. R. F., Tesch, H. *et al.* Monoclonal B cell proliferation in lymphoproliferative disease associated with herpesvirus type 6 infection. *Anticancer Res.* **9**: 1511; 1989.
22. Josephs, S. F., Buchbinder, A., Streicher, H. Z. *et al.* Detection of human B-lymphotropic virus (human herpesvirus 6) sequences in B cell lymphoma tissues of three patients. *Leukemia* **2**: 132; 1988.
23. Jarrett, R. F., Gledhill, S., Qureshi, F. *et al.* Identification of human herpesvirus 6-specific DNA sequences in two patients with non-Hodgkin's lymphomas. *Leukemia* **2**: 496; 1988.
24. Hanto, D. W., Frizzera, G., Gajl-Peczalska, K. J. *et al.* Lymphoproliferative diseases in renal allograft recipients. *In* "Immune Deficiency and Cancer" (Ed. Purtilo, D. T.). Plenum, New York, 1984.
25. Katzenstein, A. -L. and Peiper, S. C. Detection of Epstein–Barr virus genomes in lymphomatoid granulomatosis analysis of 29 cases by the polymerase chain reaction technique. *Modern Path.* (In press.)
26. Ablashi, D. V. Interleukin-6 production by HHV–6 stimulated macrophages. (Unpublished results).
27. Lee, F., Chiu, C. -P, Wideman, J. *et al.* Interleukin-6: a multifunctional

regulator of growth and differentiation. *Ann. N. Y. Acad. Sci.* 557: 215; 1989.
28. Van Snick, J., Renault, J. -C., Simpson, R. J. *et al.* Mouse IL-6: a hybridoma growth factor with multiple effects on normal B and T cells. *Ann. N. Y. Acad. Sci.* 557: 206; 1989.
29. Van Damme, J. Biochemical and biological properties of human HPGF/IL-6. *Ann. N. Y. Acad. Sci.* 557: 104; 1989.
30. Klein, G. Epstein-Barr virus and its association with human disease: an overview. *In* "Epstein–Barr Virus and Human Disease" (Eds Ablashi, D. V., Faggioni, A., Krueger, G. R. F. *et al.*). Humana Press, Clifton, NJ; 1989.
31. Krueger, G. R. F., Ablashi, D. V., Salahuddin, S. Z. *et al.* Diagnosis and differential diagnosis of progressive lymphoproliferation and malignant lymphoma in persistent active herpesvirus infection. *J. Virol. Methods* 21: 255; 1988.
32. Wang, F., Petti, L., Braun, D. *et al.* A bicistronic Epstein–Barr virus mRNA encodes two nuclear proteins in latently infected, growth transformed lymphocytes. *J. Virol.* **61**: 945; 1987.
33. Razzaque, A., and Josephs, S. F. Oncogenic potential of human herpesvirus–6 DNA. 14th Internat. Herpesvirus Workshop, Nyborg Strand, Denmark; 1989.
34. Ablashi, D. V., Salahuddin, S. Z., Streicher, H. Z. *et al.* Elevated HBLV (human herpesvirus–6) antibody in HIV–1 antibody-positive and asymptomatic individuals. IVth Internat. Conf. AIDS, Stockholm, Sweden; 1988.
35. Krueger, G. R. F., Koch, B., Ramon, A. *et al.* Antibody prevalence to HBLV (human herpesvirus–6, HHV–6) and suggestive pathogenicity in the general population and in patients with immune deficiency syndromes. *J. Virol. Methods* 21: 125; 1988.
36. Seyda, M. and Krueger, G. R. F. Complex infectious copathogenesis of AIDS in HIV positive individuals. *Clin. Immunol. Newsletter* 881; 1987.
37. Webster, A., Lee, C. A., Cook, D. G. *et al.* Cytomegalovirus infection and progression towards AIDS in hemophiliacs with human immunodeficiency virus infection. *Lancet* 2: 63; 1989.
38. Rinaldo, C. R., Kingsley, A., Lyter, D. W. *et al.* Association of HTLV–III with Epstein–Barr virus infection and abnormalities of T lymphocytes in homosexual men. *J. Infect. Dis.* 154: 556; 1986.
39. Sumaya, C. V., Boswell, R. N., Ench, Y. *et al.* Enhanced serological and virological findings of Epstein–Barr virus in patients with AIDS and AIDS-related complex. *J. Infect. Dis.* 154: 864; 1986.
40. Fox, R. Epstein–Barr virus and human autoimmune diseases: possibilities and pitfalls. *J. Virol. Methods* 21: 19; 1988.
41. Fox, R. I., Saito, I., Chan, E. K. *et al.* Viral genomes in lymphomas of patients with Sjoegren's syndrome. *J. Autoimmun.* 2: 449; 1989.
42. Hoffman, A., Krueger, G. R. F., Barth, A. *et al.* Active human

herpesvirus-6 infections in systemic lupus erythematosus. II. World Congr. SLE, Singapore, 1989. (In press.)

43. Ward, N. K., Gray, J. J. and Efstathiou, S. Brief report: human herpesvirus-6 infection in a patient following liver transplantation from a seropositive donor. *J. Med. Virol.* 28: 69; 1988.
44. Hanto, D. W., Frizzera, G., Purtilo, D. T. *et al.* Clinical spectrum of lymphoproliferative disorders in renal transplant recipients and evidence for the role of the Epstein–Barr virus. *Cancer Res.* **41**: 4253; 1981.
45. Lusso, P., Ensoli, B., Markham, P. D. *et al.* Productive dual infection of human CD4+ T lymphocytes by HIV–1 and HHV–6. *Nature* 337: 370; 1989.
46. Ablashi, D. V., Josephs, S. F., Buchbinder, A. *et al.* Human B lymphotropic virus (human herpesvirus–6). *J. Virol. Methods* 21: 29; 1988.
47. Suga, S., Yoshikawa, T., Asano, Y. *et al.* Simultaneous infection of human herpesvirus–6 and measles virus in infants with fever and rash. *J. Med. Virol.* 31: 306; 1990.
48. Montagnier, L., Gruest, J., Chamaret, S. *et al.* Adaptation of lymphadenopathy associated virus (LAV) to replication in EBV transformed B lymphoblastoid cell lines. *Science* 225: 63; 1984.
49. Krueger, G. R. F., Ablashi, D. V., Lusso, P. *et al.* Immunological dysregulation of lymph nodes in AIDS patients. *C. T. Pathol.* (In press.)
50. Krueger, G. R. F., Schonnebeck, M. and Braun, M. Changes in cell membrane fluidity and in receptor expression following infection with HHV–6 may influence superinfection with other viruses. *AIDS Res. Human Retrovir.* **6**: 148; 1990.
51. Schonnebeck, M., Krueger, G. R. F., Braun, M. *et al.* Human herpesvirus–6 infection may predispose cells for superinfection by other viruses. *In Vivo.* (In press.)
52. Gendelman, H. E., Phelps, W., Feigenbaum L. *et al.* Transactivation of the human immunodeficiency virus long terminal repeat sequence by DNA viruses. *Proc. Natl. Acad. Sci. USA* **83**: 9759; 1986.
53. Ensoli, B., Lusso, P., Schachter, F. *et al.* Human herpesvirus–6 increases HIV–1 expression in co-infected T cells via nuclear factors binding to the HIV–1 enhancer. *EMBO J.* **8**: 3019; 1989.
54. Kaplan, M. H. Interactions of Epstein–Barr virus with human retroviruses. *In* "Epstein–Barr Virus and Human Disease 1988" (Eds Ablashi, D. V., Faggioni, A., Krueger, G. R. F. *et al.*). Humana Press, Clifton, NJ; 1989.
55. Ablashi, D. V., Luka, J., Buchbinder, A. *et al.* Interaction of HBLV (HHV–6) with EBV and HIV. *In* "Epstein–Barr Virus and Human Disease 1988" (Eds Ablashi, D. V., Faggioni, A., Krueger, G. R. F. *et al.*). Humana Press, Clifton, NJ; 1989.
56. Salahuddin, S. Z., Ablashi, D. V., Hunter, E. A. *et al.* HTLV–III

infection of EBV genome-positive B-lymphoblastoid cells with or without detectable T4 antigen. *Int. J. Cancer* 39: 198; 1987.
57. Pagano, J. S., Kenney S., Markovitz D. *et al.* Epstein–Barr virus and interactions with human retroviruses. *J. Virol. Methods* 21: 229; 1988.
58. Straus, S. E. Treatment of persistent active herpesvirus infections. *J. Virol. Methods* 21: 305; 1988.
59. Levine, P. H., Krueger, G. R. F., Kaplan, M. *et al.* The post-infectious chronic fatigue syndrome. *In* "Epstein–Barr Virus and Human Disease 1988" (Eds Ablashi, D. V., Faggioni, A., Krueger, G. R. F. *et al.*). Humana Press, Clifton, NJ; 1989.
60. Krueger, G. R. F. and Hilgers, A. Chronic fatigue syndrome: an as yet unappreciated medical problem in Germany. *Heart of America News*. pp. 1–4; Spring/Summer 1990.
61. Shapiro, R. S. and Filipovich, A. H. Successful therapy for EBV associated B cell lymphoproliferative disorders in immunodeficiency using alpha interferon and intravenous immunoglobulin. *In* "Epstein–Barr Virus and Human Disease 1988" (Eds Ablashi, D. V., Faggioni, A., Krueger, G. R. F. *et al.*). Humana Press, Clifton, NJ: 1989.
62. Hoffman, A., Mueller, R., Krueger, G. R. F. *et al.* Erfolgreiche Therapie einer lebensbedrohlichen Infektion mit humanem Herpesvirus Typ 6 (vormals humanes B-lymphotropes Virus bezeichnet). *Med. Welt* 39: 510; 1988.
63. Stiehm, R. E. Use of IVIG in secondary immunodeficiencies. *In* "Intravenous Immunoglobulin Symposium" (Eds Imbach, P., Morell, A. *et al.*). Academic Press, London; 1990.
64. Schaad, U. B. IVIG in pediatric AIDS. *In* "Intravenous Immunoglobulin Symposium" (Eds Imbach, P., Morell, A. *et al.*). Academic Press, London; 1990.
65. Tutschka, P. J. Use of IVIG in clinical allogeneic marrow transplantation. *In* "Intravenous Immunoglobulin Symposium" (Eds Imbach, P., Morell, A. *et al.*). Academic Press, London; 1990.
66. Elfenbein, G. J. IVIG in bone marrow transplantation. *In* "Intravenous Immunoglobulin Symposium" (Eds Imbach, P., Morell, A. *et al.*). Academic Press, London; 1990.
67. Klintmalm, G. B. The use of IVIG after liver transplantation. *In* "Intravenous Immunoglobulin Symposium" (Eds Imbach, P., Morell, A. *et al.*). Academic Press, London; 1990.
68. Corvetta, A. IVIG treatment in sytemic lupus erythematosus and in lupus-like syndromes. *In* "Intravenous Immunoglobulin Symposium" (Eds Imbach, P., Morell, A. *et al.*). Academic Press, London; 1990.
69. Shulman, S. T. Kawasaki disease and IVIG treatment. *In* "Intravenous Immunoglobulin Symposium" (Eds Imbach, P., Morell, A. *et al.*). Academic Press, London; 1990.

70. Meyers, J. D. Management of cytomegalovirus infection. *Am. J. Med.* 85 (Suppl. 2A): 102; 1988.
71. Anderson, J. and Ernberg, I. Management of Epstein–Barr virus infections. *Am. J. Med.* 85 (Suppl. 2A): 107; 1988.
72. Winston, D. J., Eron, L. J., Monto, H. V. *et al.* Recombinant interferon alpha 2a for treatment of herpes zoster in immunosuppressed patients with cancer. *Am. J. Med.* 85: 147; 1988.
73. Ablashi, D. V., Salahuddin, S. Z., Josephs, S. F. *et al.* Human herpesvirus–6 (HHV–6). 2nd Natl. Virol. Congr., Valladolid, Spain, 1990. *In Vivo* (In press.)
74. Biberfeld, P., Petren, A. -L., Eklund, A. *et al.* Human herpesvirus–6 (HHV–6, HBLV) in sarcoidosis and lymphoproliferative disorders. *J. Virol. Methods* 21: 49; 1988.
75. Krueger, G. R. F., Papadakis, T. and Schaefer, H. J. Persistent active Epstein–Barr virus infection and atypical lymphoproliferation. *Am. J. Surg. Pathol.* 11: 972; 1987.
76. Epstein, M. A. and Achong, B. G. The relationship of the virus to Burkitt's lymphona. *In* "The Epstein–Barr virus (Eds Epstein, M. A. and Achong, B. G.). Springer, Berlin; 1979.
77. DuBois, R. E., Seeley, J. K., Brus, I. *et al.* Chronic mononucleosis syndrome. *South. Med. J.* 77: 1376; 1984.
78. Tobi, M. and Morag, A. Chronic mononucleosis. *In* "Immune Deficiency and Cancer" (Ed. Purtilo, D. T.). Plenum, New York; 1984.
79. Honda, K., Yoshioki, M. and Nakamura, M. A case of Castleman lymphoma (plasma cell type) in retroperitoneum with higher titer of EBV virus antibodies. *Nippon Shokakibyo Gakkai Zasshi* 81: 1083; 1984.
80. Weiss, L. M., Movahed, L. A., Warnke, R. A. *et al.* Detection of Epstein–Barr virus genomes in Reed-Sternberg cells of Hodgkin's diseases. *N. Engl. J. Med.* 320: 502; 1989.
81. Jones, J. F., Shurin, S., Abramovsky, C. *et al.* T-cell lymphomas containing Epstein–Barr viral DNA in patients with chronic Epstein–Barr virus infections. *N. Engl. J. Med.* 318: 733; 1988.

Discussion

P. F. Strembers

When there are so many diseases correlated with herpesviruses, as you described, but the incidence of the viruses in the human population is high too (up to 90%). I would like to know what your definition is of "association"? Have you just found the virus in the cells of the affected organ or is there evidence of the virus as an etiologic agent in this disease?

G. Krueger
In these diseases caused by or related to viruses with a high prevalence (latency), we consider a certain pathologenic association to exist between virus and disease if (a) serology indicates active infection (demonstration of replication-associated antigens, e.g. anti-EA in EBV etc., or IgM antibodies); (b) there is increased load of viral antigen (by immunohistology and monoclonal antibodies) and/or viral genome (in situ hybridization) in tissues; and (c) virus isolation from diseased patients and/or tissues signal persistent viral activity.

U. Nydegger
The main rationale to prophylaxis and treatment of viral diseases by IVIG is neutralization and enhancement of antibody-dependent cellular cytotoxicity by virus-infection-specific antibodies contained in IVIG. However, some *in vitro* evidence has accumulated that antiviral antibodies favor infection of target cells by opsonizing virus. Do you believe that this concern applies to at least some herpesvirus infections?

G. Krueger
I believe that there may be no significant risk of reactivating latent viruses by this treatment, since cells latently infected don't express (at least not quantitatively) the necessary surface antigens. Cells with replicating virus do, and these you want to destroy. Virus reactivation rather seems to occur after non-specific stimulation (non-specific with regard to the virus antigens), i.e. by anti-IgM autoantibodies latent EBV in IgM-positive B lymphocytes may be reactivated. Infecting cells by 'opsonization' is still disputable. Phagocytes may take up virus by this way, but it has not been convincingly shown that virus may replicate or latently infect these cells by this mechanism.

Viruses and immunodeficiency

A. D. B. WEBSTER and A. SA'ADU

Immune Deficiency Diseases Research Group, Clinical Research Centre, Watford Road, Harrow, UK

Introduction

Since this symposium is mainly concerned with dysregulation of antibody production and the effects of immunoglobulin replacement therapy, I shall concentrate on the virus infections that are associated with hypogammaglobulinemia (HGG). I will first discuss enteroviral and hepatitis virus infections in HGG patients, which are either clearly secondary to the antibody deficiency or iatrogenically acquired from contaminated gammaglobulin. Finally, I will discuss our current view of the pathogenesis of "common variable" hypogammaglobulinemia (CVH) and our attempts to implicate viruses in this process.

Enteroviruses

These comprise a large group of RNA viruses (coxsackie, polio, echoviruses) which spread through the community via fecal/oral or pharyngeal droplet contamination. Coxsackie and echoviruses usually cause an acute self-limiting gastroenteritis or mild meningitis in immunocompetent subjects. These viruses are genetically unstable

Immunotherapy with Intravenous Immunoglobulins
ISBN 0-12-370725-0

and in persistent infections mutations may give rise to variants, with the possibility that a more pathogenic virus may become dominant.

Polio virus

Children with either severe combined immunodeficiency or severe HGG may develop paralytic poliomyelitis following immunization with live polio vaccines, which consequently are contraindicated (1). There is anecdotal evidence that HGG patients excrete vaccine strains in their feces for prolonged periods following oral immunization, and there is concern that new mutations may lead to the emergence of pathogenic strains which would be a risk to both the patient and others in the community (2). Polio virus replicates in the small bowel, and is excreted for about 6 weeks following routine oral immunization. HGG patients should theoretically be at risk from infection with vaccine strains in the community, and a study to assess this risk would be worthwhile.

Echo and coxsackie viruses

Chronic echovirus infections of the central nervous system and muscles became a recognized complication in HGG patients in the mid-1970s (3). Patients with X-linked agammaglobulinemia were particularly at risk. The expression of the disease was variable, but common features were eighth nerve deafness, headaches, convulsions and a gradual fibrosis in the limb muscles. There is evidence of a chronic vasculitis affecting the small vessels in the muscles and the meninges. The disease is insidious, sometimes with slow progression for up to 10 years, death being due to involvement of a major brainstem center. Echoviruses can be readily cultured from the CSF, and/or the muscles in most cases. More than one strain may be isolated from a single patient, implying multiple infection or the development of new strains by mutation (4).

The disease can be stabilized by giving specific antibodies, either as plasma from immune donors, or as IVIG which in some cases has been given directly into the cerebral spinal fluid (5). Alpha-interferon, given systemically or into an Ommaya reservoir was of no benefit in one of our cases.

Since 1980 we have not diagnosed a new case of echovirus disease. However, HGG patients still develop chronic central nervous system disease, sometimes with similar features to the classical echovirus syndrome. Table 1 outlines our recent experience, highlighting the

Table 1
Chronic CNS disease in UK HGG patients during the last decade (CSF viral cultures negative)

Age of onset of HGG	Duration of CNS symptoms	CNS signs: Cerebella ataxia	CNS signs: Dementia	Other features
2	9	+	+	Limb spasticity Brain biopsy = encephalitis
23	10[a]	+	+	Optic atrophy Convulsions
53	5[a]	+	+	Limb spasticity
27	3	+		Limb spasticity
7	2			Myeloradiculopathy Bilateral 8th nerve deafness Mild myositis
26	6[a]			Paraparesis

[a] Died.

dementia as a new feature not previously associated with echovirus disease. Brain biopsy from one of these patients strongly suggests a chronic infection, but frequent attempts in all cases to culture viruses from the CSF, which usually contains a slightly raised protein and cell count, has proved negative. There are similar patients in New York (Dr C. Cunningham-Rundles) and Barcelona (Dr T. Espanol) where again no virus has been cultured.

It is likely that this variable CNS disease is due to chronic enteroviral infection, perhaps modified by the regular use of intravenous gammaglobulin therapy which probably contains a wide spectrum of low titer specific antibodies to echoviruses. The inability to culture virus from the CSF may reflect the very small number of viral particles present due to partial neutralization by antibody. This scenario could theoretically be confirmed by utilizing oligonucleotide primers, common to all enteroviruses, in a polymerase chain reaction to amplify the viral RNA from brain, muscle or CSF cells (6).

Hepatitis viruses

Non-A non-B hepatitis

There have been clusters of non-A non-B (NANB) hepatitis in HGG patients following treatment with contaminated batches of gammaglobulin (7). In general, the prognosis is poor and apparently worse than that associated with factor VIII therapy in hemophiliacs. Liver failure and/or cirrhosis has already caused or contributed to the death of 7 out of 13 patients in our clinic who were infected in 1983. These deaths are confined to CVH patients; two out of three XLA patients infected at the same time have completely recovered, with the third having a subclinical mild hepatitis. CVH patients with splenomegaly prior to infection usually develop hypersplenism (see below) which contributes to the morbidity. It is our impression that NANB hepatitis accelerates the hypersplenic "syndrome" in CVH patients, possibly through the release of immune mediators and portal hypertension.

It is recommended that patients on intravenous gammaglobulin therapy are regularly monitored for elevation of serum alanine transferase as a marker for NANB hepatitis. Difficulties in interpretation may arise in HGG patients who develop chronic inflammatory bowel disease or granulomatous hepatitis, the latter being confined to CVH patients. The advent of tests which recognize hepatitis C RNA should clarify the issue and demonstrate whether there is low-level contamination of IVIG preparations which might be responsible for some of the unexplained liver abnormalities.

Treatment

In our experience, HGG patients with NANB hepatitis have been unexpectedly intolerant to alpha-interferon therapy, in contrast to immunocompetent subjects who have acquired the disease from blood transfusions (8, 9). Although the hepatitis improved on this therapy, only one out of four patients managed to tolerate the treatment for more than 6 months, with fever, headache, myalgia and malaise being the main complications. All relapsed after discontinuing therapy. Liver transplantation has been considered in some patients, but none have yet been suitable because of additional complications.

Hepatitis B

HGG patients are probably more prone to hepatitis B virus infection than normal subjects, and we are aware of five patients with chronic antigenemia in the UK, all having evidence of chronic hepatitis. Furthermore, it is clearly undesirable for patients requiring regular blood tests and replacement therapy to be infectious to others. Effective treatment is now possible with a mouse monoclonal antibody to the surface antigen of hepatitis B virus. HGG patients can tolerate repeated injections of animal protein, and the virus appears to have been eliminated in a pilot study on two patients (15).

Viral etiology for CVH

Lymphadenopathy, associated with a glandular fever-like illness precedes the diagnosis of hypogammaglobulinemia in about 10% of CVH patients; this suggests a viral infection. There is a genetic predisposition to CVH, linked to the Class II or Class III region on chromosome 6, which may predispose to persistent viral infection (10). More recently, we have studied the spleens and abdominal lymph nodes removed from two CVH patients with hypersplenism. These contained lymphoid follicles with normal architecture and sIgM-positive B cells were present in normal numbers, but there were no plasma cells. These B cells secrete IgM *in vitro* when stimulated with anti-IgM-coated Sepharose beads and IL–2, indicating that there is a block in the differentiation of B cells to secreting plasma blasts *in vivo* (16).

There is now good evidence in the majority of CVH patients, but particularly in those with splenomegaly and liver granulomas, of persistent immune hyperactivity involving T cells and macrophages, in that serum neopterin (14), soluble CD8 and soluble IL–2 receptor levels are very high (M. North, in preparation). These findings are consistent with a chronic viral infection involving lymphocytes and/or macrophages, perhaps with release of down-regulatory signals for B-cell differentiation. However, formal evidence for persistent viral infection in these patients is weak (11). The isolation of HIV–1 viruses from two "not at risk" CVH patients by us in 1982 has not been repeated in other patients. Furthermore, a recent search for HIV–1 pro-viral DNA in peripheral blood mononuclear cells of 12 CVH patients, using a variety of conserved oligonucleotide primers in polymerase chain reactions failed to produce evidence of HIV–1 infection. This suggests that our two patients may have acquired the HIV infection in 1981 from intravenous gammaglobulin, which at that time was obtained from donors who were not screened for HIV infection.

Further evidence against the involvement of an HIV–1-like virus is the finding that hypogammaglobulinemia can be reversed following HIV–1 infection in CVH patients. This has occurred in at least three patients whose immunoglobulin levels steadily increased, sometimes to very high levels, with some recovery in specific antibody production (12). The mechanism is obscure, but we have shown that intact virus, and more recently recombinant gp120 representing part of the HIV–1 envelope, can increase IgM and IgG production *in vitro*, but only as a co-stimulus with IL–2 (13). Furthermore, there is marked subject variability in this response, suggesting that genetic factors determine the response; Class II molecules are possible candidates.

We continue our search for viruses in CVH; persistent CMV or EBV infection is unlikely in view of negative tests with appropriate monoclonal antibodies; HSV–6 remains a possible candidate. The common occurrence of granulomas in CVH suggests that the putative virus may reside within macrophages, and perhaps a better approach is to attempt culture of an agent from splenic tissue using macrophage growth factors and supporting cell lines.

Summary

Virus infections associated with hypogammaglobulinemia (HGG) are discussed. Chronic central nervous system disease remains a significant problem. This is probably due to echovirus infection, but there is currently an unexplained difficulty in culturing the agent from cerebrospinal fluid. Non-A non-B hepatitis, probably due to Hepatitis C virus (HCV) is still a potential problem in patients receiving regular intravenous gammaglobulin therapy. Once infected, the prognosis is very poor in HGG patients. However, it appears that chronic hepatitis-B infection can be effectively treated with monoclonal antibodies to HBs. There is still no formal evidence for a viral etiology for "common variable" hypogammaglobulinemia, but indirect evidence is discussed.

References

1. Wyatt, H. V. Poliomyelitis in hypogammaglobulinaemia. *J. Infect. Dis.* 128: 802, 1973.
2. MacCallum, F. O. Antibodies in hypogammaglobulinaemia. *In* "Hypogammaglobulinaemia in the United Kingdom". Medical Research Council SRS 310. Her Majesty's Stationery Office, London; 1971.
3. Wilfert, C. M., Buckley, R. H., Mohanakumar, T. *et al.* Persistent and fatal central-nervous-system echovirus infections in patients with agammaglobulinaemia. *N. Engl. J. Med.* **296**: 1485; 1977.
4. Webster, A. D. B. Echovirus disease in hypogammaglobulinaemic patients. *Clin. Rheum. Dis.* 10: 189; 1984.
5. McKinney, R. E. Jnr., Katz, S. L. and Wilfert, C. M. Chronic

enteroviral meningoencephalitis in agammaglobulinaemic patients. *Rev. Infect. Dis.* **9**: 334; 1987.
6. Cova, L., Kopecka, H., Aymard, M. and Girard, M. Use of cRNA probes for the detection of enteroviruses by molecular hybridization. *J. Med. Virol.* **24**: 11; 1988.
7. Cunningham-Rundles, C. Immunoglobulin replacement therapy. *In* "Immunodeficiency and Disease" (Ed. Webster, A. D. B.). Kluwer Academic, London; 1988.
8. Thomson, B. J., Doron, M., Lever, A. M. L. and Webster, A. D. B. Alpha interferon therapy for non-A non-B hepatitis transmitted by gammaglobulin replacement therapy. *Lancet* **1**: 539; 1987.
9. Jacyna, M. R., Brooks, M. G., Loke, R. H. T. *et al.* Randomized controlled trial of interferon alpha in chronic non-A non-B hepatitis. *Br. Med. J.* **289**: 80; 1989.
10. Schaffer, F. M., Palmeros, J., Zhu, Z. B. *et al.* Individuals with IgA deficiency and common variable immunodeficiency share polymorphisms of major histocompatibility complex class III genes. *Proc. Natl. Acad. Sci. USA* **86**: 8015; 1989.
11. Spickett, G. P., Millrain, M., Beattie, R. *et al.* Role of retroviruses in acquired hypogammaglobulinaemia. *Clin. Exp. Immunol.* **74**: 177; 1988.
12. Webster, A. D. B., Lever, A., Spickett, G. *et al.* Recovery of antibody production after HIV infection in "common" variable hypogammaglobulinaemia. *Clin. Exp. Immunol.* **77**: 309; 1989.
13. Spickett, G., Beattie, R., Farrant, J. *et al.* Assessment of responses of normal human B lymphocytes to different isolates of human immunodeficiency virus (HIV–1): role of normal donor and of cell line used to prepare viral isolate. *AIDS Res. Hum. Retrovir.* **5**: 355; 1989.
14. Harland, T., Shah, T., Webster, A. D. B. and Peters, T. J. Serum neopterin in patients with X-linked and acquired "common variable" hypogammaglobulinaemia. *Int. Arch. Allergy Appl. Immunol.* **88**: 1989.
15. Lever, A. M. L., Waters, J., Brook, M. G. *et al.* Monoclonal antibody to HBsAg for chronic hepatitis B virus infection with hypogammaglobulinaemia. *Lancet* **335**: 1529; 1990.
16. Bryant, A., Calver, N. C., Toubi, E. *et al.* Classification of patients with Common Variable Immunodeficiency by B cell secretion of IgM and IgG in response to anti-IgM and Interleukin-2. *Clin. Immunol. Immunopath.* **56**: 239–248; 1990.

Discussion

R. E. Stiehm
In agammaglobulinemia with hepatitis-B antigenemia, why not use HBIG, or IVIG which also has anti-HBs in it?

A. D. B. Webster
IVIG does not work because there is not enough anti-HBs present. Hyperimmune HBIG has not been tried and may work. Monoclonal antibodies will have a much more powerful effect and prevent the possibility of resistant HBV strains emerging.

E. Gelfand
The patients with CNS disease are intriguing. Do you have additional information concerning clustering and whether they have been on the same type of IVIG?

A. D. B. Webster
Five of the six patients in our group have been on Sandoglobulin for between 1 and 5 years, four developed CNS signs when they were on IVIG. Two had some plasma therapy prior to the CNS disease. These data, and those from similar patients elsewhere in the world, show no consistent pattern of therapy or the onset of CNS disease, although the subsequent use of IVIG in some patients may have modified the natural history.

R. Schiff
Classic echovirus meningoencephalitis occurs primarily in X-linked or females lacking B cells. Does this new syndrome occur in CVID or in X-linked primarily?

A. D. B. Webster
Although the early descriptions of echovirus meningitis were in XLA patients, the condition does occur in those with "common variable" hypogammaglobulinemia with circulating B cells. Four of the patients with the "new" CNS syndrome(s) I have described had CVH.

J. M. Dwyer
A number of viral infections may be associated with a poor T-cell response, and T-cell function is often depressed in hypogammaglobulinemia. Has any intrathecal IVIG been given to patients with your "new" syndrome?

A. D. B. Webster
There was no evidence of a significant consistent T-cell defect in our group of patients; two had XLA where T-cell responses are characteristically normal. We have not tried intrathecal IVIG in this group of patients because the experience worldwide in echovirus infection is not very encouraging, although there have been a few apparent successes.

The role of IVIG in pediatric HIV infection

URS B. SCHAAD

Division of Pediatric Infectious Diseases, Department of Pediatrics, University of Bern, Bern, Switzerland

Introduction

In 1982, soon after the acquired immunodeficiency syndrome (AIDS) had been observed in homosexual men and intravenous drug users, some children were described presenting a disease entity suggestive of AIDS (1). In the following years, much new information about AIDS became available, including landmark reports of the syndrome in children by Oleske *et al.* (2), Rubinstein *et al.* (3) and Scott *et al.* (4), and the discovery of the etiologic agent, the human immunodeficiency virus (HIV), by the research groups of Gallo (5) and Montagnier (6).

Pediatric HIV infection has emerged as a leading cause of immunodeficiency in infants and children. The major route of infection is vertical HIV transmission from mother to child during pregnancy. Characteristics of pediatric HIV infection include defective humoral immunity leading to recurrent or serious bacterial infections, development of various opportunistic infections despite still normal absolute number of helper T lymphocytes, failure to thrive, and rather typical findings such as lymphoid interstitial pneumonitis and encephalopathy (7). Major problems arising are the difficulty of establishing, unequivocally, the diagnosis during the first 18 months of life, the

Immunotherapy with Intravenous Immunoglobulins
ISBN 0–12–370725–0

relative lack of knowledge concerning mother-to-child transmission of HIV, the only partially understood, special immunopathogenesis of pediatric HIV disease, and the lack of clear prognostic markers and accepted, optimal treatment recommendations. Adequate research is drastically limited because of uneven geographic distribution of the disease, its associated social, legal and ethical complexities, and the absence of sufficient funds (8). The ultimate goal consists of prevention, effective treatment and eradication of HIV infection in children. High-quality and coordinated contributions from the disciplines of basic research, pediatrics, nursing, social work and public health are the basis for this optimistic future.

In the meantime, the current mainstays for the individual care of HIV-infected children are supportive management, immunizations and antimicrobial agents. In this context, the prophylactic use of regular intravenous immunoglobulins (IVIG) deserves serious consideration.

Rationale for IVIG use

Substitution

In HIV-infected children, defects in B-cell function are generally apparent earlier than those of cell-mediated immunity, and recurrent or serious bacterial infections are the result and represent an important cause of morbidity (9). Most probably, B-cell function is compromised by loss of antigen-specific T helper cells and by direct effect of HIV on B-cell maturation (10). It is likely that children are more prone than adults to have problems with bacterial infections because they lack pre-existing development of primary humoral immune response. *In vitro* and *in vivo* studies have shown that antibody responses of children with AIDS are functionally impaired (11, 12). The B cells are polyclonally activated by Epstein–Barr virus or HIV, and frequently elevated serum immunoglobulin levels are observed early in pediatric HIV infection (7).

Therefore, clinical presentations of infants with AIDS often resemble patients with primary humoral immunodeficiency. Considering the well-documented benefit of IVIG prophylaxis in these patients, continuous substitution with IVIG seems a promising therapeutic modality in pediatric AIDS despite its hypergammaglobulinemic state.

Immunomodulation

Several studies have shown that periodic IVIG treatment can favorably influence impaired HIV-associated immunity. Such immunologic improvements included stabilizations or even increases in helper T lymphocytes and lymphocyte proliferative mitogenic responses, decreases in circulating immune complex and lactate dehydrogenase values, and normalization of suppressor T-cell function (13, 14, 15). These immunomodulatory effects of IVIG may be due in part to neutralization and elimination of infective agents, thus reducing antigenic stimulation of B cells. Feedback inhibition of B-cell proliferation by anti-idiotypic antibodies passively infused with IVIG represents another possible mechanism. Removal of antigen–antibody-complement complexes, normalization of suppressor T-cell function, and possible direct virus-neutralizing effect by HIV-specific antibodies could all contribute to control HIV infection by diminishing virus propagation in CD4-positive cells.

Suppression of autoimmunity

HIV infection is associated with a variety of presentations which in part are autoimmune phenomena (16). These findings include fever, lymphadenopathy, rash, renal dysfunction, and neurological and hematological disorders. Thrombocytopenia is an increasing problem with pediatric HIV infection. Immune-mediated platelet destruction presenting with high levels of platelet-associated IgG and circulating immune complexes seems to be the most common pathogenesis, and initial treatment with high-dose IVIG is indicated (17). However, other mechanisms for thrombocytopenia, such as severe bone marrow aplasia and complicating infections, and also additional functional platelet defects, certainly do occur (17, 18, 19). Moreover, the exact mode of action of high-dose IVIG in immune-mediated thrombocytopenia without HIV infection is not yet completely understood (20, 21).

Clinical experience

The relevant published data on IVIG use in pediatric AIDS are summarized in the Table 1 (13–15, 22–26). So far, no randomized, controlled trials have been published; such a double-blind, placebo-controlled multicenter study sponsored by the US National Institute of

Table 1
Results of IVIG treatment in pediatric AIDS

	Oleske *et al.* (22, 23)		Rubinstein *et al.* (13–15)		Schaad et al. (24)	Williams et al. (25)	Hunziker et al. (26)
	IVIG (n = 19)	Controls (n = 12)	IVIG (n = 14)	Controls (n = 27)	IVIG (n = 7)	IVIG (n = 5)	IVIG (n = 2)
Observation period (months)	≥24	≥24	12–24	12–24	6–24	3–13	12–15
Monthly dose of IVIG (g/kg)	0.2	—	0.6	—	0.4–0.8	0.3	0.4
Infectious episodes	Decrease	Increase	21%	96%	Decrease	Decrease	Decrease
Lymphoid interstitial pneumonitis	?	?	5× stable	5× deterioration	2× deterioration	?	—
HIV encephalopathy	?	?	?	?	2× stable	1× improvement	2× improvement
Clinical condition	Improvement	Deterioration	Improvement	Deterioration	Improvement	Improvement	Improvement
Mortality (%)	16	83	14	48	0	0	0

Child Health and Human Development is still in progress. The control groups included in the present synopsis were non-randomly selected, untreated patients (13, 23). The majority of these patients also received antimicrobial prophylaxis.

The monthly IVIG dose was 0.2–0.8 g/kg body weight and the observation period ranged from 3 to ≥ 24 months. In all series, the IVIG-treated children had fewer infectious episodes including episodes of fever and proven sepsis, and showed clear overall clinical improvement. Also mortality decreased or was absent during regular IVIG administration. Moreover, lymphoid interstitial pneumonitis and HIV encephalopathy tend to respond favorably to IVIG. As mentioned before, the majority of these beneficial effects can be explained with antibody substitution and immunomodulation by IVIG treatment. A well-documented case of specific antibody substitution had been published by Woods *et al.* (27). In this 2-year-old, HIV-infected infant, monthly injections of IVIG stopped her recurrent episodes of pneumococcal bacteremia, and increased her serum concentrations of type-specific pneumococcal antibodies stepwise.

High-dose IVIG (1–2 g/kg body weight over 4–5 days) is effective in restoring platelet counts in only about one-third of the pediatric AIDS cases with immune-mediated thrombocytopenia, and the majority of attained remissions are temporary only (17, 19). As stated before, additional functional platelet defects are usually present. Optimal therapy for HIV-associated thrombocytopenia is not yet established. Therapies currently being investigated include steroids, steroids plus IVIG, steroids plus danazol, danazol alone, anti-Rh immunoglobulins, and zidovudine (28, 29).

Conclusions

The available data clearly demonstrate that IVIG treatment is of substantial clinical benefit for symptomatic HIV-infected pediatric patients. Periodic administration of 0.4.–0.8 g IVIG per kg body weight every month will prevent or markedly reduce infectious episodes and improve overall clinical conditions. Additional advantages regarding HIV-associated immunodeficiency and organ involvement are possible. The ultimate outcome of HIV infection, however, is not altered by IVIG and long-term prognosis may be unchanged. Nevertheless, I strongly believe that IVIG therapy should be part of standard supportive care for pediatric AIDS, with and without concomitant specific antiviral treatment. I am convinced that the currently conducted double-blind, placebo-controlled, multicenter trial will confirm the utility of IVIG. It is possible that in the future specific indications to start IVIG therapy in pediatric HIV infection can be formulated based on clinical (e.g. recurrent bacterial infections) and/or laboratory markers (e.g. impaired antibody response to vaccination). Optimal commencement, dose and interval of IVIG administration in pediatric HIV infection need to be defined.

The development of specific anti-HIV antibody preparations for the prophylaxis and treatment of HIV infections is currently a very active area of research (30). Such passive immunoneutralization of HIV represents an additional, attractive role of immunoglobulin preparations in HIV infection.

Summary

IVIG therapy should be part of standard supportive care for pediatric AIDS. Mechanisms of action include substitution of functionally impaired antibody response and modulation of HIV-associated immunodeficiency. The principal benefits of periodic IVIG administration in symptomatic pediatric HIV infection are reduction of infectious episodes and improvement of general clinical conditions. The efficacy of IVIG in suppressing HIV-associated autoimmune phenomena including thrombocytopenia is clearly limited.

References

1. Anon. Unexplained immunodeficiency and opportunistic infections in infants —New York, New Jersey, California. *Morb. Mort. Wkly Rep.* 31: 665–667; 1982.
2. Oleske, J., Minnefor, A., Cooper, R. *et al.* Immune deficiency syndrome in children. *J. Am. Med. Assoc.* **249**: 2345–2349; 1983.
3. Rubinstein, A., Sicklick, M., Gupta, A. *et al.* Acquired immunodeficiency with reversed T4/T8 ratios in infants born to promiscuous and drug-addicted mothers. *J. Am. Med. Assoc.* **249**: 2350–2356; 1983.
4. Scott, G. B., Buck, B. E., Leterman, J. G. *et al.* Acquired immunodeficiency syndrome in infants. *N. Engl. J. Med.* **310**: 76–81; 1984.
5. Gallo, R. C., Sarin, P. S., Gelmann, E. P. *et al.* Isolation of human T-cell leukemia virus in acquired immune deficiency syndrome (AIDS). *Science* **220**: 865–867; 1983.
6. Barré–Sinoussi, F., Chermann, J. C., Rey, F. *et al.* Isolation of a

T-lymphotropic retrovirus from a patient at risk for acquired immune deficiency syndrome (AIDS). *Science* **220**: 868–871; 1983.

7. Falloon, J., Eddy, J., Wiener, L. and Pizzo, P. A. Human immunodeficiency virus infection in children. *J. Pediatr.* **114**: 1–30; 1989.
8. Nicholas, S. W., Sondheimer, D. L., Willoughby, A. D. *et al.* Human immunodeficiency virus infection in childhood, adolescence, and pregnancy: a status report and national research agenda. *Pediatrics* **83**: 293–308; 1989.
9. Krasinski, K., Borkowsky, W., Bonk, S. *et al.* Bacterial infections in human immunodeficiency virus-infected children. *Pediatr. Infect. Dis. J.* **7**: 323–328; 1988.
10. Ochs, H. D. Intravenous immunoglobulin in the treatment and prevention of acute infections in pediatric acquired immunodeficiency syndrome patients. *Pediatr. Infect. Dis. J.* **6**: 509–511; 1987.
11. Bernstein, L. J., Ochs, H. D., Wedgwood, R. J. and Rubinstein, A. Defective humoral immunity in pediatric acquired immune deficiency syndrome. *J. Pediatr.* **107**: 352–357; 1985.
12. Borkowsky, W., Steele, C. J., Grubman, S. *et al.* Antibody responses to bacterial toxoids in children infected with human immunodeficiency virus. *J. Pediatr.* **110**: 563–566; 1987.
13. Calvelli, T. A. and Rubinstein, A. Intravenous gamma-globulin in infant acquired immunodeficiency syndrome. *Pediatr. Infect. Dis. J.* **5**: S207–S210; 1986.
14. Silverman, B. A. and Rubinstein, A. Serum lactate dehydrogenase levels in adults and children with acquired immune deficiency syndrome (AIDS) and AIDS-related complex: possible indicator of B cell lymphoproliferation and disease activity. Effect of intravenous gammaglobulin on enzyme levels. *Am. J. Med.* **78**: 728–736; 1985.
15. Gupta, A., Novick, B. E. and Rubinstein, A. Restoration of suppressor T-cell functions in children with AIDS following intravenous gamma globulin treatment. *Am. J. Dis. Child.* **140**: 143–146; 1986.
16. Kopelman, R. G. and Zolla-Pazner, S. Association of human immunodeficiency virus infection and autoimmune phenomena. *Am. J. Med.* **84**: 82–88; 1988.
17. Ellaurie, M., Burns, E. R., Bernstein, L. J. *et al.* Thrombocytopenia and human immunodeficiency virus in children. *Pediatrics* **82**: 905–908; 1988.
18. Weinblatt, M. E., Scimeca, P. G., James-Herry, A. G. and Pahwa, S. Thrombocytopenia in an infant with AIDS. *Am. J. Dis. Child.* **141**: 15; 1987.
19. Weinblatt, M. Thrombocytopenia and pediatric patients with AIDS. *Pediatrics* **84**: 401–402; 1989.
20. Imbach, P., Barandun, S., d'Apuzzo, V. *et al.* High-dose intravenous gammaglobulin for idiopathic thrombocytopenic purpura in childhood. *Lancet* **1**: 1228–1231; 1981.
21. Kawada, K. and Terasaki, P. I. Evidence for immunosuppression

by high-dose gammaglobulin. *Exp. Hematol.* 15: 133–136; 1987.
22. Siegal, F. P. and Oleske, J. M. Management of the acquired immune deficiency syndrome: is there a role for immune globulins? *In* "Clinical Use of Intravenous Immunoglobulins" (Eds Morell, A. and Nydegger, U. E.), pp. 373–383. Academic Press, London; 1986.
23. Oleske, J. M., Connor, E. M., Bobila, R. *et al.* The use of IVIG in children with AIDS. *Vox Sang.* 52: 172; 1987.
24. Schaad, U. B., Gianella-Borradori, A., Perret, B. *et al.* Intravenous immune globulin in symptomatic paediatric human immunodeficiency virus infection. *Eur. J. Pediatr.* 147: 300–303; 1988.
25. Williams, P. E., Hague, R. A., Yap, P. L. *et al.* Treatment of human immunodeficiency virus antibody positive children with intravenous immunoglobulin. *J. Hosp. Infect.* 12: (Suppl. D): 67–73; 1988.
26. Hunziker, U. A., Nadal, D., Jendis, J. J. *et al.* Stable human immunodeficiency virus encephalopathy in two infants receiving early intravenous gammaglobulin plus antimicrobial prophylaxis. *Eur. J. Pediatr.* 148: 417–422; 1989.
27. Woods, C. C., McNamara, J. G., Schwarz, D. F. *et al.* Prevention of pneumococcal bacteremia in a child with acquired immunodeficiency syndrome-related complex. *Pediatr. Infect. Dis. J.* 6: 654–656; 1987.
28. Schreiber, A. D., Chien, P., Tomaski, A. and Cines, D. B. Effect of danazol in immune thrombocytopenic purpura. *N. Engl. J. Med.* 316: 503–508; 1987.
29. Oksenhendler, E., Bierling, P., Brossard, Y. *et al.* Anti-Rh immunoglobulin therapy for human immunodeficiency virus-related immune thrombocytopenic purpura. *Blood* 71: 1499–1502; 1988.
30. Yap, P. L. and Williams, P. E. Immunoglobulin preparations for HIV-infected patients. *Vox Sang.* 55: 65–74; 1988.

Discussion

R. Stricker
You mentioned that only one-third of patients with thrombocytopenia respond to IVIG. Do you have any data on clinical indications on which patients will respond to IVIG and which patients will not?

U. B. Schaad
There are no clinical or laboratory findings that would predict the response of HIV-associated immune-mediated thrombocytopenia to IVIG. It is evident that other mechanisms for thrombocytopenia such as post-infectious bone marrow aplasia must be excluded.

A. Brand
Is there any correction of oligoclonal hypergammaglobulinemia after IVIG substitution indicating immunomodulation?

U. B. Schaad
According to our studies, the polyclonal hypergammaglobulinemia is not clearly altered by IVIG substitution. However, we have observed a decrease of total serum IgG concentrations after years of regular IVIG treatment in some AIDS patients, but detailed analyses have not yet been performed.

C. J. Baker
It has been observed that pediatric patients with HIV infection are a heterogeneous group in their clinical manifestations. For example, those with lymphoid interstitial pneumonitis have an indolent course in which bacterial or opportunistic infections are rare. It is quite likely, therefore, that the large, multicenter trials in the USA comparing either IVIG to placebo or zidovidine (AZT) plus IVIG or placebo will show efficacy only in a select group of patients with repeated bacterial infections. Would you comment on this please?

U. B. Schaad
I fully agree with these statements. The indication for IVIG treatment in pediatric AIDS should most probably include clinical or laboratory evidence of impaired functional antibody response to bacterial and/or viral antigens.

Intravenous immunoglobulin in marrow transplantation

NEENA KAPOOR

The Ohio State University, Bone Marrow Transplantation Division, Columbus, Ohio, USA

Bone marrow transplantation in the last two decades has evolved from experimental therapy to accepted frontline treatment for many lethal and sublethal disorders. An increasing number of patients are undergoing allogeneic matched related and unrelated bone marrow transplant, autologous bone marrow transplant, mismatched related marrow transplant, and autologous and allogeneic peripheral stem cell transplant. To prepare for the acceptance of marrow graft, the prospective patient is given an aggressive myeloablative and immunosuppressive regimen or they already are immunocompromised due to their underlying disease such as classical severe combined immunodeficiency. The preparative regimen markedly weakens the physical barriers such as the skin, mucosal membrane of the gastrointestinal tract, and bronchial mucosa. In addition, the conditioning regimen invariably leads to complete aplasia and virtually total immune deficiency. Restoration of lymphohematopoietic function through donor graft occurs in stages (1, 2). Though granulocytopenia and lymphopenia generally last for 3–4 weeks after marrow transplant, functions of these hematopoietic elements are not evident for several months and often not completed until 1–2 years after transplantation.

Immunotherapy with Intravenous Immunoglobulins
ISBN 0–12–370725–0

The bone marrow transplant recipient initially has combined immunodeficiency, progressing later to a T-cell deficiency. This immunodeficiency has somewhat predictable time kinetics, starting with the conditioning regimen which eliminates all the host hematopoietic and immunological system for several weeks, when bone marrow function begins to return with increase in leukocytes in peripheral blood. Even though peripheral neutrophil count may become greater than 5×10^8/l, the functional capacity of these cells such as chemotaxis, phagocytosis, and intracellular kill is significantly compromised for a period of 3–6 months. Initially, with the reconstitution of the lymphoid system, there is a predominance of CD8-positive lymphocytes. CD4-positive cell recovery is delayed in almost all types of transplantation irrespective of conditioning regimen or preparation of bone marrow inoculum.

The lymphocyte blast transformation in response to mitogens, antigens, and allogeneic cells is suppressed for 3–9 months post-transplant. There is decreased production of IL-2 and this defect is further perpetuated by the use of cyclosporine and steroid for the prevention of graft-versus-host disease (GVHD). In the event of the development of acute or chronic GVHD there is injury to various tissues, and to control GVHD more aggressive immunosuppressive therapy is needed which in turn worsens the immunocompetence of the patient.

Through the initial stages of transplantation patients also have poor humoral immunity. Serum immunoglobulin levels fall due to the decline in production because of the elimination of functional B cells following immunosuppressive regimen and the delay in functions of newly engrafted B cells due to the lack of helper T cells. Such immune status may last for 1–2 years post-transplant, even in cases where no other transplant-related complication is noted. During initial stages patients also have high catabolism of immunoglobulin. A significant amount may be lost due to protein loss through the enteral route because of diarrhea secondary to chemotherapy, radiation therapy, graft-vs-host disease, or due to infectious gastroenteritis. During this period not only is there disruption of the mucosal barrier but also the disappearance of IgA and IgM plasma cells from lamina propria due to mucosal injury. Thus, no secretory antibodies are produced to neutralize the microorganisms in the gut lumen to prevent their entry through the mucosal surface and production of invasive systemic disease. Even if there is a normal uncomplicated course following marrow transplant, patients serum immunoglobulin level declines to less than 50% of the normal level by 3 weeks after transplant, and these levels fall further in ensuing months. Though B-cell function of donor origin can be seen as early as 1 month post-transplant, T-cell-helper function for the production of immunoglobulin starts returning during the second month. Normal immunoglobulin is not reached until at least 4 months after marrow grafting and does not return to a full complement of subclasses until approximately 1 year post-grafting. During the first year post-transplant period these patients continue to show the clinical features similar to patients with primary hypogammaglobulinemia or common variable immunodeficiency.

Considering the profound and global defects in host defenses accompanying bone marrow transplantation, infectious complications such as sepsis, interstitial pneumonia, cystitis, enteritis, and triggering of GVHD following infection are well-recognized causes of morbidity and mortality in bone marrow transplant recipients (3–4). Attempts are made to prevent these complications by nursing the patient in protected isolation, laminar air flow room, complete or selective decontamination, and by providing passive immunity with intravenous gammaglobulin (5).

Since the availability of intravenous preparation of gammaglobulin, various studies have been carried out to determine its role in prevention of infections, especially CMV and interstitial pneumonia which had invariably fatal outcome once established in the marrow transplant recipients (6).

The prophylactic trials have been carried out with standard preparations of IVIG and with hyperimmune gammaglobulin (7). Consensus of data is that in CMV-seronegative recipients who receive CMV-seronegative bone marrow and CMV-seronegative blood products, IVIG can prevent acquisition of new infection. In CMV-seropositive recipients patient may develop infection but have decreased incidence of CMV pneumonia.

At our institution, patients are generally prepared for bone marrow transplant with a combination regimen of Busulfan and cyclophosphamide and patients receive cyclosporine and methylprednisolone as GVHD prophylaxis (8). As a part of passive immunity, patients are given IVIG 500 mg/kg every 2 weeks. Average trough level of serum IgG in these patients is 600 mg/dl. This regimen of gammaglobulin infusion every 2 weeks is carried out for 4 months post-transplant. By that time the patient's catabolism of immunoglobulin is decreased and we are able to maintain normal physiological levels of serum immunoglobulin by monthly infusion. This is in contrast to some of the other studies, where an initial weekly infusion of intravenous gammaglobulin appeared necessary to maintain protective levels of serum immunoglobulin. The difference is probably related to conditioning regimen.

With our regimen we have had a 2% incidence of documented bacteremia within the first 30 days post-transplant (our median discharge time is 25 days). In the CMV-negative patients who received CMV-negative or -positive bone marrow and CMV-negative blood products 3% developed CMV infection. None developed CMV pneumonia. The study suggests that prophylactic immunoglobulin administered to CMV-seronegative bone marrow transplant recipients prevents CMV infection. Furthermore, even in CMV-seropositive bone marrow recipients IVIG appears to reduce the incidence of interstitial pneumonia (9). In established invasive systemic disease, interstitial pneumonia, IVIG alone is not very effective in the treatment; however, in combination with gancyclovir IVIG can effectively treat 50% of the cases of CMV disease (10). Of course early institution of such therapy is the key factor for successful outcome.

Improvement of survival with the institution of IVIG is not only related to decreased incidence of CMV infections but it also prevents other viral and bacterial infections by providing neutralizing antibodies and opsonizing antibodies even during the time when the patient is away from the protective environment during the post-transplant period for almost 1 year or longer. Rationale for such therapy came from observations made by us and others. IgG subclasses IgG_2 and IgG_4 may be quite deficient for a period of time, predisposing the patients to the infections related to encapsulated organisms, such as step pneumoniae or hemophilus influenza (11). This subclass deficiency was noted in spite of a normal serum IgG level. Again in this circumstance immunoglobulin provided the specific and opsonizing antibodies, however, the prevention of such infection is still best achieved with the combination of IVIG and prophylactic antibiotics. Antibiotics alone have not provided adequate protection. In a few patients the IgG subclass deficiency is persistent even 4 years after transplant and the continuation of replacement therapy is necessary.

As mentioned earlier, during the early post-transplant period the gastrointestinal tract is severely affected by the preparative regimen for bone marrow transplant with the development of ulcers, denudation of mucosal membranes, disappearance of plasma cells from Peyer's patches, and lack of neutralizing antibodies. In such instances, replication of viruses and other organisms can occur unrestricted. This further accentuates the mucosal injury and invasion of mucosal membranes by these microorganisms.

On the basis of several animal studies we presume that IgG might be effective in modifying rotovirus infection in humans. Having studied the degradation of IgG given orally, it has been shown that IgG antibody survives passage through the gastrointestinal tract and emerges as intact molecules. In a pilot study at our institution where 30 patients were given IVIG preparation orally in doses of 50 mg/kg/day for 4 weeks. Prior to administration of oral gammaglobulin, no IgG could be demonstrated in the stool. Following an approximate 3-week period, two-thirds of the patients had levels up to 400 mg/dl in the stool. In this pilot study only one patient developed adenovirus gastroenteritis (12). Subsequently, a double blood study has been carried out to determine the efficacy of such therapy in prevention of enteritis in the immediate post-transplant period when morbidity related to such disease processes is highest.

The role of IVIG in the prevention and treatment of GVHD is most intriguing. Such effect of IVIG could be because of its role in prevention of infection and treatment of infection. Infections do set the stage for the development of GVHD by turning on cytotoxic cells which, in turn, could become alloreactive and effector cells in the process of GVHD. Whether IVIG has a role in causing direct immunomodulation and thus prevents or treats GVHD remains to be determined.

There are many steps in bone marrow transplantation where IVIG has played a big role singularly or in combination with another therapeutic agent in improving the survival of transplant recipients. As we are learning more about transplantation immunology, the role of these biological agents, such as gammaglobulin, needs to be further explored so that such agents can be utilized judiciously and effectively.

Summary

Bone marrow transplantation recipients develop combined immunodeficiency due to the myeloablative and immunosuppressive pretransplant conditioning regimen. Following marrow transplant, it takes 1–2 years for complete restoration of immune competence. During this immunocompromised state, patients are at high risk to develop infectious complications. Passive immunity with intravenous gammaglobulin has significantly reduced the infection related morbidity and mortality during all phases of the post transplant period. The full contribution of IVIG in modulating transplant biology is being evaluated.

References

1. Witherspoon, R. P. Suppression and recovery of immunologic function after bone marrow transplantation. *J. Natl. Cancer Inst.* **76**: 1321–1329; 1986.
2. Lum, L. G., Orcutt-Thordasson, N. and Seihneuret, M. C. The regulation of IG synthesis after marrow transplantation. *J. Immunol.* 129: 113; 1982.
3. Winston, D. J., Gale, R. P., Meyer, D. V. and Young, L. S. Infectious complications human bone marrow transplantation. *Medicine (Baltimore)* **58** (1): 1; 1979.
4. Pollard, M., Chang, C. F. and Shrivasta, K. U. The role of microflora in development of graft-vs-host disease. *Transplant. Proc.* **8**: 533; 1976.
5. Peterson, F. B., Bowden, R. A., Thornquist, J. D. *et al.* The effect of prophylactic intravenous immune globulin on the incidence of septicemia in marrow transplant recipients. *Bone Marrow Transplant.* **2**: 141; 1987.
6. Winston, D. J., Ho, W. G., Lin, C.-H. *et al.* Intravenous immune globulin for prevention of cytomegalovirus infection and interstitial pneumonia after bone marrow transplantation. *Ann. Intern. Med.* **106**: 12; 1987.
7. Reed, E. C., Bowden, R. A., Dandliker, P. S. and Meyers, J. D. Efficacy of cytomegalovirus immunoglobulin in marrow transplant recipients with cytomegalovirus pneumonia. *J. Infect. Dis.* **156**: 641; 1987.
8. Tutschka, P. J., Copelan, E. A. and Kline, J. Bone marrow transplantation for leukemia following new busulfan and cyclophosphamide regimen. *Blood* **70**: 1382; 1987.
9. Kapoor, N., Copelan, E. A. and Tutschka, P. J. Cytomegalovirus infection in bone marrow transplant recipients: Use of intravenous gammaglobulin as prophylactic and therapeutic agent. *Transplant. Proc.* **XXI**: 3095; 1989.
10. Emanuel, D., Cunningham, I., Jules-Elysee, K. *et al.* Cytomegalovirus pneumonia after bone marrow transplantation successfully treated with the combination of gancyclovir and high-dose intravenous gammaglobulin. *Ann. Intern. Med.* **109**: 777; 1988.
11. Sheridan, J. F., Tutschka, P. J., Sedmak, D. D. and Copelan, E. A. Immunoglobulin G subclass deficiency and pneumococcal infection after allogeneic bone marrow transplantation. *Blood* 75(7): 1583; 1990.
12. Copelan, E. A., Sheridan, J. F., Neff, J. C. *et al.* Oral administration of immunoglobulin in marrow transplant recipients. *Exp. Hemat.* 12(5): 362; 1985.

Discussion

G. Lanzer
Is the relapse rate in the IVIG-treated group changed (graft-vs.-leukemia reaction)?

N. Kapoor
In our study, high disease-risk patients with GVHD had a lower incidence of relapse, but the overall survival was not changed, because of fatal complications related to infections. In the standard disease-risk group, GVHD decreased the overall survival, due to infections. Patients without GVHD in this group had a better survival. At present our assumption is that IVIG is only one of many contributing factors playing a role in GVHD.

G. Krueger
Can you please more specifically identify the type of GVHD which is influenced by IVIG? Is it the classical acute GVHD (i.e. cytotoxic T-cell response against epidermal–mucosal–hepatic cells, etc.), or is it rather the chronic GVHD (i.e. wasting, SLE-type changes, interstitial pneumonia), which has probably a different mechanism?

N. Kapoor
Infections play a role both in acute and chronic forms of GVHD. Concomitant with infection, generation of CD8 cells occurs, which probably function as cytotoxic cells. As I mentioned earlier, the effect of IVIG on GVHD is primarily by controlling infections. The possible modulatory influence of IVIG on functions of cytotoxic T cells, on blocking of Fc receptors and on interference with immune responses are topics of upcoming investigations.

Intravenous immunoglobulin for cytomegalovirus pneumonia

GERALD ELFENBEIN[1], JEFFREY KRISCHER[2], JOHN GRAHAM-POLE[2], RICHARD HONG[3], JAN JANSEN[4], HILLARD LAZARUS[5], ELLIOT WINTON[6] and RONALD BABINGTON[7]

The Bone Marrow Transplantation Programs of [1] University of South Florida, Tampa, Florida, USA; [2] University of Florida, Gainesville, Florida, USA; [3] University of Wisconsin, Madison, Wisconsin, USA; [4] Indiana University, Indianapolis, Indiana, USA; [5] Case Western Reserve University, Cleveland, Ohio, USA; [6] Emory University, Atlanta, Georgia, USA; [7] Sandoz Pharmaceuticals, Hanover, New Jersey, USA

Introduction

In the 1990s we now feel confident that allogeneic bone marrow transplantation (BMT) is a curative procedure for severe aplastic anemia, acute myelogenous leukemia, acute lymphoblastic leukemia, chronic myelocytic leukemia, and a growing list of miscellaneous malignant and non-malignant lymphohematopoietic diseases and inherited disorders of metabolism. Approximately 5000 allogeneic BMTs are performed annually worldwide. There still remain a number of clinical problems which limit the ultimate success of BMT. Chief among these are relapse of the malignant disease and infection either in the setting of acute or chronic graft-versus-host disease (GVHD) or not. One of the most common infections experienced by allogeneic BMT recipients is caused by cytomegalovirus (CMV)

Immunotherapy with Intravenous Immunoglobulins
ISBN 0-12-370725-0

and the most severe form of CMV disease is interstitial pneumonitis (IP).

In 1985 we designed a prospective, multicenter, single-arm clinical trial to address this problem. The study was based upon the results of three randomized controlled trials performed over the preceding 5 years which had shown that pooled human intravenous immunoglobulin (IVIG) effectively prevented CMV IP after allogeneic BMT (1–3). Each of these studies had enrolled only a small number of patients and none of the studies used an IVIG preparation which was commercially available in the United States at the time our study was conducted. Also, at the time of study development there was no effective therapy for CMV IP; usually, 90% of affected patients died. Thus, the principal objective of our study was to prevent CMV IP and, hence, prevent death from CMV IP after allogeneic BMT in a large number of patients at five institutions using five different non-prescreened lots of a commercially available IVIG product. The intent was to simulate the conditions of clinical practice. The hope was that the data would provide useful information for rational decision-making about the use of IVIG for allogeneic BMT recipients in a variety of clinical settings.

Methods

All enrolled patients gave informed consent to participate in this study which was approved and reviewed annually by the institutional review boards of each of the five treating institutions, which were the Universities of Florida and Wisconsin and Case Western Reserve, Emory, and Indiana Universities. The study commenced in November 1985, and closed in June 1988. Consecutive eligible patients were enrolled at each institution. Entry criteria included disease and BMT preparative regimen including at least 450 cGy of total body irradiation (TBI). Balanced accrual was obligatory and total accrual was limited to 182 patients.

Each patient received 500 mg/kg of IVIG (Sandoglobulin®) beginning 8 days before BMT and continuing weekly for a total of 16 doses. Every patient was followed for 150 days after BMT for survival, development of any form of IP, development of CMV IP, and death due to CMV IP. Data concerning donor–recipient HLA matching, acute GVHD prophylaxis, and supportive care were reported on forms designed by the statistics office. When a case of IP was detected, aggressive invasive methods for the diagnosis of the etiologic agent were mandated by the protocol which required histopathologic, cytologic and viral culture studies for CMV. Other outcome data were collected, including the development of acute GVHD and all documented infections. A second report was filed for each patient at least one year after the close of the study at which time data concerning chronic GVHD, relapse, and late infections were reported. This communication is a final report for the first 150 days after BMT for all 182 patients (4, 5). The remainder of the data collected by this study will be reported in full detail elsewhere.

Results

Enrolled in the study were 107 male and 75 female, 170 white and 12 non-white patients. There were 22 patients aged 0–9 years, 32 aged 10–19, 49 aged 20–29, 55 aged 30–39, 23 aged 40–49, and 1 patient over 50. The diagnosis was acute myelogenous leukemia in 57 patients of whom 37 were in first remission, chronic myelocytic leukemia in 56 patients of whom 47 were in first chronic phase, or acute lymphoblastic leukemia in 40 patients of whom 31 were in first ($n = 10$) or second ($n = 21$) remission. The remainder of the patients had severe aplastic anemia ($n = 12$), myelodysplastic syndrome ($n = 5$), or miscellaneous disorders ($n = 12$) including lymphomas, neuroblastoma, biphenotypic acute leukemia, and multiple myeloma. The Karnofsky performance score was 90–100% for 154, 70–89% for 22, and 30–69% for 6 patients.

Donors were genotypically HLA identical siblings for 165 patients and at-least-one-haplotype-identical relatives for 17 patients. TBI cumulative doses were 450–600 cGy for 38, 601–900 cGy for 37, 901–1200 cGy for 66, and 1320–1375 cGy for 41 patients. Acute GVHD prophylaxis was methotrexate ± prednisone for 28, cyclosporine ± methotrexate for 99, *ex vivo* T-cell depletion ± cyclosporine and methotrexate for 35, and cyclophosphamide ± methotrexate for 3 patients. Seventeen recipients of genotypically HLA identical sibling grafts received no prophylaxis for acute GVHD. The development, time to onset and maximum grade of severity of acute GVHD was recorded for all patients. We observed acute GVHD of grade 0 in 93, grade 1 in 26, grade 2 in 23, grade 3 in 11 and grade 4 in 29 patients.

CMV serology was recorded for all patients, donors and blood products transfused. In 51 cases the patient, donor and blood products were all CMV seronegative. In 38 cases the patient was CMV seronegative but either the donor was CMV seropositive or the blood products were unscreened for CMV serostatus. In the remaining 103 cases the recipient was CMV seropositive. Within the first 150 days after allogeneic BMT there were 39 cases of IP of which 14 were identified to be associated with CMV. The attack rate of any IP was 21%, the attack rate of CMV IP was 7.7%. CMV was associated with 36% of the cases of IP.

Using a time-dependent, proportional hazards, general linear model, multivariate analyses were performed using the variables discussed above where the independent variable was CMV IP within 150 days after allogeneic BMT. From this analysis the following variables were found to be independently associated with the development of CMV IP in the setting of prophylaxis with IVIG: (1) age over 40 ($P = 0.04$), (2) diagnosis of acute lymphoblastic leukemia ($P = 0.02$), (3) recipient CMV seropositivity ($P = 0.04$), (4) acute GVHD grades 3 and 4 ($P = 0.02$), (5) cumulative dose of TBI more than 1300 cGy ($P = 0.01$) and (6) *ex vivo* T-cell depletion to prevent acute GVHD ($P = 0.02$). For these variables the following are the hazard ratios with the 95% confidence intervals given in parentheses: (1) age over 40: 3.9 (1.0–14.5), (2) acute lymphoblastic leukemia: 4.9 (1.2–19.3), (3) more than 1300 cGy TBI: 4.4 (1.4–14.0), (4) more than grade 2 acute GVHD: 3.8 (1.2–12.0), (5) T-cell depletion to prevent acute GVHD: 3.9 (1.0–12.4), and (6) CMV seropositivity of patient: 3.6 (1.0–12.3).

Discussion

One of the major objectives of this prospective, multicenter, single-arm trial was to simulate the conditions encountered in the clinical practice of allogeneic BMT. We feel that this objective has admirably been met as shown by the diversity of patient ages, diagnoses, disease stages, BMT preparative regimens in terms of TBI dosages, genetics of HLA matching, techniques to prevent acute GVHD, development of acute GVHD, and CMV serostatus of the patient, donor and blood products. Although some investigators may consider this lack of homogeneity a weakness of this study, we consider this diversity a strength as it gives broader limits for the study permitting interpolations rather than extrapolations, which narrowly designed homogeneous studies mandate, when trying to determine what to do for individual patients in the future.

A second criticism which may be leveled at this study is that it is not a placebo-controlled trial. We believe that the indication for using IVIG to prevent CMV IP after allogeneic BMT was established by the three previous controlled trials (1–3), and confirmed by a subsequent study of our own (6). Our purpose, then, was to establish the frequency of CMV

IP when a new human IVIG was used as prophylaxis in the setting of allogeneic BMT. For a period of time during the study, Sandoglobulin® was the only FDA-approved product that had any data (or was under study) to support its (potential) role in BMT recipients. The large size of our patient population studied lends confidence to the finding of a low attack rate of CMV IP when Sandoglobulin® is used as prophylaxis. This is all the more meaningful when one recalls that five different non-prescreened lots of Sandoglobulin® were utilized (7).

The most remarkable finding of our study is that the attack rate of CMV IP was only 7.7% when weekly, large (500 mg/kg) doses of Sandoglobulin® were employed from one week before through 14 weeks after allogeneic BMT. In the subset of our patients who were CMV seropositive (n = 103), the attack rate of CMV IP was only 9.1%. This certainly compares favorably with the attack rate for high-dose acyclovir-treated (n = 86) as well as for control subjects (n = 65) in a recent, dual institution report where the attack rates for CMV IP in the first 100 days after allogeneic BMT were 19% and 31%, respectively (8).

Critics of the role for IVIG as prophylaxis for CMV IP highlight not only the acyclovir trial mentioned above but also two other studies. The first trial (9) demonstrated nicely the role of CMV-seronegative blood products as prophylaxis for CMV IP when both the patient and the donor were CMV seronegative. However, as our study with consecutive entry of non-preselected patients shows, this fortunate circumstance occurred unfortunately for only 28% of our patients. Thus, the use of CMV-seronegative blood products would not have been indicated for 72% of our patients. The second trial (10) failed to demonstrate the value of an IVIG preparation in a controlled study. In this trial the untreated group was rather small (n = 27) and the attack rate of CMV IP for this group was uncharacteristically low (11%). Moreover, the dose of IVIG was low and the interval between infusions was long. We (11) and others (12) have demonstrated that the half-life of transfused IgG anti-CMV antibodies is rather brief when the source of antibodies is from a pooled donor preparation of IVIG. Thus, to our thinking this negative report (10) does not vitiate against the value of IVIG as prophylaxis for CMV IP after allogeneic BMT.

Two new risk factors for CMV IP after allogeneic BMT have surfaced from the multivariate analysis of our data. They are T-cell depletion of the donor marrow to prevent acute GVHD and the diagnosis of acute lymphoblastic leukemia. For acute lymphoblastic leukemia we have no explanation to offer why this may be an independent risk factor. For T-cell depletion, however, we may speculate why this may be an independent risk factor. Perhaps, the donor marrow does, indeed, confer some level of protective cellular immunity against CMV, i.e. adoptive immunity, that T-cell depletion selectively removes. Under appropriate circumstances (13, 14) adoptive immunity can be demonstrated after allogeneic BMT and, at least, one other group of investigators (15) have reported that T-cell depletion to prevent acute GVHD may increase rather than decrease the attack rate of CMV IP. Furthermore, another group of investigators (M. Trigg, *et al.*, personal communication) have reported increased opportunistic viral and fungal infections after T-cell-depleted bone marrow transplants. The other significant risk factors that were detected in this study have already been described or have long been suspected, e.g. moderate to severe acute GVHD, patient CMV seropositivity, high-dose TBI, and patient age (16, 17).

There is one more area that deserves a brief discussion before closing, even though it does not bear directly on CMV IP. That is the topic of additional benefits that IVIG may bring to the allogeneic BMT patient when it is being employed to prevent CMV IP. IVIG has been reported not only to decrease the death rate from CMV IP but also from all other infectious causes of death (18–20). IVIG has also been reported to decrease the incidence of acute GVHD (3, 20). Finally, IVIG has sometimes been useful in the therapy of platelet transfusion refractory states (21). For all its high dollar costs, IVIG is essentially non-toxic and has a variety of positive benefits for the allogeneic BMT recipient. It is not yet clear, however, that IVIG has any beneficial role in autologous BMT.

Summary

This communication reports the results of a prospective, multicenter, single-arm trial of intravenous immunoglobulin as prophylaxis against cytomegalovirus pneumonia after allogeneic bone marrow transplantation. The results for a total of 182 consecutively enrolled, eligible patients, who received at least 450 cGy of total body irradiation as part of their preparation for bone marrow transplantation, are reported. The attack rate for cytomegalovirus pneumonia in the entire population was only 7.7% during the first 150 days after allogeneic bone marrow transplantation when 500 mg/kg intravenous immunoglobulin was given weekly beginning one week before transplant through 14 weeks after transplant. In the subpopulation of 103 patients who were cytomegalovirus seropositive prior to allogeneic bone marrow transplantation, the attack rate was only 9.1%. From a time dependent, multivariate analysis, six independent risk factors for cytomegalovirus pneumonia were identified in this study. They are: (a) age over 40

($P = 0.04$), (b) diagnosis of acute lymphoblastic leukemia ($P = 0.02$), (c) patient seropositive for cytomegalovirus ($P = 0.04$), (d) moderate to severe acute graft-versus-host disease ($P = 0.02$), (e) cumulative dose of total body irradiation over 1200 cGy ($P = 0.01$), and (f) *ex vivo* T-cell depletion of donor marrow to prevent acute graft-versus-host disease ($P = 0.02$).

References

1. Condie, R. M. and O'Reilly, R. J. Prevention of infection by prophylaxis with an intravenous hyperimmune, native, unmodified cytomegalovirus globulin. *Am. J. Med.* 76 (Suppl. 3A): 134; 1984.
2. Kubanek, B., Ernst, P., Ostendorff, P. *et al.* Preliminary data of a controlled trial of intravenous hyperimmune globulin in the prevention of cytomegalovirus infection in bone marrow transplantation. *Transplant. Proc.* 17: 468; 1985.
3. Winston, D. J., Ho, W. G., Lin, C. H. *et al.* Intravenous immunoglobulin for prevention of interstitial pneumonia after bone marrow transplantation. *Ann. Intern. Med.* 106: 12; 1987.
4. Elfenbein, G. J., Krischer, J., Rand, K. H. *et al.* Preliminary results of a multicenter trial to prevent death after cytomegalovirus pneumonia with intravenous immunoglobulin after allogeneic bone marrow transplantation. *Transplant. Proc.* 19: 138; 1987.
5. Elfenbein, G. J., Krischer, J., Babington, R. *et al.* Interim results of a multicenter trial to prevent cytomegalovirus pneumonia after allogeneic bone marrow transplantation. *Transplant. Proc.* 21: 3099; 1989.
6. Elfenbein, G. J., Siddiqui, T., Rand, K. H. *et al.* Successful strategy for preventing cytomegalovirus interstitial pneumonia after HLA-identical bone marrow transplantation. *Rev. Infect. Dis.* 12: S805; 1990.
7. Chehimi, J., Peppard, J. and Emanuel, D. Selection of an intravenous immunoglobulins for the immunoprophylaxis of cytomegalovirus infections: An *in vitro* comparison of currently available and previously effective immunoglobulins. *Bone Marrow Transplant.* 2: 395; 1987.
8. Meyers, J. D., Reed, E. C., Shepp, D. H. *et al.* Acyclovir for prevention of cytomegalovirus infection and disease after allogeneic marrow transplantation. *N. Engl. J. Med.* 138: 70; 1988.
9. Bowden, R. A., Sayers, M., Flournoy, N. *et al.* Cytomegalovirus immune globulin and seronegative blood products to prevent cytomegalovirus infection after marrow transplantation. *N. Engl. J. Med.* 314: 1006; 1986.
10. Ringden, O., Pihlstedt, P., Volin, L. *et al.* Failure to prevent cytomegalovirus infection by cytomegalovirus hyperimmune plasma: A randomized trial by the Nordic Bone Marrow Transplantation Group. *Bone Marrow Transplant.* 2: 299; 1987.

11. Rand, K. H., Houck, H., Ganju, A. *et al.* Pharmacokinetics of cytomegalovirus specific IgG antibody following intravenous immunoglobulin in bone marrow transplant patients. *Bone Marrow Transplant.* 4: 679; 1989.
12. Hagenbeck, A., Brummelhuis, G. J., Donkers, A. *et al.* Rapid clearance of cytomegalovirus-specific IgG after repeated intravenous infusions of human immunoglobulin into allogeneic bone marrow transplant recipients. *J. Infect. Dis.* 155: 897; 1987.
13. Drummond, J. E., Shah, K. V., Saral, R. *et al.* BK virus specific humoral and cell mediated immunity in allogeneic bone marrow transplantation (BMT) recipients. *J. Med. Virol.* 23: 331; 1987.
14. Donnenberg, A. D., Hess, A. D., Noga, S. J. *et al.* Regeneration of genetically restricted immune functions after human bone marrow transplantation: Influence of four different strategies for graft-v-host disease prophylaxis. *Transplant. Proc.* 19: (Suppl. 7): 144, 1987.
15. Engelhard, D., Or, R., Strauss, N. *et al.* Cytomegalovirus infection and disease after T cell depleted allogeneic bone marrow transplantation for malignant hematologic diseases. *Transplant. Proc.* 21: 3101; 1989.
16. Meyers, J. D., Flournoy, J. C. and Wade, M. C. Biology of interstitial pneumonia after marrow transplantation. *In* "Recent Advances in Bone Marrow Transplantation" (Ed. Gale, R. P.), p. 405. Alan R. Liss, New York; 1983.
17. Weiner, R. S., Bortin, M. M., Gale, R. P. *et al.* Interstitial pneumonitis after bone marrow transplantation. *Ann. Intern. Med.* 104: 168; 1986.
18. Graham-Pole, J., Camitta, B., Casper, J. *et al.* Intravenous immunoglobulin may lessen all forms of infection in patients receiving allogeneic bone marrow transplantation for acute leukemia. *Bone Marrow Transplant.* 3: 559; 1988.
19. Graham-Pole, J., Elfenbein, G., Amylon, M. *et al.* The use of intravenous immunoglobulin for preventing systemic infections after allogeneic marrow transplantation: A randomized comparison of two dose regimens. *Am. J. Pediatr. Hemat. Onc.* (In press).
20. Sullivan, K. M., Kopecky, K., Jocom, J. *et al.* Antimicrobial and immunomodulatory effects of intravenous immunoglobulin in bone marrow transplantation. *Blood* 72: 410a; 1988.
21. Kekomaki, R., Elfenbein, G. J., Gardner, R. *et al.* Improved response of patients to random-donor platelet transfusions by intravenous gammaglobulin. *Am. J. Med.* 76(3A): 199; 1984.

Discussion

V. Blanchette

Can you comment on the use of extreme leukodepletion by filtration of transfused blood products to prevent or reduce the incidence of CMV infection in the setting of bone marrow transplantation?

G. Elfenbein
Leukodepletion may prevent the transfer of CMV viral genome to the BMT recipient. It will take a carefully designed trial of CMV-seronegative blood products versus leukodepleted CMV-seropositive blood products in the setting that both the BMT donor and recipient are CMV seronegative to prove the point.

D. Engelhard
1. What were your criteria for CMV pneumonia?
2. How many patients had CMV viremia, and how many of these developed CMV pneumonia?
3. How many patients died of other causes than CMV pneumonia during the study period, and how many of those had CMV disease such as enteritis?
4. If I understood you well, you had a relatively high number of patients who developed CMV pneumonia although they, the donors and the blood products, were seronegative!

G. Elfenbein
1. The diagnosis of CMV IP was made by lung biopsy or broncho-alveolar lavage with positive cytology, immunofluorescence, histopathology, and/or culture for CMV.
2. The incidence of CMV viremia was low. I cannot, at this time, recall the incidence of CMV IP (intestitial pneumonia) in this setting.
3. From our long-term follow-up, we know that the long-term survival of our patients at 3 years is 41–50% for standard risk (early) disease and 30% for high risk (more advanced) disease. CMV IP was a minor cause of death in this series. I do not recall CMV as a significant cause of death other than by pneumonia.
4. It is true that the incidence of CMV IP was about 6% in the setting where the patient, donor and transfused blood products were all CMV seronegative. It is possible that the serologic techniques used failed to pick up all individuals who had prior exposure to CMV.

J. Kadar
To what extent did high-dose IVIG suppress or delay the antibody and IgG production of patients during the treatment period?

G. Elfenbein
Although not presented in this report, we have found in our institution five or six of 36 patients who clearly produced endogenous IgG anti-CMV antibodies with rapid and sustained rises of antibody levels far above that achieved by IVIG. At this point of our evaluation we cannot yet speak to the possible clinical correlates of this observation. To answer the question, but perhaps only indirectly, a significant proportion of our patients made antibodies to CMV while receiving IVIG. We do not know, however, the denominator, i.e.

how many should have made antibodies, to address the question of IVIG suppression of antibody production.

S. Graphakos
Your results concerning the incidence of CMV pneumonitis in T-cell depleted bone marrow transplant recipients are surprising. Did you deplete only T cells or the whole lymphocyte population from bone marrow?

G. Elfenbein
Indeed our observations concerning T-cell depletion are surprising, but were confirmed independently by Engelhard *et al.*, *Transplantation Proceedings*, 1989. I cannot comment on what additional subsets of cells were removed from the mononuclear cell population of the marrow graft as each institution performing T-cell depletion did so with their intra-institutional technology.

J. Schifferli
If there is a lot-to-lot variation of antibody titer (anti-CMV) in IVIG, did you analyze your results according to specific antibody contents? If not, you should. This might answer an important question, i.e. is IVIG effective by its specific antibody content, or by other immunomodulatory reactions.

G. Elfenbein
First, we are in the process of preparing the final report of the study for publication. We will evaluate the incidence of CMV IP by lot number to see if variability of anti-CMV antibodies from lot to lot may be correlated with the incidence of CMV IP. Second, it is possible that IVIG diminishes CMV IP by modulating (decreasing) acute GVHD. However, we must point out that in our own institutional experience IVIG did not modulate acute GVHD. From this study, we report that T-cell depletion (the best prophylaxis for acute GVHD) resulted in increased rather than decreased acute GVHD. Thus, the prevention of acute GVHD by T-cell depletion did not decrease CMV IP, and, whether or not IVIG modulates acute GVHD is not entirely clear.

The effect of prophylactic immune globulin on cytomegalovirus infection in liver transplants

JOSEPH B. COFER, CHRISTINE A. MORRIS, WILLIAM L. SUTKER,[1] BO S. HUSBERG, ROBERT M. GOLDSTEIN, THOMAS A. GONWA and GORAN B. KLINTMALM

Transplantation Services and [1]Department of Internal Medicine, Baylor University Medical Center, Dallas, Texas, USA

Introduction

Cytomegalovirus (CMV) is a common cause of infection in the liver transplant recipient, reportedly occurring in 39–57% (1, 2) of patients. The impact of CMV can be severe, leading to fatal pneumonitis or hepatitis, or impairing the immune system (3, 4) so as to increase bacterial infections and possibly triggering rejection (2, 5, 6). Prevention and treatment of CMV infections are of utmost importance in transplantation.

Passive immunoglobulin (IgG) infusion has been shown to be helpful in treating renal transplant recipients (7, 8), bone marrow recipients (9), and selected groups of liver transplant recipients (10–13). The purpose of this study was to assess the efficacy of intravenous immunoglobulin (IVIG) in decreasing the incidence and severity of CMV infection in the liver transplant recipient.

Immunotherapy with Intravenous Immunoglobulins
ISBN 0–12–370725–0

Materials and methods

From 7 September 1988 to 21 May 1989, 64 orthotopic liver transplants (OLT) were performed at Baylor University Medical Center. Of these, 53 were primary OLT. Fifty of these 53 patients were entered into the study. Three patients were excluded because of inability to obtain consent in two, and the presence of Bruton's agammaglobulinema in the third, requiring biweekly IgG injection. The 50 remaining patients were randomly assigned to either the study or control group. The groups were double-blinded. The patients were followed for 12 weeks.

The study group received 500 mg/kg of human immune globulin (Sandoglobulin®) IV as a 6% solution on post-operative days 1, 7, 14, 21, 28, 42, 56, 70 and 84. The control group received albumin in a similar concentration on the same days.

Viral cultures of the throat, urine and blood were taken per protocol pre-operatively and on post-operative days 7, 14, 21, 56, 84, and when clinically indicated. All liver biopsies were submitted for viral culture. Titers of IgM and IgG for CMV were measured pre-operatively and on post-operative days 7, 14, 21, 42, and 84, similarly for EBV pre-operatively and on post-operative days 42 and HSV–1, HSV–2, and VZV pre-operatively and on post-operative day 7 and 14.

The patients were monitored for any adverse effects of solution administration, and were closely observed for any clinical or laboratory indications of viral infection.

Patients with documented CMV infections of a clinically significant nature were treated with gancyclovir (DHPG) at a dose of 5 mg/kg every 12 h, adjusted for renal function. All infections were graded for severity as outlined in Table 1.

Table 1
Scoring system for severity of CMV disease

	CMV disease score			
	1	2	3	4
Hepatitis	SGOT* < 400	400–600	> 600	Death
Pneumonitis	Positive bronchial lavage $P_AO_2 > 70$	$P_AO_2 < 70$ on room air	Intubation	Death
Enteritis	Pain, N/V	Bleeding	Bleeding and/or surgery	Death

* SGOT, Serum glutamic oxaloacetic transaminase.

Standard immunosuppressive induction includes CyA 1–1.5 mg/kg IV every 12 h with transition to 5–7.5 mg/kg po every 12 h when tolerated. The desired CyA 12-h whole-blood trough level is 250–400 ng/ml by a monoclonal radioimmune assay. Azathioprine was routinely used for the first week as 1–2 mg/kg/day and discontinued if there was no rejection. Methylprednisolone was given as a tapering dose, 200 mg/day to 20 mg/day over 5 days and then oral prednisolone at 20 mg/day was continued. Liver biopsies were performed weekly while the patient was in the hospital, and when clinically indicated. Rejection when diagnosed and confirmed by biopsy was treated with a steroid recycle, and OKT-3 was used for steroid-resistant rejections (14).

Results

In the study group there were 9 males and 16 females with a mean age of 47.7, the control group had 8 males and 17 females with a mean age of 41.5 (NS).

There were 17 patients in the study group who were CMV-positive pre-transplant, 10 of these received a CMV-positive liver and 7 received a CMV-negative graft. Eight patients were CMV-negative pre-transplant, 4 received CMV-positive grafts and 4 CMV-negative.

In the control group 22 recipients were CMV-positive and 3 CMV-negative pre-transplant. Of the positive patients 9 received CMV-positive grafts and 13 received CMV-negative allografts. All of the CMV-negative recipients received CMV-negative allografts.

Of the 25 patients entered into each group, two died in each group prior to completing the study. In the study group, one died of primary non-function and staphylococcal sepsis before he could be retransplanted and one died of a ruptured hepatic artery anastamosis associated with a pancreatic abcess. Neither of these patients had any CMV infections.

In the control group, one died of sepsis associated with a preoperative infected sternal wound and a thrombosed portal vein, and one died of post-transplant malignant lymphoproliferative disorder (LPD) prior to completing the study. The first patient had a positive blood culture for CMV but with no clinical symptoms, and had a positive lung tissue culture for CMV on autopsy. The patient who died with LPD had a positive liver culture for CMV and was on DHPG but CMV was not felt to be a significant contributing factor to his death, as the acute terminal event was sepsis and hemorrhage related to a liver biopsy.

In the study group there were 11 patients with positive CMV cultures and 8 of these developed a clinical infection requiring DHPG. There were 14 patients with positive CMV cultures in the control group with 5 patients with 6 infections requiring DHPG (NS) (Table 2). The mean severity score in the study group was 1.7 and was 2.0 in the control group (NS).

Table 2
Comparison between groups of incidence, type and severity of CMV disease

	Disease (severity)		
	Hepatitis	Pneumonitis	Enteritis
Study	5 (1, 1, 1, 2, 3)	3 (1, 1, 2)	2 (1, 3)
Control	4 (1, 1, 1, 3)	1 (3)	1 (3)

In the study group 9 patients had one rejection during the study period with 2 of these patients requiring OKT–3 after failure of steroid rejection therapy; 3 patients had 2 rejections with clearing between, one eventually receiving one course of OKT–3 and another receiving OKT–3 once and antilymphocyte globuline once. In the control group 11 patients had one rejection with 3 of these needing OKT–3 because of steroid failure, and 2 patients had 2 rejections, with one requiring OKT–3 (NS).

The groups were compared with respect to incidence of infection including bacterial and viral. In the study group there were 5 pneumonias, 1 case of urosepsis, 5 wound infections, 1 case of intra-abdominal sepsis, and 3 cases of bacteremia and the numbers in the control group were 4, 1, 3, 2, 0 respectively (NS). Finally, the two groups were compared with respect to hospital days and ICU days. The mean total hospital day stay in the study group was 36.6 days and 34.7 days in the control group (NS). The mean total time spent in ICU was 9.2 days in the study group and 9.3 days in the control group (NS).

Intra-operative packed red blood cell (PRBC) transfusions were 9.5 in the study group and 6.0 in the control group (NS) and units of fresh frozen plasma used intra-operatively were 10.1 in the study group and 5.28 in the control group ($P = 0.047$). The mean operating time was 10.0 h in the study group and 9.7 h in the control group (NS).

Comparing viral serology for CMV in the patients pre-operatively and the donor population revealed 4 CMV-negative patients in the control group and 3 CMV-negative patients in the study group who received a CMV-negative graft. All seven of these patients did not develop clinical CMV disease. There were only 4 CMV-negative recipients in the control group and none in the study group who received CMV-positive grafts. Therefore, no comparison between these groups was possible. But 3 of these 4 patients did develop significant CMV disease. The difference in the incidence of disease between CMV-negative patients who received CMV-positive livers and those who received CMV-negative livers was significant ($P = 0.02$).

Discussion

The incidence of CMV infection in our liver transplant population has been demonstrated to be 39.1% (2). CMV can cause severe hepatitis, pneumonitis, enteritis, endometritis and encephalitis, and can depress the bone marrow, impair the immune system so as to increase other bacterial infections and possibly trigger rejection (2–6). Prevention and treatment of CMV infection is a major goal in liver transplantation. Since the advent of gancyclovir, we have had an effective agent for treatment of CMV infection (15, 16). Prophylactic IV infusion of IgG has shown promise in preventing or treating CMV in some renal transplant recipients (7, 8) and bone marrow recipients (9).

Similarly IgG has been used prophylactically in treating liver transplant recipients (10–13) with good results in groups of patients. On the other hand, Rakela *et al.* (17) showed no benefit in using IgG in preventing CMV infection or decreasing severity. A difference between these studies and ours was the use of CMV hyperimmune globulin in these studies as opposed to standard pooled human IgG in our study.

Our study was designed to answer the question of efficacy of human IgG infusion in decreasing the incidence and severity of CMV disease. We were unable to demonstrate any difference between the two randomly assigned groups. None of the four deaths were attributable to CMV. The incidence of infections as measured by positive cultures or disease as measured by occurrence of signs and symptoms together with the appropriate tissue positivity for CMV were not significantly different. There was also no effect on bacterial infections or incidence of rejection. There were only four patients who were CMV-negative originally and received positive allografts, and unfortunately no counterparts in the other group existed for comparison. The high (75%) incidence of significant disease in this group though is interesting, especially when compared with the 0% incidence in the seven patients who were CMV negative pre-operatively and received negative grafts, and this difference was significant. This is especially interesting in that no effort was made to control the CMV status of blood products used in any patient.

In conclusion, we were unable to demonstrate clinical efficacy of human immune IgG used in a prophylactic fashion. We were unable to comment on that crucial group of patients who are CMV negative pre-transplant but receive a CMV-positive allograft. Based on the work of others (10–13), and our clinical experience, perhaps this selected group of liver transplant recipients would benefit from prophylactic IgG infusion. The ultimate answer though would probably be to reserve use of only CMV-negative allografts and blood products for these patients. Unfortunately, the problem with allograft supply severely limits this option.

Summary

Fifty orthotopic liver transplant recipients were entered into a randomized double blind study to test the efficacy of prophylactic human immune globulin (IgG) on preventing cytomegalovirus (CMV) infection in liver transplant recipients. The study group received 500 mg/kg of IgG in weekly doses, the control group albumin. There was no significant difference in the incidence or severity of CMV disease in the two groups. Neither was the incidence or severity of rejection, or other infections affected.

References

1. Ho, M. Infections in liver transplant recipients, *In* "Hepatic Transplantation" (Eds Winter, P. and Kang, Y. G.), p. 202. Praeger, New York; 1986.
2. Sayage, L. H., Gonwa, T. A., Goldstein, R. M., Husberg, B. S. and Klintmalm, G. B. Cytomegalovirus infection in orthotopic liver transplantation. *Transplant Int.* 2: 96–101; 1989.
3. Ware, A. J., Luby, J. P., Hollinger, B. *et al.* Etology of liver disease in renal transplant patients. *Ann. Intern. Med.* 91: 364; 1979.
4. Rand, K. H., Pollard, R. B. and Merigan, T. C. Increased pulmonary superinfection in cardiac transplant patients undergoing primary cytomegalovirus infection, *N. Engl. J. Med.* **298**: 951; 1978.
5. Lopez, C., Simmons, R. L., Mauer, S. M. *et al.* Association of renal allograft rejection with virus infections. *Am. J. Med.* **56**: 280; 1974.

6. Simmons, R. L., Weil, R., Tallent, M. B. *et al.* Do mild infections trigger the rejection of renal allografts? *Transplant Proc.* 2: 419; 1970.
7. Snydman, D. R., Werner, B. G., Heinze-Lacey, B. *et al.* Use of cytomegalovirus immune globulin to prevent cytomegalovirus disease in renal-transplant recipients. *N. Eng. J. Med.* 317: (17): 1049–1054; 1987.
8. Fassbinder, W., Ernst, W., Hanke, P. *et al.* Cytomegalovirus infections after renal transplantation: Effect of prophylactic hyperimmunoglobulin. *Transplant Proc.* 18 (5): 1393–1396; 1986.
9. Myers, J. D., Leszczynski, J., Zaia, J. A. *et al.* Prevention of CMV infection by CMV immune globulin after marrow transplantation. *Ann. Intern. Med.* 98: 442–446; 1983.
10. Saliba, F., Gugenheim, J., Samuel, D. *et al.* Incidence of cytomegalovirus infection and effects of cytomegalovirus immune globulin prophylaxis, after orthotopic liver transplantation. *Transplant Proc.* 19(5): 4081; 1987.
11. Dusaix, E. and Wood, C. Cytomegalovirus infection in pediatric liver recipients. *Transplantation* 48: 272; 1989.
12. Saliba, F., Arunaden, J. C., Gugenheim, J. *et al.* CMV hyperimmune globulin prophylaxis after liver transplantation: a prospective randomized controlled study. *Transplant Proc.* 21(1): 2260–2262; 1989.
13. Bell, R., Shei, A. G. R., McDonald, J. A. and McCaughan, G. W. The role of CMV immune prophylaxis in patients at risk of primary CMV infection following orthotopic liver transplantation. *Transplant Proc.* 21(5): 3781–3782; 1989.
14. Klintmalm, G. B. G., Nery, J. R., Husberg, B. S., Gonwa, T. A. and Tillery, G. W. Rejection in liver transplantation. *Hepatology* 10(6): 978–985; 1989.
15. Harbison, M. A., De Girolami, P. C., Jenkins, R. L. and Hammer, S. M. Gancyclovir therapy of severe cytomegalovirus infections in solid-organ transplant recipients. *Transplantation* 46: 82–88; 1988.
16. Mai, M., Nery, J., Sutker, B. *et al.* DHPG (gancyclovir) improves survival in CMV pneumonia. *Transplant Proc.* 21: 2263–2265; 1989.
17. Rakela, J., Wiesner, R. H., Taswell, H. F. *et al.* Incidence of cytomegalovirus infection and its relationship to donor–recipient serologic status in liver transplantation. *Transplant Proc.* 19(1): 2399–2402; 1987.

Part IV
Autoimmune disorders

New clinical aspects of immune thrombocytopenic purpura (ITP)

P. IMBACH

Central Laboratory of the Swiss Red Cross Blood Transfusion Service, Bern, Switzerland

Within the last decade the definition of ITP has changed from idiopathic to immune or autoimmune thrombocytopenic purpura, and the new possibility of intravenous immunoglobulin (IVIG) treatment has altered the therapeutic procedure. In this article we will focus on these two issues. The mechanism of action of IVIG and its implication to a wide range of immune-related disorders are described in several other contributions of this volume.

The change of definition from idiopathic to immune or autoimmune thrombocytopenic purpura

ITP is a bleeding disorder characterized by increased destruction and normal or enhanced production of circulating platelets. Since 1950, clinical evidence has been found indicating antiplatelet factors in the pathogenesis of ITP. Since then, the active factor causing thrombocytopenia was found to be present in the IgG of blood plasma and on the platelets. Recently, sensitive assays using monoclonal autoantibodies against platelet glycoprotein IIb/IIIa and glycoprotein Ib/IX have been

Immunotherapy with Intravenous Immunoglobulins
ISBN 0–12–370725–0

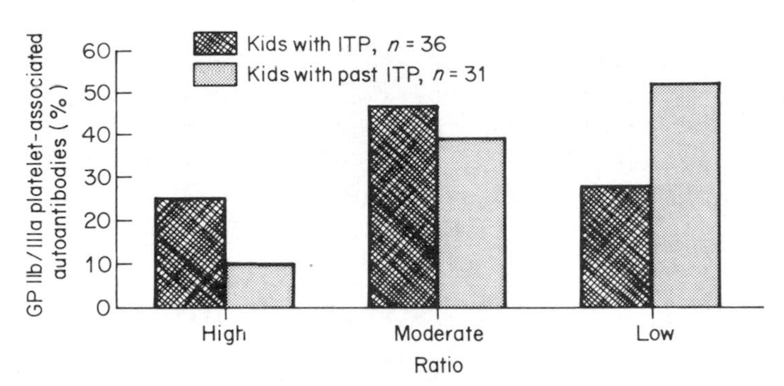

Figure 1. Percentage of children with high, moderate and low levels of platelet-associated autoantibody and chronic ITP (for details see text).

developed (1, 2). In adults with chronic ITP, platelet-associated autoantibodies were found in 79.7% of cases and plasma autoantibodies were noted in one-half of them (3). In children with chronic ITP platelet-associated and plasma autoantibodies were detected (Fig. 1) using the same immunobead assay (1, 3, 4). Results were considered positive if > 3 times the standard deviation above controls and were divided into high, moderate or low positives if > 5 times, 2–5 times or 1–2 times the control means plus 3 standard deviations, respectively. In thrombocytopenic children with chronic ITP 72.2% patients had high (25%) or moderate (47.2%) levels of platelet-associated autoantibodies. High autoantibody levels (> 5 times) were noted more frequently in older children and plasma autoantibodies was demonstrable only when platelet-associated autoantibodies were high. Of children with chronic ITP in the past but with normal counts ($>150 \times 10^9$/l) at the time of study, 48.4% had elevated platelet-associated autoantibodies (9.7% high, 38.7% moderate levels) but negative plasma autoantibodies. Thus, the detection of autoantibodies against platelet glycoprotein changed the definition of ITP from idiopathic to immune or auto-immune thrombocytopenic purpura. Patients with negative results may have autoantibody against other platelet antigens or may have thrombocytopenia based on a different immune or non-immune mechanism. In children the results of determination of platelet autoantibodies suggest that different forms of ITP exist. Future studies aimed at serial autoantibody determination throughout the patient's course may define better ITP subgroups.

Therapy with ITP

In 1980 it was observed in a child with ITP that IVIG was followed by a rapid increase of platelet count. Following this observation, first a pilot study (5) and then controlled clinical IVIG multicenter studies separating children with newly diagnosed ITP from those with chronic ITP unresponsive to previous treatment were organized (6, 7). The main conclusions from these studies were the following:

— A rapid increase of platelet counts within 24–76 h in the majority of patients with acute or chronic ITP could be observed.

— In children with chronic ITP, 62% displayed long-term improvement (no more bleeding, platelet count $> 20 \times 10^9$/l) (7).

— The side effects of IVIG treatment were mild and consisted of headache, fever, chills, rash, vomiting or malaise in about 25% of patients or in 1–2% of all IgG infusions.

— Under study condition, the patients received 0.4 g IVIG/kg body weight on 5 consecutive days. Two-thirds of the patients had platelet increases of over 30×10^9/l on the third day after receiving 2 times 0.4 g IVIG/kg body weight only. After termination of the studies, the reduction of the dosage of IVIG to 1×0.8 g IVIG/kg body weight showed similar effects in the majority of children. The reduced dosage markedly lowered the overall cost of the treatment (cost for IVIG, shortening of the duration of hospitalization).

— As regards the treatment schedule, three categories of severity of ITP due to bleeding symptoms (and platelet counts below 30×10^9/l) may be distinguished:

(1) Patients with severe bleeding, or at risk of bleeding (i.e. before surgery): if such a patient has infection, is at risk of infection or has a postinfectious or immunocompromised status, IVIG is recommended. Dosage: $1–2 \times 0.4–1.0$ g IVIG/kg body weight. Otherwise, corticosteroids in high doses (8–12 mg/kg weight per day) for 2–3 days may be used. In life-threatening situation, the combination of IVIG, high-dose corticosteroids and platelet transfusion may reduce bleeding.

(2) Patients at risk of spontaneous bleeding. In children with long-term bleeding problems, treatment with 0.4 g IVIG/kg body weight given at 2–8 week intervals, depending upon hemorrhagic symptoms, is recommended.

(3) Patients with occasional bleeding: no routine treatment. Some patients with special activities (i.e. sport) may need individual treatment.

The effect of IVIG is now confirmed worldwide. A review of 28 published reports including 282 patients showed an increase in platelet counts above $10 \times 10^9/l$ in 64% and above $50 \times 10^9/l$ in 83% of cases (8). Furthermore, Bussel *et al.* reported that following repeated doses of IVIG, splenectomy could be postponed (9). Newland (10) documented the existence of two distinct groups of adults with ITP in relation to their response to IVIG treatment. In particular, the response of patients treated early in the course of their disease was different from that of those treated later. Up to 50% of patients treated within the first 6 months had a long-term response to IVIG alone. Conversely, in virtually all patients treated in the chronic phase (6 months or more after onset of ITP), the response to IVIG was transient. In only occasional adult patients did the author observe prolonged or sustained responses. Following intermittent treatment with IVIG over 2–3 months, 10–15% of adult patients with ITP achieved a stable partial remission.

In the future, studies should be done to determine the minimal effective dosage of IVIG. Such a study should also include a stratification between the different, intact IgG-preparations. From the clinical data in children with ITP it would appear that IVIG treatment may also reduce the number of patients with chronic ITP. Therefore, a study to evaluate prospectively the effect of IVIG in preventing the development of chronic ITP in children should be carried out. With the low incidence of chronic ITP and in view of the heterogeneity of ITP, it is apparent that large numbers of patients are needed in order to evaluate the efficacy of a chosen treatment. A further problem lies in the fact that at the beginning of the disease there are so far no criteria to recognize the children at risk for chronic ITP; determination of antiplatelet autoantibodies may be useful in selecting different forms of ITP in children.

Summary

Determinations of autoantibodies to platelet glycoproteins have changed the definition of ITP from idiopathic to immune or autoimmune thrombocytopenic purpura. In the future, studies of serial autoantibody determination may better define ITP subgroups, which would provide the possibility of screening the patients for prognostic factor. The now well-accepted new possibility of intravenous immunoglobulin treatment has altered the therapeutic procedure of bleedings or of prevention of bleedings in patients with ITP. As a conclusion, from our IVIG multicenter studies appropriate dosages of IVIG and treatment schedules in the different categories of severity of ITP are proposed.

References

1. McMillan, R., Tani, P., Millard, F. *et al.* Platelet-associated and plasma antiglycoprotein autoantibodies in chronic ITP. *Blood* 70: 1040–1045; 1987.
2. Kiefel, V., Santoso, S., Weisheit, M. and Mueller-Eckhardt, C. Monoclonal antibody-specific immobilization of platelet antigens (MAIPA); a new tool for the identification of platelet-reactive antibodies. *Blood* 70: 1722–1726; 1987.
3. Tani, P., Berchtold, P. and McMillan, R. Autoantibodies in chronic ITP. *Blut* 59: 44–46; 1989.
4. Imbach, P., Tani, P., McMillan, R. *et al.* Different forms of chronic ITP in children defined by antiplatelet autoantibodies. *J. Pediatr.* (In press.)
5. Imbach, P., Barandun, S., d'Apuzzo, V. *et al.* High dose intravenous gammaglobulin for idiopathic thrombocytopenic purpura in childhood. *Lancet* 1: 1128, 1981.
6. Imbach, P., Wagner, H. P., Berchtold, W. *et al.* Intravenous immunoglobulin versus oral corticosteroids in acute immune thrombocytopenic purpura in childhood. *Lancet* 2: 464–468; 1985.
7. Imholz, B., Imbach, P., Baumgartner, C. *et al.* Intravenous immunoglobulin (i.v. IgG) for previously treated acute or for chronic idiopathic thrombocytopenic purpura (ITP) in childhood; a prospective multicenter study. *Blut* 56: 63–68; 1988.
8. Bussel, J. B. and Pham, L. C. Intravenous treatment with gammaglobulin in adults with immune thrombocytopenic purpura; review of the literature. *Vox Sang.* 52: 206–211; 1987.
9. Bussell, J. B., Schulmann, I., Hilgartner, M. W. and Barandum, S. Intravenous use of gammaglobulin in the treatment of chronic immune thrombocytopenia as a means to defer splenectomy. *J. Pediatr.* 103: 652–654; 1983.
10. Newland, A. C. Clinical and therapeutic aspects and treatment with IV IgG. *In* "Idiopathic Thrombocytopenia-Proceedings of a Workshop" (Ed. Imbach, P.), pp. 63–72. Pharmanual, Pharmalibra; 1986.

Intravenous immunoglobulin: new aspects of mechanism of action in chronic ITP

PETER BERCHTOLD[1] and ROBERT McMILLAN[2]

[1]*Department of Medicine, University of Bern, Bern, Switzerland*
[2]*Department of Molecular and Experimental Medicine, Research Institute of Scripps Clinic, La Jolla, California, USA*

Introduction

Chronic immune thrombocytopenic purpura (ITP) is an autoimmune disease characterized by increased platelet destruction due to anti-platelet autoantibodies (1). In 75% of patients with chronic ITP, platelet-associated antibodies to platelet glycoprotein (GP) IIb/IIIa and GPIb/IX have been demonstrated. Circulating plasma autoantibodies against the same antigens have been shown in 58% of these patients (2).

The beneficial short-term effect of high-dose intravenous immunoglobulin (IVIG) in childhood and adult chronic ITP has been shown in a large number of studies (3–5). Moreover, recent reports have suggested that long-term therapy with IVIG may result in remission or stabilization of the disease in some patients (6–8). However, the mechanism of action is still unknown. Fehr *et al.* (4) showed that administration of IVIG was followed by Fc-receptor blockade resulting in a decreased clearance of antibody-coated platelets. However, a response to IVIG has also been reported in patients without prolongation

Immunotherapy with Intravenous Immunoglobulins
ISBN 0–12–370725–0

of Fc-receptor-mediated clearance (9). Other possibilities include enhancement of suppressor T-cell function in responding patients (10) or suppression of the production of antiplatelet autoantibody (11). Finally, recent studies have suggested that the response to IVIG may be due to the effect of anti-idiotypic antibodies present in IVIG preparations (12).

There is increasing evidence that anti-idiotypic antibodies may play an essential role in regulating the immune system and it has been suggested that autoimmunity may arise from disturbance of the idiotypic network (13). In patients with systemic lupus erythematosus, anti-idiotypes to anti-DNA autoantibodies were found in remission but not during the active phase of the disease (14). A similar relationship between disease activity and occurrence of anti-idiotypes to autoantibodies has also been shown in patients with autoimmune dysfibrinogenemia and autoimmunity to factor VIII (15, 16). It has been speculated that the expression of autoantibodies in healthy persons and in patients who have revcovered from autoimmune diseases may be down-regulated by anti-idiotypic antibodies (16).

Results and discussion

Several reports have indicated that IVIG, prepared from pooled normal plasma, contain anti-idiotypic antibodies against autoantibodies to factor VIII, DNA and thyroglobulin (17, 18). We have evaluated the ability of IVIG to inhibit the *in vitro* binding of autoantibodies from patients with chronic ITP to platelet glycoprotein IIb/IIIa (12). This inhibition is most likely due to anti-idiotypic antibodies present in IVIG.

Prior to measurement of antiplatelet antibodies, plasma samples or purified autoantibody eluates, known to contain antibodies to glycoprotein IIb/IIIa, were preincubated with different concentrations of IVIG or bovine serum albumin (BSA control). If present, anti-idiotypes would bind to the autoantibodies and reduce the amount detectable in the following radioimmunoassay specific for antibodies to platelet glycoprotein IIb/IIIa, as has been described in detail elsewhere (2). The results are expressed as percentage inhibition of control autoantibody results obtained using BSA instead of IVIG.

We studied nine patients with chronic ITP and autoantibodies to the GPIIb/IIIa complex. As shown in Fig. 1, binding of plasma autoantibody to GPIIb/IIIa was reduced by pre-incubation with IVIG in all patients. Using IVIG at a 3.2% final concentration in the pre-incubation

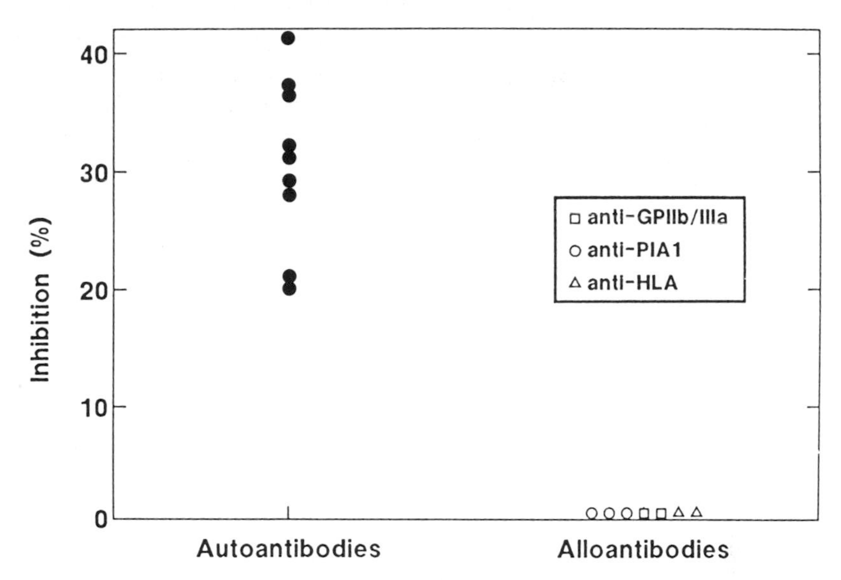

Figure 1. Inhibition of antiplatelet autoantibody binding by IVIG.

mixture, which is comparable to *in vivo* levels attained during treatment with IVIG, a mean decrease of autoantibody binding ranging from 20.2% to 41.3% was noted (Fig. 1). In contrast, no inhibitory effect by IVIG was seen when plasma from seven patients with antiplatelet alloantibodies was tested (Fig. 1). These alloantibodies, induced by transfusion of blood products, were directed in five patients to GPIIb/IIIa (2 Glanzmann's thrombasthenia, 3 post-transfusion purpura) and in two patients against HLA antigens. Inhibition of autoantibody binding to platelets was proportional to the IVIG concentration used during the pre-incubation and there was no significant difference between three commercial IVIG preparations (Fig. 2).

$F(ab')_2$ fragments of IVIG were also examined for inhibitory activity. Table 1 shows that both $F(ab')_2$ fragments and undigested IVIG blocked the binding of plasma autoantibodies as well as the binding of purified autoantibodies, prepared by elution from antigen affinity columns. The reason for the lesser inhibition of $F(ab')_2$ fragments is not known, but it could be due to damage during the procedure of low pH and pepsin digestion. However, these results suggest that the inhibitory activity of IVIG is mediated by the variable region of IVIG.

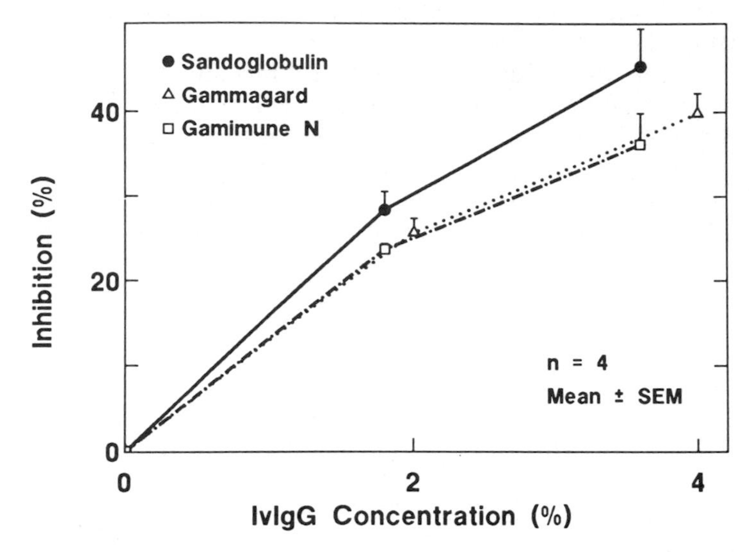

Figure 2. Inhibition of antiplatelet autoantibody binding by different IVIG preparations. N = numbers of separate experiments. The plasma from each case came from the same patient.

Table 1
Inhibition of plasma and purified autoantibody binding by IVIG and $F(ab')_2$ fragments of IVIG

	IVIG	$F(ab')_2$
	(% Inhibition)	
Plasma autoantibodies	37.3±8.7%	23.5±6.3%
Purified autoantibodies	37.6±8.0%	18.7±4.7%

This dose-dependent inhibition of autoantibody binding to platelet GPIIb/IIIa indicates that IVIG contains anti-idiotypic antibodies directed against idiotypes on antiplatelet autoantibodies but not to idiotypes on alloantibodies against the same or different molecules. The finding that IVIG inhibits different autoantibodies to a varying degree suggests heterogeneity among the idiotypes located on autoantibodies.

Administration of IVIG in patients with chronic ITP is usuallly followed by a rapid but transient rise of the platelet count. In addiiton to blocking of Fc-receptor-mediated clearance of platelets, this short-term effect may involve inhibition of autoantibody binding to platelet glycoproteins by anti-idiotypic antibodies. *In vivo*, anti-idiotypes may bind to idiotype-bearing autoantibodies and thus block their combining site for the platelet antigen. This may explain the response to IVIG in some patients without detectable Fc-receptor-blockade and the decrease in platelet-associated antibody reported after IVIG (9, 11).

In some patients with chronic ITP, prolonged remissions have been reported after repeated maintenance infusions of IVIG. This long-term effect may be due to a down-regulation of the immune reponse by anti-idiotypic antibodies. Anti-idiotypes may inactivate idiotype-bearing B lymphocytes and therefore inhibit autoantibody-producing B-cell clones or they may have a beneficial effect on immunoregulatory T lymphocytes. This is consistent with findings after IVIG treatment where it has been suggested that production of antiplatelet antibodies may decrease and impaired suppressor T-cell function may be corrected (11, 19, 20).

A quarter of patients with chronic ITP do not respond to IVIG. Several reasons may account for unresponsiveness to anti-idiotypic antibodies: although IVIG preparations contain millions of anti-idiotypic specificities, some may be under-represented for an auto-antibody of a non-responding patient with chronic ITP; immunosuppressive therapy prior to treatment with gammaglobulin may interfere with the therapeutic effect of intravenous IgG by rendering the patients immunoregulation unresponsive for anti-idiotypic antibodies (21). As a third possibility, infusion of anti-idiotypes may increase in some instances the pathological immune response in patients with chronic ITP (22).

Conclusions

In summary, we think that IVIG contains anti-idiotypic antibodies directed against anti-GPIIb/IIIa autoantibodies from patients with chronic ITP. These anti-idiotypes could inhibit the *in vivo* binding of autoantibodies to platelet antigens and may down-regulate the pathological immune response in patients with chronic ITP.

Summary

Intravenous immunoglobulin (IVIG) causes an acute rise in the platelet count in most patients with chronic immune thrombocytopenic purpura (ITP), but the mechanism of action is still unknown. We observed that the *in vitro* binding of autoantibodies from nine patients with chronic ITP to platelet glycoprotein (GP) IIb/IIIa was inhibited by IVIG. This inhibitory effect of IVIG was dose-dependent. $F(ab')_2$ fragments of IVIG also inhibited the binding of both plasma autoantibodies as well as purified anti-GPIIb/IIIa antibodies. In contrast, no inhibition by IVIG of alloantibody binding to the same or different molecules was detected (five patients with anti-GPIIb/IIIa and two anti-HLA alloantibodies). We concluded that IVIG cotains anti-idiotypic antibodies to anti-GPIIb/IIIa autoantibodies. These anti-idiotypes may inhibit the *in vivo* binding of autoantibodies to platelets and in some cases suppress the pathological immune response in patients with chronic ITP.

References

1. McMillan, R. *N. Engl. J. Med.* **304**: 1135–1147; 1981.
2. McMillan, R., Tani, P., Millard, F., Berchtold, P., Renshaw, L. and Woods, V. L. *Blood* **70**: 1040–1045; 1987.
3. Imbach, P., Barandun, S., d'Apuzzo, V. and Baumgartner, C. *Lancet* **1**: 1228–1231; 1981.
4. Fehr, J., Hofmann, V. and Kappeler, U. *N. Engl. J. Med.* **306**: 1254–1258; 1982.
5. Newland, A. C., Treleaven, J. G., Minchinton, R. M. and Waters, A. H. *Lancet* **1**: 84–87; 1983.
6. Bierling, P., Divine, M., Farcet, J. P., Wallet, P. and Duedari, N. *Am. J. Hematol.* **25**: 271–275; 1987.
7. Bussel, J. B., Pham, L. C., Aledort, L. and Nachman, R. *Blood* **72**: 121–127; 1988.
8. Imholz, B., Imbach, P., Baumgartner, C., Berchtold, W., Gaedicke, G., Gugler, G., Hirt, A., Hitzig, W., Mueller-Eckhardt, C. and Wagner, H. P. *Blut* **56**: 63–68; 1988.
9. Budde, U., Auch, D., Niese, D. and Schaefer, G. *Scand. J. Haemat.* **37**: 125–129; 1986.
10. Delfraissy, J. F., Tchernia, G., Laurian, Y. and Wallon, C. *Br. J. Haemat.* **60**: 315–322; 1985.
11. Bussel, J. B., Kimberly, R. P., Inman, R. D. and Schulman, I. *Blood* **62**: 480–486; 1983.
12. Berchtold, P., Dale, G. L., Tani, P. and McMillan, R. *Blood* **74**: 2414–2417; 1989.
13. Burdette, S. and Schwartz, R. S. *N. Engl. J. Med.* **317**: 219–224; 1987.
14. Abdou, N. I., Wall, H., Lindsley, H. B., Halsey, J. R. and Suzuki, T. *J. Clin. Invest.* **67**: 1297–1302; 1981.
15. Sultan, Y., Rossi, F. and Kazatchkine, M. D. *Proc. Natl. Acad. Sci. USA* **84**: 828–831; 1987.
16. Ruiz-Arguelles, A. *J. Clin. Invest.* **82**: 958–963; 1988.

17. Sultan, Y., Kazatchkine, M. D., Maisonneuve, P. and Nydegger, U. E. *Lancet* 2: 765–768; 1984.
18. Rossi, F. and Kazatchkine, M. D. *J. Immunol.* 143: 4104–4109; 1989.
19. Tsubakio, T., Kurata, Y., Katagiri, S. and Kanakura, Y. *Clin. Exp. Immunol.* 53: 697–702; 1983.
20. Dammaco, F., Iodice, G. and Campobasso, N. *Br. J. Haemat.* 62: 125–135; 1986.
21. Nydegger, U. E., Sultan, Y. and Kazatchkine, M. D. *Clin. Immunol. Immunopathol.* 53: S72–S82; 1989.
22. Cleveland, W. L., Wassermann, N. H., Sarangarajan, R., Penn, A. S. and Erlanger, B. F. *Nature* 305: 56–57; 1983.

Discussion

R. Stricker

The concept of autoantibody binding to GPIIb/IIIa is problematic since Karpatkin has recently shown that GPIIIa contains an IgG receptor (perhaps an Fc receptor). These immune complexes may bind to GPIIIa. Do you think that IVIG could compete for this binding? Are you sure that your patients had autoantibodies?

P. Berchtold

Fc receptors have been proposed on a variety of platelet glycoproteins and it has been reported that binding of immune complexes to platelets may be important in HIV-related immune thrombocytopenia. In contrast, there is little evidence that patients with autoimmune thrombocytopenia have circulating immune complexes. In the majority of these patients, we have shown antibodies reactive with GPIIb/IIIa or GPIb/IX and their specificity has been evaluated by elution studies, immunoblotting and immunoprecipitation. These antibodies most likely represent autoantibodies rather than alloantibodies, since most of the patients had no history of either transfusion or pregnancy.

G. Gaedicke

Clinical experience makes me doubt the importance of anti-idiotype mechanisms as a basic mode of action in IVIG in the various immune thrombocytopenias. I have two objections:

(1) For the anti-idiotype mechanism you need a Fab-to-Fab interaction. Fab-fragmented IVIG preparations, however, do not work in patients with acute or chronic ITP.

(2) You said you couldn't observe anti-idiotype-related inhibitory

effects on PLA-1 alloantibodies. Therapy of choice in alloimmune thrombocytopenias (in newborns as well as in post-transfusion purpura) is—besides maternal platelets—high-dose IVIG.

P. Berchtold

I agree that the clinical significance of these anti-idiotypes as therapeutical agent remains to be determined. On the other hand, effectiveness of IVIG in alloimmune thrombocytopenia or ineffectiveness of Fab-fragmented IVIG does not rule out this possibility. I think that the effect of IVIG in chronic ITP is mediated by several mechanisms, such as infusion of anti-idiotypic antibodies or delayed clearance of antibody-coated cells due to Fc-receptor blockade. The latter could be involved in the initial response in chronic ITP and in alloimmune thrombocytopenia, whereas long-term remissions observed after IVIG in some patients with chronic ITP may be due to a beneficial effect of anti-idiotypes on immunoregulation.

Treatment effects on chronic idiopathic thrombocytopenia purpura

JAMES B. BUSSEL

New York Hospital and Cornell Medical College, New York, USA

Introduction

Idiopathic thrombocytopenia purpura (ITP) has been classically characterized as a disease whereby platelet destruction results from antiplatelet antibodies binding to platelets. This was initially demonstrated by Harrington (1) and confirmed and extended by Shulman (2) in studies in which plasma from ITP patients transfused into normal recipients caused a marked thrombocytopenia. This resolved a debate over whether the problem was in the bone marrow, i.e. platelet production, or more peripherally, i.e. accelerated destruction.

Platelet antibodies

Circulating

The great bulk of the subsequent study of ITP has revolved around the "destroying (effector) agent": the platelet antibody. Considerable research has attempted to define and thereby classify the disease by measuring the level of antiplatelet antibody. Initial work involved

Immunotherapy with Intravenous Immunoglobulins
ISBN 0–12–370725–0

serum or plasma and measurements were made of "free", "circulating", "indirect" or "serum" antibody. The stickiness of platelets and the occurrence of such antibodies for other reasons (previous transfusions or pregnancy) made such testing difficult. In addition approximately one-third of patients with unquestioned ITP failed to reveal any antibody on testing.

Bound

The first study describing antibody on platelets (platelet-associated IgG) was by Dixon and Rosse in 1973 (3). Other investigators developed similar techniques and were able to show that platelet-associated IgG was elevated in > 90% of patients with ITP (4).

Subsequently several studies appeared indicating that not all platelet-associated IgG was specific antiplatelet antibody. Shulman emphasized that the amount of antibody required to destroy equivalent numbers of platelets, when injected into rabbits, was several orders of magnitude less than that being measured on the platelets of patients with ITP (5). Kelton demonstrated that platelet-associated albumin

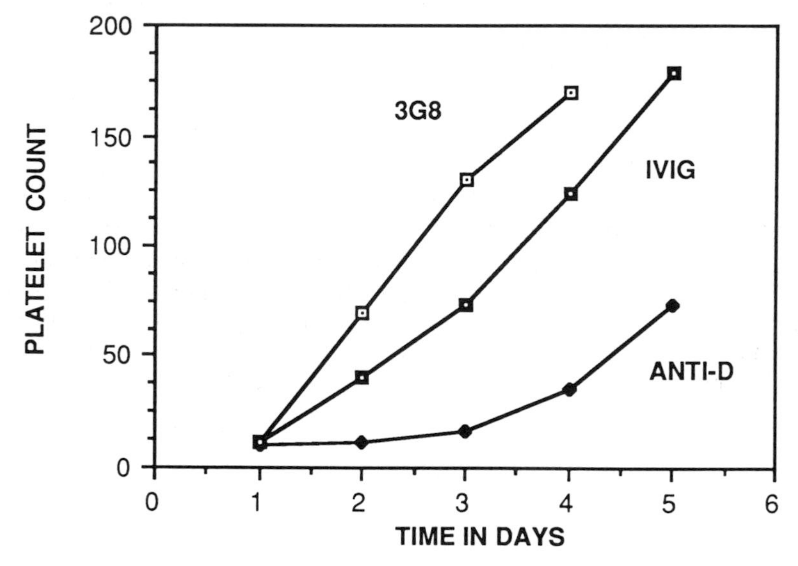

Figure 1. Comparative platelet increases following initiation of treatment on day 1 for three treatments which all appear to have as an initial mechanism Fc-receptor blockade. The IVIG and IV anti-D data are composite information representing typical (average) responses. The 3G8 data represent the response of one of the patients with the best response to illustrate the potential of a treatment having only one possible acute mechanism of effect for blockade.

increased when platelet-associated IgG increased (6). Finally, George provided at least a partial explanation for this phenomenon by showing that platelet alpha granules contain IgG which could be released when platelets were activated (7). Various attempts were made, most notably by LoBuglio (8), to improve the technique of measuring platelet-associated IgG and thereby reduce the background, but the situation remains currently unresolved.

Currently, techniques have shifted from using the whole platelet to specific antigen targets, i.e. GPIIb/IIIa (9, 10) but the results of this newer strategy are not yet clearly different from older work. Hopefully this work will soon lead to a more specific marker of the "activity" of the disease. In turn this might lead to a better understanding of the natural history of ITP and different therapies could be better monitored in regard to their effects on autoantibody levels.

Fc-receptor interactions

The advent of intravenous gammaglobulin (IVIG), as part of its therapeutic impact, focused attention on Fc-receptor (FcR) blockade as a means of elevating the platelet count in patients with ITP (see Fig. 1). This effect had originally been demonstrated for glucocorticoids, including a classic study by Stossell (11) showing a relationship of neutrophil phagocytosis with the platelet count and the prednisone dose. Subsequent study of IVIG suggested that its effects, as quantitated by the antibody-coated autologous red cell clearance, were more profound than was that of steroids (12, 13). Direct comparisons were not made but the values and uniformity of prolongation of clearance following IVIG seem clearly greater than that reported following corticosteroids. This raises the question of the predominant mechanism of effect of steroids in increasing the platelet count in ITP. Could the predominant mechanism of steroid effect be dissociation of antibody from platelets rather than Fc–receptor blockade rather than paralysis of phagocytosis?

IVIG

The suggestion that the initial effect of IVIG to raise the platelet count occurred via FcR blockade was originally made by Imbach (14) based on work by Fehr which was published the following year. Imbach *et al.* also hypothesized that long-term responses were due to a decrease in the level of auto-antiplatelet-antibodies. Fehr *et al.* not only demonstrated the occurrence of FcR blockade but also that it returned to baseline with a time course approximating the return to baseline of the platelet count. This raised two important questions which are still incompletely answered.

1. Mechanism of FcR blockade

The first was how IVIG infusion caused FcR blockade. Possibilities initially considered included the tripling of the IgG monomer level, and the infusion of dimers and trimers and aggregates, but the apparent rapid recycling of surface Fc-receptors on mononuclear phagocytes was originally thought to render these effects less likely. Salama and Mueller-Eckhardt suggested in 1983 that perhaps FcR blockade was mediated by anti-red cell antibodies contained in low levels in the IVIG (15). They "confirmed" their hypothesis by injecting anti-D into D^+ patients and demonstrating a platelet increase in most recipients (Fig. 1). However, at the present time it appears that the mechanism of causation of FcR blockade by anti-D and by IVIG may be different for the following reasons: (1) IVIG is effective in splenectomized patients whereas anti-D is not; (2) IVIG is effective independent of patient blood type whereas for anti-D the patient must be Rh+; (3) the platelet count increase following IVIG is usually immediate, i.e. begins within 48 h, whereas with anti-D the first increase in responsive patients is not until 72 h; (4) the Coombs test is not usually positive following IVIG; and (5) certain patients respond to IVIG but not to anti-D and vice versa.

Therefore, if sensitization of red cells by IVIG is not the sole mechanism of FcR blockade seen following IVIG, how does FcR blockade develop? The answer is unclear but seems to relate to an initial occupancy/down-modulation of FcR without rapid recirculation. The pathobiology contributing to the lack of immediate recirculation of Fc receptors remains uncertain, although presumably it is regulated by cytokines. Whether the level of immune complexes/aggregates in the preparations plays a role assumes greater importance in understanding the effects of anti-D. The entire effect of this treatment is apparently caused by large immune complexes which are created following infusion. Nonetheless, the effects of treatment are still delayed, i.e. until 72 h.

2. FcR blockade and platelet increase

Given that FcR blockade occurs following IVIG infusion and that the mechanism of this effect is not clear, can this effect underlie a platelet increase in patients with ITP? The best "proof" demonstrating this effect is the use of an anti-FcRIII monoclonal antibody in the treatment of refractory ITP (16, 17; see Fig. 1). Its success in elevating the platelet count dramatically in the majority of 15 treated patients strongly implies that FcR blockade alone is sufficient to result in a dramatic albeit transient increase in the platelet count. The increase in the platelet count following infusion of anti-D, where 1/1000th as much IVIG is infused and which is ineffective in Rh− patients, also confirms the central role of FcR blockade.

Other effects of FcR interaction

Of great importance for the future is understanding the implications and possibilities of FcR blockade. Expressed crudely, is FcR blockade merely "putting the lid on the garbage pail for a while" so that antibody-coated platelets do not get "thrown out"? There are suggestions but no hard evidence that FcR interaction may indeed play a role in long-term effects of a therapy. For example, patients have been noted, in uncontrolled trials, to apparently have beneficial long-term effects of IVIG treatment (18, 19). In general this is attributed to effects on platelet antibodies, perhaps mediated directly via anti-idiotypic antibodies. However, another contributing possibility is FcR interaction. The full panoply of mediators that can be released, especially by intense *in vivo* stimulation of FcRs, is not known nor are the exact effects of known mediators completely understood. There probably are widespread immune effects resulting from IVIG stimulation of FcRs which generally "dampdown" rapidly. However, repeated stimulation may gradually achieve a "long-term effect". This has also been suggested in the studies of monoclonal anti-FcRIII infusion where several patients either developed perceptible long-term improvement without the need for further treatment and/or became responsive to conventional treatments to which they were previously refractory (17). One possible mechanism whereby both IVIG and the monoclonal anti-FcRIII antibody could create such an effect would be by interaction with FcRIII on natural killer cells. These studies all imply the possibility of Fc-mediated effects that, if better understood, could be used in conjunction with other treatments, for example serving to diminish the level of antiplatelet antibodies and to allow development of new therapeutic strategies in ITP.

Summary

ITP is a disease mediated by antiplatelet antibodies which result in destruction of platelets via Fc receptors in the mononuclear phagocyte system. The difficulty in quantitating specific antiplatelet antibody has impaired a better understanding of therapeutic responses to date. IVIG appears to work initially via FcR blockade. This is confirmed by studies of anti-D and infusion of an anti-FcRIII monoclonal antibody. Whether lasting effects of any of these therapies may be generated via FcR-mediated immunomodulation remains open to question.

References

1. Harrington, W. J., Minnich, V. *et al.* Demonstration of a thrombocytopenic factor in the blood of patients with thrombocytopenic purpura. *J. Lab. Clin. Med.* **38**: 1; 1951.
2. Shulman, N. R., Weinrach, R. S., Libre, E. P. and Andrews, H. L. The role of the reticuloendothelial system in the pathogenesis of idiopathic thrombocytopenic purpura. *Trans. Assoc. Am. Physicians* **78**: 374; 1965.
3. Dixon, R. and Rosse, W. Platelet antibody in autoimmune thrombocytopenia. *Br. J. Haemat.* **31**: 129; 1975.
4. McMillan, R. Chronic idiopathic thrombocytopenic purpura. *N. Engl. J. Med.* **304**: 1135–1147; 1981.
5. Shulman, N. R., Leissinger, C. A., Hotchkiss, A. J. and Kautz, C. A. The nonspecific nature of platelet-associated IgG. *Trans. Assoc. Am. Physicians* **95**: 213–220; 1982.
6. Kelton, J. G. and Steeves, K. The amount of platelet-bound albumin parallels the amount of IgG on washed platelets from patients with immune thrombocytopenia. *Blood* **62**: 924; 1983.
7. George, J. N., Saucerman, S., Levine, S. P. and Knieriem, L. K. Immunoglobulin G is a platelet alpha granule-secreted protein. *J. Clin. Invest.* **76**: 2020–2025; 1985.
8. LoBuglio, A. F. *et al.* Immune thrombocytopenic purpura: Use of a 1251 labeled anti-human IgG monoclonal AB to quantify platlelet bound IgG. *New. Engl. J. Med.* **308**: 459; 1983.
9. Beardsley, D. S., Spiegel, J. E., Jacobs, M. M., Handin, R. I. and Luz, S. E. 4th Platelet membrane glycoprotein IIIa contains target antigens that bind anti-platelet antibodies in immune thrombocytopenias. *J. Clin. Invest.* **74**: 1701–1707; 1984.
10. McMillan, R., Tani, P., Millard, F., Berchtold, P., Renshaw, L. and Woods, V. L. Jr. Platelet-associated and plasma anti-glycoprotein autoantibodies in chronic ITP. *Blood* **70**: 1040–1045; 1987.

11. Robson, H. N. and Duthie, J. J. R. Capillary resistance and adrenocortical activity. *Br. Med. J.* 2 971; 1950.
12. Fehr, J., Hoffman, V. and Kappeler, U. Transient reversal of thrombocytopenia in idiopathic thrombocytopenia purpura by high dose intravenous gammaglobulin. *N. Engl. J. Med.* **306**: 1254–1258; 1982.
14. Imbach, P., Barandun, S., D'Apuzzo, V., Baumgartner, C., Hirt, A., Morell, A., Rossi, E., Scholini, M., Vest, M. and Wagner, H. P. High-dose intravenous gammaglobulin for idiopathic thrombocytopenic purpura in childhood. *Lancet* 1: 1228–1231; 1981.
15. Salama, A., Mueller-Eckhart, C., and Kiefel, V. Effect of intravenous immunoglobulin in immune thrombocytopenia. *Lancet* 2: 193; 1983.
16. Clarkson, S. B., Bussell, J. B., Kimberly, R. P., Valinsky, J. E., Nachman, R. L. and Unkeless; J. C. Treatment of refractory immune thrombocytopenic purpura with an anti Fc gamma receptor antibody. *N. Engl. J. Med.* **314**: 1236–1239; 1986.
17. Bussel, J., Kimberly, R., Clarkson, S., Nochman, R., Valinsky, J. and Unkeless, J. C. Infusion of a monoclonal anti-FcR III in patients with refractory ITP. *Neo-Adjuvant Chemother.* **169**: 883–887; 1988.
18. Hollenberg, J. P., Suback, L. L., Ferry, J. J. and Bussel, J. B. Cost effectiveness of splenectomy versus intravenous gammaglobulin in treatment of chronic immune thrombocytopenic purpura in childhood. *J. Pediatr.* 112: 530–539; 1988.
19. Bussell, J. B., Pham, L. C., Aledort, L. and Nachman, R. Maintenance treatment of adults with chronic refractory immune thrombocytopenic purpura using repeated intravenous infusions of gammaglobulin. *Blood* 72: 121–127; 1988.

Kawasaki disease and IVIG: what's going on here?

STANFORD T. SHULMAN

Department of Pediatrics, Northwestern University Medical School, Chicago, Illinois, USA

Kawasaki disease (KD) was described in 1967 by Dr Tomisaku Kawasaki, a Tokyo pediatrician (1). This illness predominately affected young children and was characterized by high fever, rash, injected conjunctivae, erythema of lips and oral mucosa, swollen and red hands and feet with subsequent periungual desquamation, and non-suppurative cervical adenopathy (2), features since incorporated into diagnostic criteria. After several sudden deaths occurred in children with prior KD, it was apparent that severe or even fatal coronary artery aneurysms and/or stenotic lesions with resultant myocardial infarction sometimes occurred (3). Since Kawasaki's description, this illness has become a major pediatric disorder, with about 100 000 cases recorded in Japan to date, approximately 3 000 cases annually in the US, and cases are reported worldwide. KD rivals or exceeds acute rheumatic fever as the leading cause of acquired heart disease in children in the US and probably in Europe. Coronary artery involvement is apparent by echocardiogram in 20–25% of untreated patients (4).

Epidemiologic studies of KD indicate characteristic findings, including median age of 2 years, male:female ratio of 3:2, endemic occurrence with superimposed time–space clusters or epidemics at

Immunotherapy with Intravenous Immunoglobulins
ISBN 0–12–370725–0

roughly $2\frac{1}{2}$–$3\frac{1}{2}$ year intervals with (in Japan) apparent wave-like spread through contiguous areas, only rare evidence for person–person spread, and highest incidence among Japanese or Korean ethnicity (5). The clinical and epidemiologic features strongly suggest an infectious etiology. However, efforts to implicate a specific etiologic agent have failed to date. A proposed retroviral etiology (6, 7) has not been confirmed (8, 9).

The pathogenesis of this disease can be inferred only from limited autopsy material and from demonstrated immunologic phenomena. The earliest cardiac findings are a diffuse interstitial pancarditis, initially with predominance of granulocytes and then with mononuclear cells. Indeed, many patients have some degree of clinically apparent myocarditis initially, and small pericardial effusions are very common. This inflammatory process over 1–2 weeks concentrates perivascularly, initially involving the coronary arterial walls, some believe particularly from the adventitial side, but frequently with granulocytes affecting the intima, resulting in destruction of the media and internal elastic lamina (10). During the second to fifth weeks after onset, granulocytes are replaced by mononuclear cells that are LEU M3–positive and acid phosphatase-positive, or LEU 3a–positive (helper cells) and DR-positive, and striking intimal thickening develops (10, 11). This is comprised primarily of activated myocytes that have migrated from the media through the disrupted internal elastic lamina to the intima.

These events lead to weakening of the arterial wall with aneurysm formation and/or to development of stenotic lesions resulting from intimal proliferation and fibrosis. Immunoglobulin deposition in vessel walls is minimal, and there is little or no evidence of complement deposition. Involvement of non-coronary medium-sized arteries occurs but with much lower frequency. Histologically and clinically, KD cannot be distinguished from a sporadic disease termed infantile periarteritis nodosa (IPAN), that dates at least to 1870 (12). IPAN was long known to be characterized by a peculiar predilection to coronary involvement in infants, and most old case reports describe an initial illness resembling acute KD.

A variety of immune perturbations are present during acute KD, most strikingly involving immunoregulatory lymphocyte numbers and function. Patients manifest diminished circulating T cells, with decreased numbers of suppressor CD8 cells and only slightly decreased or normal helper CD4 cell numbers (13). Consequently, the CD4/CD8 ratio is elevated. However, there is a striking increase in the number of activated CD4 cells expressing Ia and DR antigens (13) and a very marked increase in circulating B cells actively producing immunoglobulin. In addition, in the presence of rabbit complement, acute KD sera are cytolytic to cultured human umbilical vein endothelial cells but only if the endothelial cells are pretreated with gamma-interferon (14), IL–1 or TNF (15). This effect is specific to endothelial cells, resides in the IgM fraction of sera, and appears related to the induction of endothelial cell neo-antigens. Additional immune abnormalities reported in KD include circulating immune complexes that peak at about the third week of illness (16), cryoglobulinemia (17), increased PMN oxygen intermediate generation (18), and impaired granulocyte chemotaxis (19). The relevance of any of these immune phenomena to the pathogenesis of KD is unclear at present.

Despite the uncertain etiology and pathogenesis of KD, remarkably effective therapy to prevent coronary artery abnormalities exists. In the early 1980s, Furusho in Japan organized a multicenter controlled trial of IVIG in patients with acute KD after observing apparent benefit in an open trial. His hypotheses were: (1) that circulating immune complexes containing house dust-mite antigens are important in the pathogenesis of KD, and (2) that exogenous IVIG blocks tissue receptors and could prevent deposition of such complexes. Furusho's results, published in late 1984, suggested that 400 mg/kg/day IVIG for 5 days with aspirin was superior to aspirin alone with respect to development of echocardiographic coronary abnormalities (20).

Because of several potential design flaws, including unblinded echocardiogram readings and patients enrolled but excluded from analysis, a US group organized a multicenter randomized trial to compare IVIG at 400 mg/kg/day for 4 days plus aspirin (80–100 mg/kg/day) to aspirin alone. The results of this NIH-sponsored trial were published in the *New England Journal of Medicine* in 1986 (21). The chief and rather dramatic findings were that: (1) coronary artery abnormalities were detected by echocardiography at 7 weeks after enrolment in 14 of 79 (18%) aspirin-treated patients, but in only 3 of 79 (4%) of IVIG-plus-aspirin-treated patients ($P = 0.005$), and (2) significantly more rapid resolution of fever and laboratory indices of inflammation occurred in the IVIG-treated group. A phase II trial of 548 patients comparing a single 2000 mg/kg IVIG dose plus aspirin to 400 mg/kg/day × 4 plus aspirin regimen has just been completed and shows more rapid decrease in fever and laboratory parameters in the single dose group, with a slightly lower rate of coronary abnormalities in the single dose recipients (22). Thus, single-dose IVIG with aspirin is the current treatment of choice.

A compilation of clinical trials of IVIG initiated within 7–10 days of onset of KD suggests that a total IVIG dose in excess of 1000 mg/kg is necessary to prevent coronary abnormalities. The extent to which IVIG is now used in KD was reflected in our survey of pediatric training programs in North America only 15 months after the *New England Journal of Medicine* report (23). Ninety-five per cent of responding programs reported treatment of at least the large majority of KD patients with IVIG.

What do we know of the mechanism of the dramatic effect of IVIG in KD? Unfortunately, very little. The following are well established:

1. IVIG induces a very prompt and dramatic anti-inflammatory effect that is frequently apparent within a few hours of initiation of IVIG infusion.
2. Coronary abnormalities are largely prevented when IVIG is initiated within the first 7–10 days of illness. Whether microscopic coronary changes develop despite IVIG is unknown.
3. Pepsin-digested gammaglobulin is ineffective, as demonstrated in a limited number of Japanese studies, indicating that intact IgG is necessary.

However, we do not understand the precise mechanism by which large amounts of exogenous pooled adult IgG in KD, an illness with excessive spontaneous immunoglobulin synthesis, results in dramatic clinical improvement. Some have reported IVIG to be associated with prompt changes toward normal in the decreased numbers of cytotoxic/suppressor T cells, the increased number of DR+ activated helper/inducer T cells, and the spontaneous production of IgG and IgM by circulating B cells (24). Others have not, however, found such effect with IVIG therapy (25). A very recent report suggests that IVIG results in marked increase in NK cell activity in KD (26).

A possibly beneficial effect of blockade or modulation of Fc-receptor function is difficult to envision in KD, particularly since there is so little evidence that circulating immune complexes are important in its pathogenesis. Although such complexes are readily demonstrable in the third and fourth weeks of illness, they are more difficult to detect earlier when coronary changes are evolving. In addition, Mason was unable to find evidence of an effect of IVIG on circulating complexes in KD (27). Neither the protective coronary artery effect nor the prompt anti-inflammatory effect of IVIG is easily explained by Fc-receptor blockade.

For those of us convinced that KD is caused by a specific unknown infectious agent or agents, it is tempting to hypothesize that pooled adult IgG contains neutralizing antibody to a putative causative agent(s), or perhaps against a toxin elaborated by the inciting microbe(s).

The age-distribution of KD is certainly consistent with the notion that its rarity in individuals over the age of 10 years indicates acquired immunity and that its frequency in those under 2 years reflects lack of immunity. Thus, a beneficial effect of pooled adult IgG can be rationalized. It is more difficult to explain the rapid anti-inflammatory effect, although neutralization of a short-acting toxin or toxins is possible. At this time, no data exist to support this possibility.

Immunomodulation by IVIG mediated by an anti-idiotypic mechanism, resulting in suppression of antibody function and/or synthesis, has been proposed in several disorders. Although an anti-idiotype(s) could possibly account for the effect of IVIG in KD, no supportive data exist at present, and the rapidity of the observed response is difficult to explain on this basis. Without more precise information regarding the etiology and/or pathogenesis of KD, this and the previous possible mechanism are essentially untestable.

Perhaps the most attractive hypothesized mechanism for the effect of IVIG in KD relates to the previously discussed down-regulation by IVGG of activated CD4 helper T cells and activated B cells. This effect may in turn down-regulate cytokine production that, at least *in vitro*, induces expression of neo-antigens that may serve as targets for cytolytic antibody on activated endothelial cells. The relatively prompt anti-inflammatory effect of IVIG might reflect decreased elaboration of short-lived cytokines. One study found decreased spontaneous *in vitro* IL–1 release by peripheral blood cells after IVIG treatment compared to release prior to IVIG therapy. Sparing of the coronary arteries could result if the immune responses that involve cytokine-dependent neo-antigens are indeed important in the pathogenesis of coronary artery changes. Considerable additional supportive data will be needed to confirm these events.

In summary, KD is one of the very few disorders in which IVIG has been demonstrated to be unequivocally beneficial in carefully designed prospective controlled trials. Nevertheless, like the etiology and the pathogenesis of this fascinating illness, the mechanism by which IVIG exerts its powerful influence has yet to be elucidated.

Summary

Kawasaki disease has become a major pediatric disorder throughout the developed world, including the US, where it is now the leading cause of acquired heart disease in children. Approximately 20–25% of patients develop coronary arteritis leading to abnormalities that may result in myocardial ischemia and/or infarction. Although epidemiologic and clinical findings strongly suggest an infectious etiology, the etiology of Kawasaki disease remains unknown. Marked immune activation is present in acute Kawasaki disease. Investigators in Japan and a US multi-center investigative group have demonstrated in controlled studies that early administration of IVIG is associated with (a) a striking anti-inflammatory effect, and (b) marked reduction in the development of coronary abnormalities. The mechanism(s) by which IVIG produces these dramatic effects is unclear. Possible mechanisms include (a) Fc receptor blockade, (b) a direct anti-etiologic agent (neutralization) effect, (c) an anti-toxic effect, (d) an immunomodulating effect possibly mediated either by anti-idiotypic antibodies or by induction of suppressor T cells, and (e) downregulation of cytokine production by activated immune cells. Clarification of the mechanism of the dramatic effect of IVIG in Kawasaki Disease would provide insights into the pathogenesis and the etiology of this important pediatric illness.

References

1. Kawasaki, T. Acute febrile mucocutaneous syndrome with lymphoid involvement with specific desquamation of the fingers and toes in children. *Jap. J. Allergology* **16**: 178–222; 1967.
2. Kawasaki, T., Kosaki, F., Shigematsu, I., Okawa, S. and Yanagawa, H. A new infantile acute febrile mucocutaneous lymph node syndrome (MLNS). *Pediatrics* **54**: 271–276; 1974.
3. Japan Research Committee on Kawasaki Disease: Report of fatal cases of Kawasaki Disease. Japanese Ministry of Health and Welfare, 1971.
4. Kato, H., Ichinose, E., Takechi, T., Yoshioka, F., Suzuki, K. and Rikitake, N. Fate of coronary aneurysms in Kawasaki Disease. *Am. J. Card.* **49**: 1758–1766; 1982.
5. Rowley, A., Gonzalez-Crussi, F. and Shulman, S. Kawaski syndrome: A review. *Rev. Infect. Dis.* **10**: 1–15; 1988.
6. Shulman, S. T. and Rowley, A. H. Does Kawasaki disease have a retroviral aetiology? *Lancet* **II**: 545–546; 1986.
7. Burns, J. C., Geha, R. S., Schneeberger, E. E., Newburger, J. N., Rosen, F. S., Glezen, L. S., Huang, A. S., Natale, J. and Leung, D. Y. M. Polymerase activity in lymphocyte culture supernatents from patients with Kawasaki Disease. *Nature* **323**: 814–816; 1986.
8. Melish, M., Marchette, N., Kaplan, J., Kihara, S., Ching, D. and Ho, D. Absence of significant RNA-dependent DNA polymerase activity in lymphocytes from patients with Kawasaki Syndrome. *Nature* **337**: 288–290; 1989.

9. Rowley, A., Castro, B., Levy, J., Sullivan, J., Koup, R., Fresco, R. and Shulman, S. Failure to confirm the presence of a retrovirus in cultured lymphocytes from patients with Kawasaki Syndrome. (Submitted for publication).
10. Kyogoku, M. A pathological analysis of Kawasaki Disease with some suggestions of its etio-pathogenesis, *in* "Kawasaki Disease" (Ed. Shulman, S. T.), pp. 257–275. Alan R. Liss, New York; 1987.
11. Tarai, M., Kohno, Y., Namba, M. *et al.* Class II major histocompatibility antigen expression on coronary arterial endothelium in a patient with Kawasaki disease. *Hum. Pathol.* 21: 231–234; 1990.
12. Gee, S. St Bartholomew's Hospital Reports, 1871.
13. Leung, D. Y. M., Siegel, R. L., Grady, S., Krensky, A., Meade, R., Reinherz, E. and Geha, R. S. Immunoregulatory abnormalities in mucocutaneous lymph node syndrome. *Clin. Immunol. Immunopathol.* 23: 100–112; 1982.
14. Leung, D. Y. M., Collins, T., Lapierre, L. A., Geha, R. S. and Pober, J. S. Immunoglobulin M antibodies present in the acute phase of Kawasaki Syndrome lyse cultured vascular endothelial cells stimulated by gamma interferon. *J. Clin. Invest.* 77: 1428–1435; 1986.
15. Leung, D. Y. M., Geha, R. S., Newburger, J. W., Burns, J. C., Fiers, W., Lapierre, L. A. and Pober, J. S. Two monokines, interleukin 1 and tumor necrosis factor, render cultured vascular endothelial cells susceptible to lysis by antibodies circulating during Kawasaki Syndrome. *J. Exp. Med.* 164: 1958–1972; 1986.
16. Mason, W. H., Jordan, S. C., Sakai, R., Takahashi, M. and Bernstein, B. Circulating immune complexes in Kawasaki Syndrome. *Pediatr. Infect. Dis. J.* 4: 48–51; 1985.
17. Herold, B. C., Davis, A. T., Arroyave, C. M., Duffy, E., Pachman, L. M. and Shulman, S. T. Cryoprecipitates in Kawasaki Syndrome: Association with coronary artery aneurysms. *Pediatr. Infect. Dis. J.* 7: 255–257; 1988.
18. Niwa, Y. and Sohmiya, K. Enhanced neutrophilic functions in mucocutaneous lymph node syndrome. *J. Pediatr.* 104: 56; 1984.
19. Ono, S., Onimaru, T., Kawakami, K., Hokonohara, M. and Miyata, K. Impaired granulocyte chemotaxis and increased circulating immune complexes. *J. Pediatr.* 106: 567–570; 1985.
20. Furusho, K., Kamiya, T., Nakano, H. *et al.* High-dose intravenous gammaglobulin for Kawasaki Disease. *Lancet* II: 1055–1058; 1984.
21. Newburger, J. W., Takahashi, M., Burns, J. C. *et al.* The treatment of Kawasaki Syndrome with intravenous gammaglobulin. *New Engl. J. Med.* 315: 341–347; 1986.
22. Newburger, J. W., for the US Multicenter Kawasaki Study Group. Preliminary results of multicenter trial of IVGG treatment of Kawasaki Disease with single infusion vs. four-infusion regimen. *Pediatr. Res.* 27: 22A (abstract no. 119); 1990.
23. Rowley, A. H. and Shulman, S. T. What is the status of intravenous

gamma-globulin for Kawasaki Syndrome in the US and Canada? *Pediatr. Infect. Dis. J.* 7: 463–466; 1988.

24. Leung, D. Y. M., Burns, J. C., Newburger, J. W. and Geha, R. S. Reversal of lymphocyte activation *in vivo* in the Kawasaki Syndrome by intravenous gammaglobulin. *J. Clin. Invest.* 79: 468–472; 1987.
25. Laxer, R. M., Schaffer, F. M., Myones, B. L., Yount, W. J. *et al.* Lymphocyte abnormalities and complement activation in Kawasaki Disease. *In* "Kawasaki Disease" (Ed. Shulman, S. T.), pp. 175–184. Alan R. Liss, New York; 1987.
26. Finberg, R. W., Newburger, J. W. and Burns, J. C. High-dose IVGG increases natural killer cell activity in patients with Kawasaki Disease. *Pediatr. Res.* 27: 156A (abstract no. 920); 1990.
27. Mason, W., Jordan, S., Sakai, R. and Takahashi, M. Lack of effect of gamma-globulin infusion on circulating immune complexes in patients with Kawasaki Syndrome. *Pediatr. Infect. Dis. J.* 7: 94–99; 1988.

Discussion

R. H. Kobayashi

The cytokine down-regulation hypothesis is attractive. Are more specific immune modulators undergoing clinical trials rather than IVIG which has a multitude of effects? This might help to dissect the possible contributory factors resulting in the pathology of Kawasaki disease.

S. T. Shulman

Our trials are only with IVIG and ASA. I am not aware of others.

High-dose intravenous immunoglobulin therapy for insulin-dependent diabetes mellitus

GARY M. LEONG,[1] ZOE THAYER,[1] GABRIEL ANTONY,[1]
STEPHEN COLAGIURI,[2] JOHN DWYER,[2] WARREN KIDSON,[2]
RICHARD FISHER,[2] and DENIS WAKEFIELD[3]

[1] Department of Paediatric Endocrinology, Prince of Wales Children's Hospital,
[2] Department of Medicine, Prince of Wales Hospital and [3] Prince Henry Hospital,
University of New South Wales, Sydney, Australia

Introduction

Insulin-dependent diabetes mellitus (IDDM) is a chronic autoimmune disorder that eventually leads to complete beta cell destruction some time after the development of glucose intolerance (1). Attempts at altering the natural course of IDDM with immunosuppressant drugs such as cyclosporin and azathioprine have been partially successful, with reports of increased remission rates (2–4). The use of these drugs in IDDM is potentially associated with serious, long-term side effects (5).

Immunomodulation, another approach to immunotherapy, carries negligible risk when compared to immunosuppression. There have been several trials with immunomodulatory agents in newly diagnosed IDDM patients. None have been shown to alter the natural course of

Immunotherapy with Intravenous Immunoglobulins
ISBN 0–12–370725–0

the disease (6). While IVIG therapy has been shown to be effective in the treatment of a number of autoimmune or immunological disorders (7–10), trials of IVIG therapy in IDDM are limited to a small number of children with newly diagnosed IDDM, who were followed for a short time and show variable results (11–14) (Table 1).

The purpose of this report is to describe IVIG therapy in 16 recently diagnosed IDDM adults and children compared to 15 control patients in a randomized, ongoing, controlled double-blind trial, in which serial C-peptide responses to i.v. glucagon and a standard meal (glucagon meal test), were used to assess beta-cell function for over 2 years.

Materials and methods

Patients

This report deals with the IVIG and control arms of a 3-arm study into which 43 IDDM patients were randomized: IVIG (n=16); controls (n=15); and transfer factor (n=12). The age and duration of diagnosis of the IVIG and control group were not significantly different (mean ± SD) (15.0 ± 7.4 years) (range 6.9–26.4) vs. (16.4 ± 5.8 years) (range 7.3–25.4) and 177 ± 154 vs. 175 ± 170 days) respectively. There were 7 males and 9 females in the IVIG group and 11 males and 4 females in the control group. All groups were subdivided according to IDDM duration: (1) $<$ 3 months (9 IVIG and 8 controls) and (2) $>$ 3 months to $<$ 2 years (7 IVIG and 7 controls). Group 2 patients were included only if their insulin dose was less than or equal to 0.5 units/kg/day, and if they had a C-peptide response to the glucagon meal test (GMT) equal to or above the 10th centile of normal controls (15).

All patients were managed by their own physicians, who determined the insulin type, dose and injection frequency. Insulin injections were given two or three times daily and home blood glucose monitoring was used to adjust the dose.

Fifteen patients in the control group and 14 patients in the IVIG group completed 6 months of the trial, 11 controls and 9 IVIG completed 12 months, 9 controls and 5 IVIG completed 18 months, and 7 controls and 2 IVIG completed 24 months, and one patient who received IVIG completed 30 months.

Table 1
Studies of IVIG therapy in IDDM

Reference	No. of subjects	Dose, frequency, duration of IVIG	Controls	Tests of beta-cell function used	Observations
Heinze *et al*. (11)	6 children age 5–14 years	2 g/kg over 5 days then 0.4 g/kg weekly, 6 months	48 conventionally treated IDDM children	i.v. glucose, arginine, standard breakfast	4/7 had demonstrable C-peptide secretion 10–30 months after diagnosis.
Pocecco *et al*. (12)	10 children aged 3–14 years	2 g/kg over 5 days, monthly, 6 months	10 age-matched, conventionally treated IDDM patients	Post-prandial C-peptide	IVIG group required less insulin than control group at 3, 6, 9 months but not at 12 months
Urakami *et al*. (13)	8 children	1.6–2 g/kg 4–5 days; 2 doses, 3–12 months	No control group	Tests not specified	Elevation of serum C-peptide in 6/8 with 1st Rx and 3/6 with 2nd Rx
Lorini *et al*. (14)	4 children mean age 9.2 years	2 g/kg for 5 days then 0.4 g/kg weekly, 4.5 months	4 age- and sex-matched IDDM patients	i.v. glucagon	No significant differences observed. No side effects.

Research protocol

After a 12 h fast, serum C-peptide responses to i.v. glucagon (10μg/kg over 30 s) given at time zero, and a standard meal given at 2 h (glucagon meal test), were measured over a 5 h period and expressed as area under C-peptide curve above zero (AUCZ) (pmol min/ml). T-cell subsets, serum immunoglobulins, complement and glycosylated hemoglobin (HbA1c) were performed at the same time and repeated with the GMT at 2, 6, 12, 18 and 24 months.

The treatment group received a total of 2 g/kg/body weight of IVIG (Sandoglobulin®, Basel, Switzerland) over 6–10 h on two consecutive days every 2 months for up to 2 years. The control group received 2 monthly i.m. normal saline as part of the double-blind, placebo-controlled arm of the trial.

Biochemical techniques

HbA1c was measured by HPLC using Biorad "Diamat" reagents (Hercules, California, USA) in an in-house assay (normal range 3.9–7.4%).

Serum C-peptide was measured by radioimmunoassay with anti-serum M-1221 (Novo, Bagsvaerd, Denmark) (16).

Immunological tests

Total T lymphocyte (T3) and subpopulations (T4 inducer and T8 supressor/cytotoxic) were determined in peripheral blood using CD3, CD4 and CD8 monoclonal antibodies (Ortho Diagnostic Systems, New Jersey, USA), using standard flow cytometric techniques (17). Serum complement (C3, C4) was determined by radial-immunodiffusion against polyspecific antisera (Dako, Copenhagen, Denmark) in 1% agarose by the technique of Mancini (18). CH50 was determined by the method of Thompson (19). Serum IgG, IgA and IGM levels were assayed by nephelometry. IgG subclasses (IGI–G4) were measured by radial-immunodiffusion using a commercially available kit (Binding Site, Birmingham, UK). The values obtained in the IgG subclass assays were compared with WHO-derived normal standards (20).

Statistical analysis

The data were examined using standard graphical methods and an analysis of co-variance was performed (21).

Results

Insulin dose and HbA1c

There were no differences in insulin dose between the IVIG and control groups. No patients in either group ceased insulin therapy during the 2-year period of the trial. Mean values of HbA1c (%) were less in the IVIG than the control group at 18 months (7.2 ± 1.1 (*n*=5) vs. 9.0 ± 2.3 (*n*=9)) and 24 months (7.1 ± 2.4 (*n*=3) vs. 9.8 ± (*n*=7)), but these differences were not significant (Table 2).

Table 2
Insulin dose, HbA1c and AUCZ control and IVIG subjects

Time (months)	Insulin dose (U/kg/day)		HbA1c (%)		AUCZ (pmol min/ml)	
	C	IVIG	C	IVIG	C	IVIG
0	0.43±0.13	0.40±0.24	7.7±1.9	8.0±3.0	132.6±53.7	126.4±64.9
2	0.43±0.24	0.39±0.19	7.8±1.3	8.7±1.9	113.6±69.4	101.1±39.6
6	0.51±0.23	0.47±0.22	7.4±1.5	8.1±2.1	94.3±63.0	90.9±60.9
12	0.60±0.20	0.53±0.23	8.8±1.9	9.0±2.5	54.2±35.8	70.0±70.3
18	0.67±0.29	0.59±0.17	9.0±2.3	7.2±1.1	45.9±54.9	44.7±18.7
24	0.54±0.11	0.49±0.09	9.8±3.1	7.1±2.4	26.1±14.1	43.9±44.0

All values are mean±SD. No. of subjects at 0–6 months *n*=15 (C), *n*=14 (IVIG); 12 months *n*=11 (C), *n*=9 (IVIG); 18 months *n*=9 (C), *n*=5 (IVIG); 24 months *n*=7 (C), *n*=3 (IVIG).

Beta-cell function

Progressive loss of beta-cell function (AUCZ) occurred in both the IVIG and control groups, and though the IVIG group had higher AUCZ at 12 months (mean ± SD) 70.0 ± 70.3 vs. 54.2 ± 35.8) and at 24 months (43.9 ± 44.0 vs. 26.1 ± 14.1), these differences were not significant (*f*-value = 1.34 on 3 and 42 degrees of freedom) (Fig. 1 and Table 2).

In Group 1 the AUCZ between the IVIG and control groups showed a non-significant difference only at 12 months (mean ± SD) IVIG 82.2 ± 91.7 (*n*=5) vs. controls 64.1 ± 40.7 (*n*=6)) (Fig. 1). In Group 2 the IVIG group had higher mean values of AUCZ at 12, 18 and 24 months than the control group: 54.7 ± 37.7 (*n*=4) vs. 36.8 ± 18.4 (*n*=4); 41.8 ± 22.9 (*n*=3) vs. 14.0± 8.4 (*n*=3); and 53.4 ± 55.6 (*n*=2) vs. 24.9 ± 5.6 (*n*=3), respectively (Fig. 1).

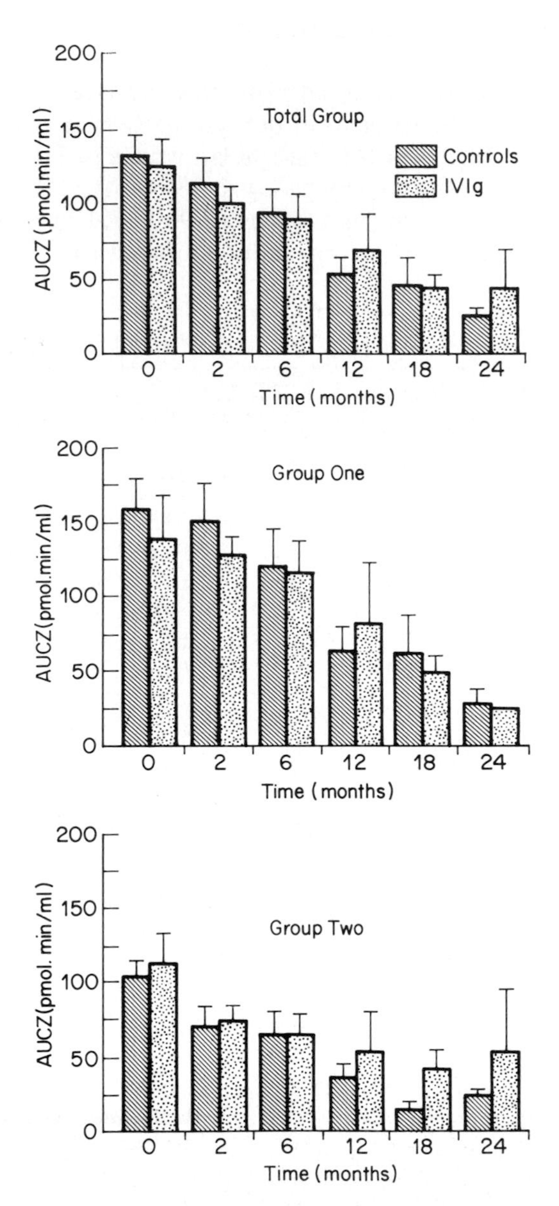

Figure 1. Beta-cell function over a 2-year period in IVIG and control group as measured by "area under the C-peptide curve" (AUCZ) in response to glucagon meal test.

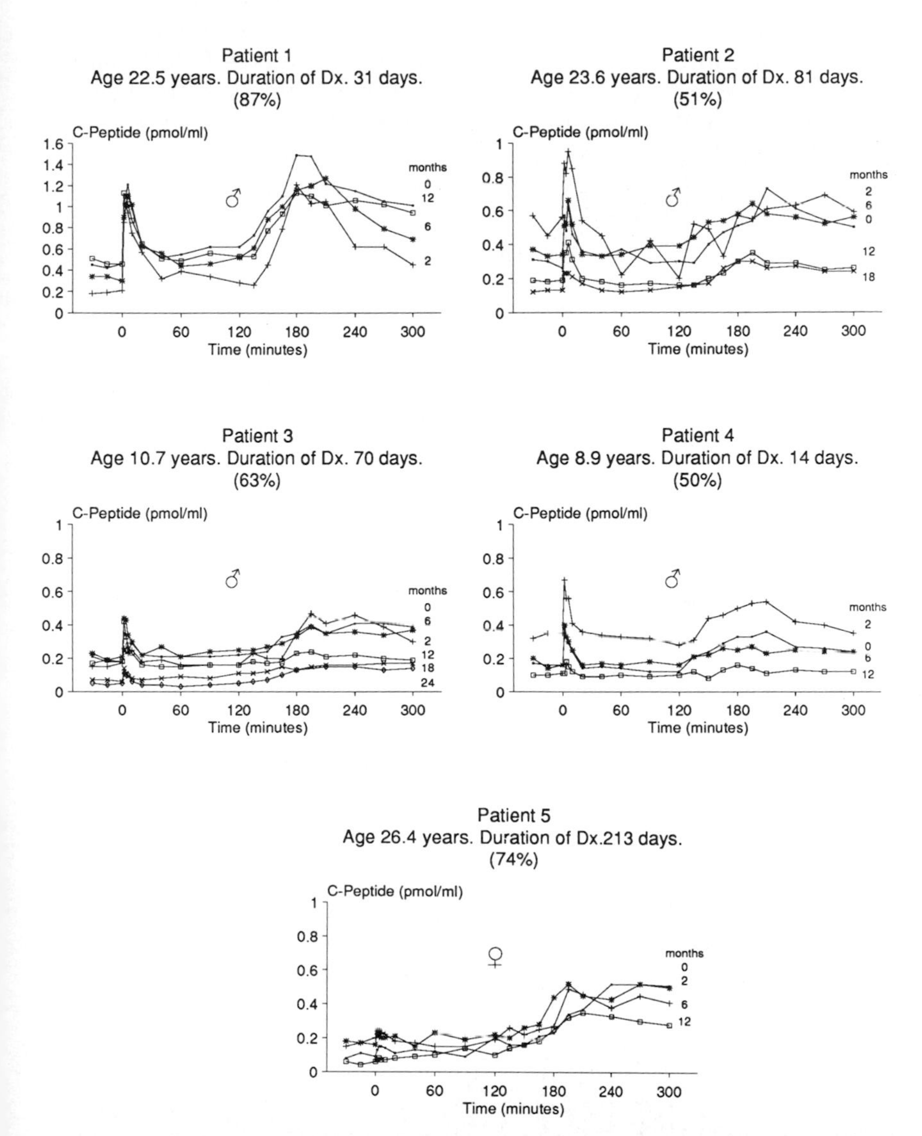

Figure 2. C-Peptide responses to GMT of five patients treated with IVIG for 12–24 months who had an AUCZ of 50% or greater than baseline at 12 months. Four of the 5 patients were male (2 adults and 2 children) and commenced IVIG treatment within 90 days of diagnosis. The other patient was an adult female who commenced IVIG treatment 213 days after diagnosis. The mean insulin dose in the 5 patients compared to the controls was less (0.43 vs. 0.60), but there were no differences in HbA1c.

Twenty patients (9 IVIG and 11 controls) were followed for at least 12 months. Of these, 5 patients, all in the IVIG group, maintained an AUCZ 50% or more of baseline at 12 months (range 14.6–87% and mean ± SD 34 ± 32) (Fig. 2), while four other patients in the IVIG group had % AUCZ of baseline at 12 months between 14 and 46% (Fig. 3). The % of baseline AUCZ at 12 months in the control patients ranged from 18% to 45% (mean ± SD 32 ± 10). Fourteen patients were followed for 18 months or more (5 IVIG and 9 controls). Of these, 7 patients (4 IVIG, 3 controls) maintained an AUCZ 25% or more of baseline at 18 and/or 24 months. In 5 patients, these data suggest IVIG may have had an effect on slowing the progressive loss of beta-cell function in the first 12–15 months after diagnosis, and in 2 other patients, prolonged C-peptide secretion to $2\frac{1}{2}$ years and 3 years after diagnosis respectively (Patients 6 and 8 in Fig. 3). Four of the 5 patients who maintained 50% of their baseline AUCZ at 12 months,

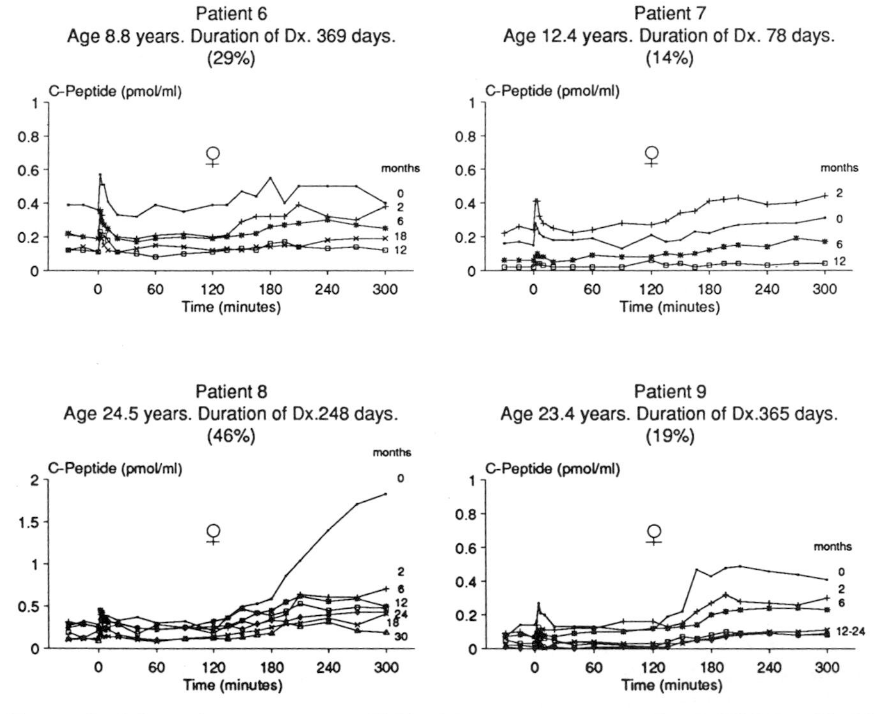

Figure 3. C-Peptide responses to GMT of four patients treated with IVIG for 12–24 months, who had an AUCZ less than 50% of baseline at 12 months. All 4 patients were females; 3 of the 4 commenced IVIG treatment more than 240 days after diagnosis.

commenced IVIG therapy within 3 months of diagnosis. No significant difference was observed in insulin doses or HbA1c in these 5 patients compared to the controls, though the mean insulin dose was less at 12 months (0.43 ± 0.23) vs. (0.60 ± 0.20). It is also of interest that 4 of these 5 patients were males (2 adults and 2 children), as adult males with IDDM treated with cylcosporin have been reported to have a higher remission rate (2).

Immunological data

T-cell subsets

Seven control patients and 7 patients in the IVIG group had abnormally low peripheral T-cell subset numbers on 2 or more occasions. Seven patients had low T3, T4 and T8 numbers (5 controls, 2 IVIG); 5 patients (4 IVIG) had low T8 numbers but normal T3 and T4 numbers, and 2 patients had low T4 and low T8 with normal T3 numbers.

Two patients had low T4/T8 ratios, one whose initial low T4/T8 ratio normalized after one IVIG infusion and remained normal, whilst the other subject had an initial normal ratio, which dropped to below normal after the second IVIG infusion.

Serum immunoglobulin levels

All patients had normal serum levels of total IgG, IgG_4 subclass, and IgA levels. IgG subclasses were abnormal in a significant number of patients in both groups, the main abnormality being low IgG_3 levels (6 control, 2 IVIG), and transiently low IgG_1 (5 controls, 1 IVIG), IgG_2 (2 controls) and IgG_3 (3 IVIG) levels. None of the patients had an increased incidence of infections.

Complement

Eleven control patients and 6 IVIG patients had either persistently or intermittently low C3 and/or C4 levels, while four control patients had low CH50 levels.

Side effects

In our study 111 infusions of IVIG were administered. The incidence of side-effects was as follows: headaches (80%), nausea (39%), vomiting (24%), lethargy (39%), pyrexia (28%), mild edema (21%), mild generalized aching (17%), transient dyspnoea (13%), while a few patients experienced anorexia and a petechial rash (Tables 3 and 4). Of

Table 3
Incidence (%) of side effects associated with IVIG

Side-effect	Mild	Moderate	Severe	Total
Headache	43	31	6	80
Nausea	23	16	0	39
Lethargy	29	10	0	39
Pyrexia	16	12	0	28
Vomiting	14	9	1	24
Edema	21	0	0	21
Generalized ache	17	0	0	17
Dyspnoea	13	0	0	13
Anorexia	4	1	0	5
Rash	2	0	0	2
Peri-orbital swelling	0	1	0	1

Table 4
Criteria used for assessing severity of side effects

Side effect	Mild	Moderate	Severe
Headache	<6 h +/− Rx	>6–24 h + Rx	>24 h + photophobia
Pyrexia (C)	37–38	38–39	>39
Nausea	No vomiting	Vomiting	
Lethargy	<48 h	>48 h	
Edema	No Rx required		

the 11 patients (6 adults and 5 children) who did not complete the trial, only one subject ceased because of side effects. This patient, an adult male, developed severe vomiting, moderate peri-orbital edema and headache near the completion of his infusion and required admission to hospital overnight, and withdrew from the study on advice from the trial investigators.

Discussion

Our data agree with previous reports that show a dramatic decrease in beta-cell function over the first 3 years after diagnosis especially in children and adolescents (22, 23). None of our patients who were followed long enough showed a clinically discernible remission. Our comprehensive immunological profiles showed the previously reported changes in T-cell subsets and immunogl'bulin subclasses (24–26) without any demonstrable clinical effect or any correlation with metabolic parameters. Using our protocol of infusing IVIG on two consecutive days, side effects were very common, although only one instance was considered to be severe, as judged by the need for an overnight hospital admission.

Though the results from this study fail to confirm any significant effect of IVIG on metabolic control and beta-cell function in IDDM, serial assessment of beta-cell function showed that an unexpected number of IVIG-treated patients, compared to our controls, maintained better C-peptide levels at 12 months and 24 months. The large majority of this subgroup of patients commenced IVIG therapy within 3 months of diagnosis, suggesting that beyond a critical time period after diagnosis, immunotherapy in IDDM has significantly less chance of success, an observation also made in the Canadian/European cyclosporin trial (2). We chose to study patients with IDDM of greater duration who had evidence of significant residual beta-cell function, as preservation of some C-peptide secretion has been shown to favorably influence the control of metabolic function and development of long-term complications (27–29). The small numbers, the wide range of ages and duration of diagnosis of the patients, and the significant incidence of side effects and subsequent high drop-out rate may have all contributed to the observed lack of significance.

To our knowledge, our data represent the longest experience and the largest numbers of patients treated to date in the only randomized, controlled trial of IVIG therapy in IDDM. A definitive evaluation of this therapy, however would require additional, long-term patient follow-up and a reducing of the side effects. Immunoglobulin therapy is rather expensive but a cost–benefit ratio cannot be determined on the basis of the available data.

Summary

Interim analysis of a controlled trial of IVIG therapy in IDDM shows a non-significant slowing compared with controls in the fall of C-peptide responses to a Glucagon Meal Test. Patient selection, small patient numbers and large individual variation in responses may account for the lack of significance. Eighty percent of the infusions caused side-effects, the majority mild. In 30% medical attention was sought. One patient was admitted to hospital overnight because of severe vomiting, headache and pyrexia. So far, under our study conditions, IVIG therapy failed to attenuate significantly the natural progression of beta cell destruction in IDDM.

Acknowledgements

We are indebted to Sr. Marie-France Ah-Lock for her expert clinical care, Mrs Lilian Tan and Ms Rohini Vikash (Endocrinology) and Mr John McShane (Immunology) for their important laboratory assistance. This work was supported by grants from Sandoz Australia Pty. Ltd., The Prince Henry Hospital Centenary Fund, Government Assistance to Medical Research Fund, Rebecca L. Cooper Medical Research Foundation, National Health & Medical Research Council of Australia, The Gavemer Foundation, and a number of other generous individuals and organizations.

References

1. Eisenbarth, G. S. Type 1 Diabetes Mellitus. A chronic autoimmune disease. *N. Engl. J. Med.* 314: 1360–1368; 1986.
2. The Canadian-European Randomized Control Trial Group. Cyclosporin-induced remission of IDDM after early intervention. *Diabetes* 37: 1574–1581; 1988.
3. Harrison, L. C., Colman, P. G., Dean, B. *et al.* Increase in remission rate in newly diagnosed Type 1 diabetic subjects treated with azathioprine. *Diabetes* 34: 1306–1308; 1985.
4. Silverstein, J., Maclaren, N., Riley, W. *et al.* Immunosuppression with azathioprine and prednisone in recent-onset insulin-dependent diabetes mellitus. *N. Engl. J. Med.* 319: 599–604; 1988.
5. Kahan, B. D. Cyclosporin. *N. Engl. J. Med.* 321: 1725–1738; 1989.
6. Pollizi, P. Immunotherapy in type 1 Diabetes. *Diab. Med.* 8: 734–735; 1988.
7. Imbach, P. Intravenous immunoglobulin therapy for idiopathic thrombocytopenic purpura and other immune-related disorders: review and update of our experiences. *Pediatr. Infect. Dis. J.* 7: S120–S125; 1988.
8. Newburger, J. W., Takahashi, M., Burns, J. D. *et al.* The treatment of Kawasaki syndrome with intravenous gammaglobulin. *N. Engl. J. Med.* 215: 341–347; 1986.
9. American Academy of Pediatrics. Committee on Infectious Diseases. Intravenous gammaglobulin use in children with Kawasaki disease. *Pediatrics* 82: 122–123; 1988.
10. Arsura, E. L., Bick, A., Brunner, N. *et al.* Effects of repeated doses of

intravenous immunoglobulin in myasthenia gravis. *Am. J. Med. Sci.* 295: 438–443; 1988.
11. Heinze, E., Zuppinger, K., Thon, A. *et al.* Gammaglobulin therapy in Type 1 Diabetes Mellitus. *In* "Pediat. Adolesc. Endocr. Vol. 15: Future Trends in Juvenile Diabetes" (Eds Laron, Z. and Karp, M.), pp. 362–370. Karger, Basel; 1986.
12. Pococco, M., Decampo, C., Cantoni, L. *et al.* Intravenous gammaglobulin therapy in newly diagnosed insulin dependent diabetes. *Helv. Paediatr. Acta* 42: 289–295; 1987.
13. Urakami, T., Hanaoka, Y., Fujita, H. *et al.* High dose gammaglobulin therapy in eight children with newly diagnosed insulin-dependent diabetes mellitus. *International Study Group of Diabetes (ISGD) Bulletin* 17: 44–45; 1987 (abstract).
14. Lorini, R., Lombardi, A., Cortona, L. *et al.* Gammaglobulin therapy in newly diagnosed children with Type 1 diabetes mellitus. *International Study Group of Diabetes (ISGD) Bulletin* 17: 48; 1987 (abstract).
15. Colagiuri, S., Antony, G., Marchant, L. *et al.* The Combined Glucagon Meal Test as a measure of beta cell function. *Diabetes Research and Clinic Practice* 5: Suppl, S509; 1988 (abstract).
16. Human C-peptide estimation by radioimmunoassay. *In* "RIA kit for Human C-peptide, antiserum M1221.1987". Supplied by Novo Research Institute, Bagsvaerd, Denmark. Catalogue no. 144.
17. Loken, M. and Herzenberg, L. Analysis of cell populations with a fluorescence-activated cell sorter. *Ann N.Y. Acad. Sci.* 254: 163–171; 1975.
18. Mancini, G., Carbonara, A. O. and Heramans, J. F. Immunochemical quantitation of antigen by single radial-immunodiffusion. *Int. J. Immunol.* 2: 235–254; 1965.
19. Thompson, R. A. and Rowes, D. S. Reactive hamolysis—a distinct form of red cell lysis. *Immunology* 14: 745–762; 1968.
20. Oxelius, V. M. IgG subclasses in infancy and childhood. *Acta Paediatr. Scand.* 68: 23–27; 1979.
21. Weisberg, S. "Applied Linear Regression", 2nd edn. Wiley, New York; 1985.
22. The DCCT Research Group. Effects of age, duration and treatment of insulin-dependent diabetes mellitus on residual beta cell function: observations during eligibility testing for the diabetes control and complications trial (DCCT). *J. Clin. Endocrinol. Metab.* 65: 30–36; 1987.
23. Schiffrin, A., Suissa, S., Poussier, P. *et al.* Prospective study of predictors of Beta cell survival in Type 1 Diabetes. *Diabetes* 37: 920–925. 1988.
24. Johnston, C., Alviggi, L., Millward, A. *et al.* Alterations in T-lymphocyte subpopulations in type 1 diabetes: exploration of genetic influence in identical twins. *Diabetes* 37: 1484–1488; 1988.

25. Tsubakio, T., Kurata, Y., Katagiri, S. *et al.* Alteration of T cell subsets and immunoglobulin synthesis in vitro during high dose gammaglobulin therapy in patients with idiopathic thrombocytopenic purpura. *Clin. Exp. Immunol.* 53: 697–702; 1983.
26. Stromquist, C., Berkel, A. I., Wilson, D. P. *et al.* Serum Immunoglobulin and IgG subclass levels in children and adolescents with insulin dependent diabetes mellitus. *Acta Paediatr. Scand.* **78**: 639–640; 1989.
27. Cahill, G. F. and McDevitt, H. O. Insulin-dependent diabetes mellitus: the initial Lesion. *N. Engl. J. Med.* **304**: 1454–1465; 1981.
28. Chase, H. P., Jackson, W. E., Hoops, S. L. *et al.* Glucose control and the renal and retinal complications of insulin-dependent diabetes. *J. Am. Med. Assoc.* **261**: 1155–1160; 1989.
29. Dahlquist, G., Blom, L., Bolme, P. *et al.* Metabolic control in 131 juvenile-onset diabetic patients as measured by HbA1; relation to age, duration, C-peptide, insulin dose, and one or two insulin injections. *Diabetes Care* 5: 399–403; 1982.

Effect of high-dose intravenous immunoglobulin in rheumatoid arthritis

A. CORVETTA, M. M. LUCHETTI, G. POMPONIO, P. J. SPAETH[1] and G. DANIELI

Department of Internal Medicine, Ancona University Medical School, Ancona, Italy
[1]Central Laboratory, Blood Transfusion Service of the Swiss Red Cross, Bern, Switzerland

Introduction

Rheumatoid arthritis (RA) is a systemic disease characterized by a chronic, recurrent, progressively destructive synovitis (1). Ten to twenty per cent of patients go into spontaneous remission. The others have a variably progressive disease leading to severe joint deformities and to extra-articular complications. The etiology of RA still remains unclear. The association of the disease with the HLA-D4 gene (2) and the observation of cellular abnormalities in the affected joints, suggest that the immune system plays a pivotal role in the onset and chronic evolution of the disease. Indeed, lymphokine-producing T cells are found in the synovial tissue and fluid during the active phases of the disease (3), and the number of MHC class II molecule-expressing cells may be increased in the synovia (4). A large number of synovial plasma cells produce rheumatoid factors, of which the IgG isotype is responsible for inducing inflammation through formation of small-size immune complexes which activate the complement system (5).

Immunotherapy with Intravenous Immunoglobulins
ISBN 0-12-370725-0

Furthermore, T helper cells recognizing "self", such as collagen, have been isolated and cloned from the joints of rheumatoid patients (6).

The present therapy for RA consists of non-steroidal anti-inflammatory drugs (NSAID), glycocorticoids, disease-modifying anti-rheumatoid drugs (DMARD) and immunosuppressive agents (Table 1).

Table 1
The classes of drugs mainly used for the treatment of rheumatoid arthritis

Class I	Class II	Class III
Analgesic	Gold salts	Azathioprine
NSAID	Antimalarian agents	Methotrexate
Glycocorticoids	d-Penicillamine	Cyclophosphamide
	Salazopyrine	Cyclosporin A

Class I drugs (NSAID and glycocorticoids) have only a temporary effect and do not limit joint destruction (7).

Class II drugs (DMARD) induce a remission of the disease in 30–60% of the patients treated. Recent studies have shown that the therapeutic maintenance rate is about 50% at 1 year and less than 20% at 5 years. The patients tend to be switched from one drug to another so that many class II drugs may have exhausted their therapeutic potential after a few years (8).

Thus, many RA patients need class III drugs (9). The major limitations of these drugs are the severity of some of their side effects, the fear of oncogenesis induction by long-term treatment, and their efficacy rate not higher than 50%.

Patients who were unresponsive to class II and class III drugs are the subject of this study.

High-dose intravenous immunoglobulin (IVIG) therapy has recently been reported to be of benefit in several autoimmune diseases, where immunomodulating and/or anti-inflammatory effects were observed (10). Several reports about preliminary experience of the IVIG therapy in patients affected by RA have been published recently (11–17). Reasons for applying IVIG to RA unresponsive to class II and class III drugs are as follows:

1. These patients usually undergo long-term immunosuppressive therapy. A potential advantage of IVIG infusion in this situation is the likely restoration of the humoral immune system.
2. The reduced galactosylation of IgG in RA may be one of the

reasons for the autosensitization to IgG. Altered IgG probably plays a role in the pathogenesis of the disease (18). It seems reasonable to interrupt such a process by substituting the patient's "abnormal" IgG with IgG derived from normal subjects, showing a normal galactosylation pattern.

3. In RA lymphocyte modulation occurring spontaneously or induced by treatment may have a beneficial effect (19). A reduction in T-helper and consequently in B-cell activity was observed in autoimmune diseases after IVIG.

Based on this rationale IVIG therapy was applied to six RA patients who failed class II and III drugs. This paper reviews the clinical and immunological results obtained.

Patients and methods

Six patients affected by classical RA according to the American Rheumatism Association criteria, 4 females and 2 males, aged 56.8 ± 8.2 years, were characterized by: (1) previous ineffective treatment with at least one class II and one class III drug; (2) long duration of the disease; (3) anatomical stage II or III; (4) "active" disease (Tables 2 and 3). IVIG therapy (0.4 g/kg/day) was applied on days 1, 3, 5 and then once a month. The treatment period ranged from 5 to 120 days. As concomitant treatment, stable doses of the NSAID used before the study was allowed. In patients 3 and 4 pulses of methyl-prednisolone followed IVIG therapy.

Table 2
Main characteristics of six patients affected by rheumatoid arthritis selected for IVIG therapy

Patient no.	Sex/age	Anatomical[a] stage	Duration of the disease (months)	Previous[b] ineffective therapy
1	F/52	III	216	GS, anti-MAL, CSA
2	F/65	III	39	GS, CSA
3	F/63	II	30	GS, CSA
4	M/61	III	66	GS, MTX
5	M/43	II	108	GS, CSA, MTX
6	F/57	III	120	GS, CSA

[a] According to Steinbrocker.
[b] GS: gold salts; anti-MAL: anti-malarian agents; CSA: cyclosporin A; MTX: methotrexate.

Table 3
Disease profiles of six patients affected by rheumatoid arthritis selected for IVIG therapy

Patient no.	ESR ≥ 60	No. of swollen joints > 9	Morning stiffness > 45 min	Active[a] disease
1	+	+	+	Yes
2	+	+	−	Yes
3	+	+	−	Yes
4	+	−	+	Yes
5	+	+	+	Yes
6	+	+	+	Yes

[a] The disease was defined as "active" when at least two of the following criteria were fulfilled: (1) ESR ≥ 30 mm.; (2) morning stiffness ≥ 45 min; (3) 9 or more swollen joints.

On each day of IVIG infusion patients underwent a complete physical examination in order to evaluate the efficacy of the treatment and signs of toxicity. Ritchie's index, grip strength, morning stiffness and number of swollen joints were used for monitoring the clinical effectiveness. Laboratory parameters studied were: blood cell counts, kidney and liver function indices, urinalysis; virus B markers.

Erythrocyte sedimentation rate (ESR) and C-reactive protein (CRP) were monitored on each day of IVIG infusion together with immunological parameters such as: IgG, IgA, IgM; rheumatoid factor (RF) titer, circulating immune complex (CIC) level as assessed by the C1q-binding assay, complement (CH50, C3 and C4), total number of peripheral blood lymphocytes, CD2, CD3, CD4, CD8, and B cells, as detected by cytofluorimetry. Interleukin 2 (IL-2), soluble IL-2 receptor (sIL-2R) and tumor necrosis factor (TNF) were detected by sandwich enzyme immunoassay, using the kits from Genzyme Corp. (Boston, MA) and from T cell Sciences (Cambridge, MA), respectively.

Results

The clinical response to IVIG treatment is summarized in Table 4. In none of the patients was there a worsening of the disease due to IVIG.

Table 4
Clinical effects of IVIG therapy in six patients affected by rheumatoid arthritis, who had been unresponsive to class II and class III drugs

Patient no.	Total number of IVIG infusions	Clinical efficacy[a] after the first 3 IVIG infusions	Clinical efficacy[a] at the end of IVIG infusions	Treatment[b] following IVIG therapy
1	6	Good	Poor	NSAID
2	5	Moderate	Poor	Oral GC
3	5	Poor	Poor	Pulses of MP
4	5	Good	Poor	Pulses of MP
5	4	Good	Poor	AZP+CTX
6	5	Poor	Poor	NSAID+oral GC

[a] Clinical efficacy was considered as good when at least three out of the following clinical parameters improved by > 30%: Ritchie's index, grip strength, morning stiffness, number of swollen joints; improvement < 30% and < 15% indicated moderate and poor efficacy, respectively.
[b] NSAID: non-steroidal anti-inflammatory drugs; GC: glycocorticoids; MP: methyl-prednisolone; AZP: azathioprine; CTX: cyclophosphamide.

No side effects were seen except in patient 1 who was sensitive to infusion rates. When these were higher than 20 drops/min of a 6% IgG solution, headache, nausea and hypotension were observed. Changes in humoral parameters which could be attributed to IVIG therapy were infrequent.

Patients 1 and 4 showed a drop in ESR after the 4th IVIG pulse (from 120 to 90 and from 80 to 25 mm, respectively), whereas in patient 3, where the ESR did not show any significant decrease after five IVIG pulses, methyl-prednisolone therapy induced a drop from 115 to 50 mm. However, an increase in ESR was observed just at the last methyl-prednisolone infusion. As expected, the IgG serum concentration reflected the amount of IgG infused, however, to a different extent from patient to patient. C1q-binding activity and CH50 values are depicted in Fig. 1. C1q-binding activity followed three different profiles: in patients 1 and 6 high baseline values did not change; in patients 3 and 4 no C1q-binding activity could be detected throughout the study; in patients 2 and 5 a significant rise in C1q-binding activity was observed after the first IgG infusion and increased values persisted thereafter. CH50 was normal or higher than normal in all patients except in patient 1. In this patient low CH50 was apparently due to the activation of the classical pathway as was indicated by low C4 and C2 concentrations. In this case three pulses of IVIG led to normalization

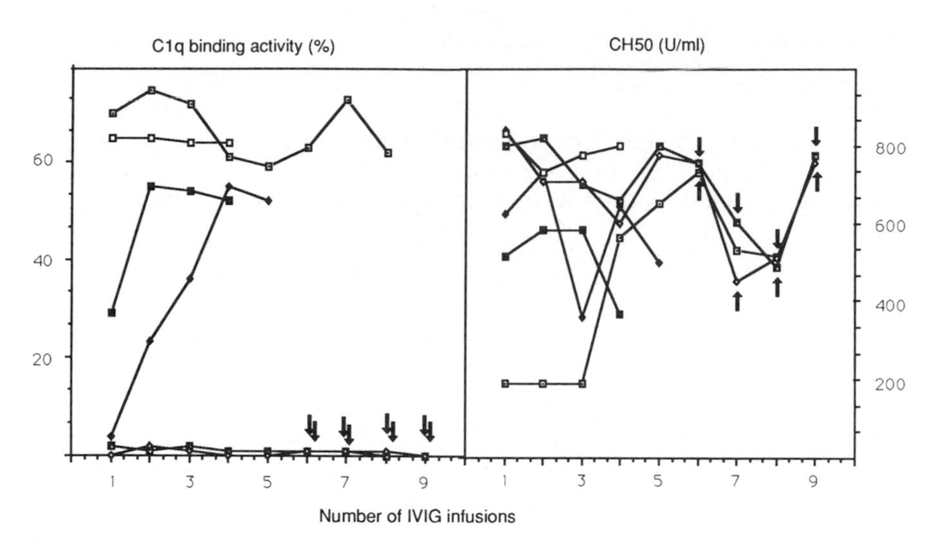

Figure 1. Profiles of C1q-binding activity and of CH50 in six patients affected by rheumatoid arthritis under IVIG therapy. (↓, Pulses of methyl-prednisolone (1 g) with no IVIG infusion.)

of C4 and CH50 values. Neither C1q-binding activity ($r = 0.071$; P = NS) nor CH50 ($r = -0.205$; P = NS), appeared to be correlated to the serum IgG level, while they were negatively correlated to each other ($r = -0.487$; P = <0.01). In three out of the four RF-positive patients IVIG infusion did not lead to any significant variation of RF titer, whereas in patient 1 a dramatic drop was observed after the first course of three IVIG pulses: indeed, RF titer fell from 10 240 U/ml to 1 035 U/ml and only minor variations were then observed during the five successive months.

Changes in cellular parameters were followed by cell counts. The baseline peripheral blood lymphocyte numbers ranged from 1.2 to 2.8 $\times 10^9$/l. In 5 out of the 6 patients the first IVIG infusion was followed by a slight drop in lymphocyte count. The successive variations of this parameter were not uniform. A further decrease was observed in patient 6, while lymphocyte counts fluctuated in all the other patients. In patients 3 and 4, pulses of methyl-prednisolone led to a 3-fold rise in the total lymphocyte numbers. However, at the end of the study, still under methyl-prednisolone therapy, their lymphocyte counts returned to the baseline values. The course of T, B, CD4 and CD8 cell counts paralleled the total lymphocyte counts (Fig. 2): early drop after the first IgG infusion in most patients, fluctuations during the next period of therapy and significant but transient increase in patients 3 and 4 while treated with methyl-prednisolone. When the correlation between IgG levels and lymphocyte counts was investigated, a general tendency towards a reduction in cell counts with increasing serum IgG was observed. The only population which was significantly correlated with serum IgG was the CD8 one ($r = -0.371$; $P < 0.05$) (Fig. 3). When analyzed after the first course of three IVIG infusions, the negative correlation between CD8 counts and IgG levels was found much more significant ($r = -0.939$; $P < 0.0001$) in patients 2, 3 and 6 who gave a moderate or poor response, compared to patients 1, 4 and 5 ($r = -0.489$; $P < 0.25$), whose clinical response was good. IL-2 was not detectable in any patient either before or during IVIG therapy, while sIL-2R showed a high baseline value in four patients with no variations during the treatment. Patient 1 was the only patient where TNF was detectable: indeed, high baseline values dropped after the first series of three IVIG pulses and persisted at low level during the next infusion period.

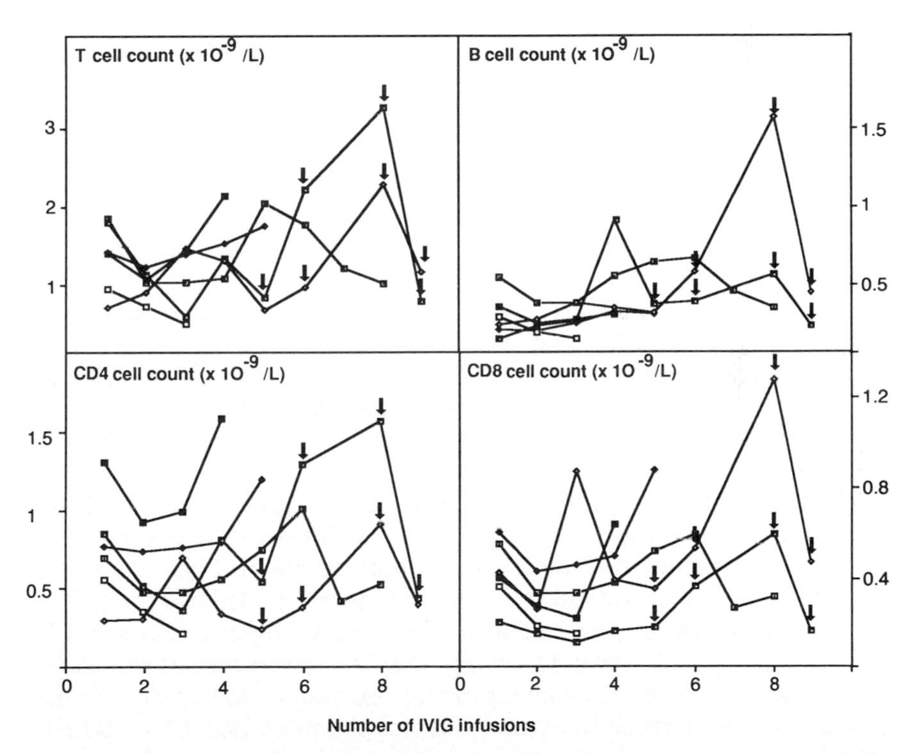

Figure 2. T, B, CD4 and CD8 cell counts in six patients affected by rheumatoid arthritis under IVIG therapy. (↓, Pulses of methyl-prednisolone (1 g) with no IVIG infusion.)

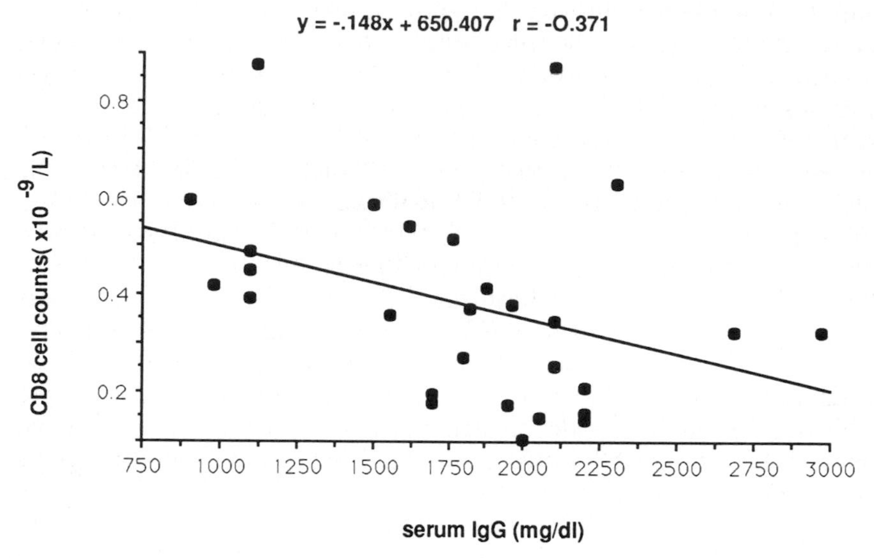

Figure 3. Statistically significant negative correlation between CD8 cell counts and IgG serum levels in six patients affected by rheumatoid arthritis under IVIG therapy.

Discussion

The patients selected for this study on effects of IVIG therapy in RA showed an advanced and active disease, characterized by severe and to a large extent irreversible joint deformities. Patients showed no response to therapeutic attempts with class II and class III drugs. In this situation good but transient clinical results with no relevant side effects were achieved in 3 out of the 6 patients treated by a polyclonal, polyvalent IgG preparation for intravenous use. The results of this study are in agreement with those reported in other observations (12–17).

High titers of RF and CIC usually characterize the more severe cases of RA. These patients often present with extra-articular complications, rheumatoid skin nodules and high levels of TNF (1, 20), a constellation which was also found in patient 1. In this patient a significant clinical improvement was accompanied by a fall in ESR, RF titer and TNF level following the first course of three IVIG infusions. Furthermore, the apparent excessive activation of the classical complement pathway could be stopped just when TNF and RF dropped. In this case IVIG obviously interfered with the mechanism(s) which apparently sustained the RF synthesis. Accelerated removal of immune complexes formed by RF and IgG (10), blockade of the complement activation, as recently observed in a guinea-pig model (21), and down-regulation of RF synthesis, are all possible explanations for the beneficial effect of IVIG therapy in patient 1. The drop in TNF, parallel to the clinical improvement, probably reflects the reduced activity of the immune complex-mediated vasculitis involving joints and skin. Although the humoral changes persisted for 3 months, the clinical remission lasted only 4 weeks. This finding suggests that the relapse was probably due to a further activation of pathogenetic mechanisms not involving RF and TNF.

A slight decrease in lymphocyte counts was another consequence of IVIG infusion. The decrease affected T and B cells to a similar extent. Sequential assessment of the relationship between serum IgG level and lymphocyte counts confirmed this behavior. The correlation between drop in cell counts and rise in IgG level was significant only for CD8 cells, especially in those 3 patients who were unresponsive to IVIG therapy. In the other 3 patients in whom IVIG showed a good effect, the above-mentioned negative correlation was not significant. Reduction in helper/inducer lymphocyte subset (CD4), accompanied by an increase in the cytotoxic/suppressor subset (CD8), was observed by Macey and Newland (22) in patients affected by idiopathic thrombocytopenic purpura (ITP) who underwent IVIG therapy. This finding has suggested that IVIG therapy may reduce autoimmune inflammatory responses by enhancing suppressor T-cell activity. However, in addition to us, others have reported a reduction both of CD4 and CD8 cell counts following IVIG therapy. Abe and Matsuda (23) observed such an effect in two hemophiliacs, while White and co-workers (24) made the same observation in nine adults affected by common variable hypogammaglobulinemia. Tsubakio and colleagues (25) reported a relative increase in the percentage of T8-positive cells in ITP patients. However, there was actually a reduction in the absolute number of OKT4- and of OKT8-positive cells following IgG therapy. The mechanism by which IgG exerts the above-mentioned effect is unclear, and doubt remains whether this effect is clinically relevant.

Our observation that the outcome of the therapy is poor in RA patients where IVIG infusion induces a significant drop in CD8 cells, supports the speculation that too low suppressor T-cell activity may hinder the remission of the disease. Indirect support for this hypothesis comes from the observation that the rise in lymphocyte counts following methyl-prednisolone therapy in patients 3 and 4 was accompanied by clinical improvement, drop in sIL-2R level and ESR. The lymphocytosis observed in patients under methyl-prednisolone is paradoxical since glycocorticoids usually induce lymphopenia. Correction of the IVIG-mediated lymphopenia or interruption of the lymphocyte migration into the affected joints may justify such a paradoxical result.

In conclusion this study indicates that IVIG therapy could be of short-term efficacy in patients affected by advanced RA, otherwise refractory to usual class II and class III drugs. A partial exception is RA characterized by extra-articular manifestations and high RF titer, where humoral immune reactions, namely immune complex-mediated vasculitis, play a crucial role in the development of the systemic manifestations. High-dose IVIG infusion proved to affect these humoral immune reactions with a transient clinical improvement. However, further studies are needed before IVIG therapy can be recommended as treatment suitable for patients affected by RA with extra-articular manifestations. Further steps to explore the potential of IVIG therapy in RA include an IgG infusion schedule other than the one used in this study and the selection of patients with a less severe and advanced disease.

Summary

High-dose intravenous immunoglobulin treatment has been applied to 6 patients affected by severe and active rheumatoid arthritis, refractory to class II and class III drugs. The infusion schedule consisted of 400 mg/kg/day on days 1, 3, 5 and then once a month. The total number of IVIG pulses was 30 and the treatment period lasted from 5 to 120 days. Three out of 6 patients experienced a partial clinical remission which was of short duration. In one patient who presented with severe arthritis, rheumatoid skin nodules and extremely high RF titer, significant drop of RF, normalization of the total complement activity and transient clinical improvement followed IgG infusion. A slight drop in lymphocyte counts was another consequence of IVIG therapy. A statistically significant negative correlation between CD8 cell counts and serum IgG levels was found in those patients who were unresponsive to IVIG.

This study shows that IVIG therapy is of limited efficacy in patients with advanced RA and suggests that a pronounced reduction in CD8 cells may be responsible for the lack of benefit, in some cases. Further studies are needed in order to explore the potential of IgG infusion in an earlier phase of the disease.

References

1. Danieli, G., Montroni, M., Corvetta, A. and Gabrielli A. "Le Connettiviti" (Ed. Gasbarrini, G.), Ed. Compositori, Bologna; 1981.
2. Strastny, P. Association of the B-cell alloantigen DRW4 with rheumatoid arthritis. *N. Engl. J. Med.* **298**: 869; 1978.
3. NIH Conference. Rheumatoid arthritis: evolving concepts of pathogenesis and treatment. *Ann. Intern. Med.* **101**: 810; 1984.
4. Burmeister, G. R., Locher, P., Koch, B. *et al.* The tissue architecture of synovial membranes in inflammatory and non-inflammatory joint diseases. The localization of the major synovial populations as detected by monoclonal reagents directed towards Ia and monocyte/macrophage antigens. *Rheumat. Int.* 3: 173; 1983.
5. Munthe, E. and Natvig, J. B. Complement-fixing intracellular complexes of IgG-Rheumatoid Factor in rheumatoid plasma cells. *Scand. J. Immunol.* 1: 217; 1972.
6. Londei, B., Grubeck-Lobenstein, B., De Bernardis, P., Greenall, C. and Feldman, M. Efficient propagation and cloning of human T cells in the absence of antigen by means of OKT3, interleukin 2, and antigen-presenting cells. *Scand. J. Immunol.* 27: 35; 1988.
7. Zoppini, A. and Spadaro, A. Uso e abuso dei farmaci antiinfiammatori. *In* "Reumatologia" (Ed. Danieli, G.) p. 519. UTET, Torino; 1989.
8. Dougados, M. and Amor, B. Cyclosporin in rheumatoid arthritis: preliminary clinical results of an open trial. *Arthr. Rheumat.* **30**: 83; 1987.
9. Corvetta, A. and Pomponio, G. Terapia della artrite reumatoide refrattaria. *In* "Reumatologia" (Ed. Danieli, G.) p. 539. UTET, Torino; 1989.
10. Nydegger, U. E. and Spycher, M. O. Polyclonal polyspecific antibody mixtures from random donors as therapeutic tools in autoimmune disease. *In* "Clinical Use of Intravenous Immunoglobulins" (Eds Morell, A. and Nydegger U. E.), p. 486. Academic Press, London; 1986.
11. Sany, J., Clot, J., Combe, B. *et al.* Traitment de le polyarthrite rheumatoide. *Presse Med.* **16** (15): 723; 1987.
12. Breeveld, F. C., Brand, A. and Aken, W. High dose intravenous gamma globulin for Felty's syndrome. *J. Rheumat.* 12(4): 700; 1985.
13. Groothoff, J. W. and Van Leeuwen, E. F. High dose intravenous gammaglobulin in chronic systemic juvenile arthritis. *Br. Med. J.* **296**: 1362; 1988.
14. Mitropoulou, J., Becker, H. and Helmke, K. High dose intravenous immunoglobulins in rheumatoid arthritis. *Clin. Exp. Rheumatol.* 5: 205; 1987.
15. Francioni, C., Materazzi, M., Megale, F. *et al.* Prospettive teraputiche delle immunoglobuline umane nelle malattie reumatiche (abstract) *Reumatismo* 41(2): 220; 1989.

16. Tumiati, B., Bellelli, A. and Veneziani, M. Immunoglobuline ad alte dosi nella terapia dell'artrite reumatoide: studio pilota di 7 casi. Proceedings of XXII Congresso Nazionale della Società Italiana di Trasfusione del Sangue, Pavia, 30–31 October 1989, p. 14.
17. Becker, H., Mitropoulou, G. and Helmke, K. Immunomodulating therapy of rheumatoid arthritis by high-dose intravenous immunoglobulin. *Klin Wochenschr.* 67: 286; 1989.
18. Parekh, R. B., Dwek, R. A., Sutton, B. J. *et al.* Association of rheumatoid arthritis and primary osteoarthritis with changes in the glycosylation pattern of total serum IgG. *Nature* **316**: 452; 1985.
19. Ichikawa, M., Yanagisawa, M., Kawai, M. *et al.* Spontaneous improvement of juvenile rheumatoid arthritis after T lymphocytosis with suppressor phenotype and function. *J. Clin. Lab. Immunol.* 27(4): 197; 1988.
20. Tracey, K. J., Vlassara, H. and Cerami, A. Cachectin/Tumour necrosis factor. *Lancet* 1: 1122; 1989.
21. Basta, M., Kirshborn P., Frank, M. M. *et al.* Mechanism of therapeutic effect of high-dose intravenous immunoglobulin. Attenuation of acute, complement-dependent immune damage in a guinea pig model *J. Clin. Invest.* **84**: 1974; 1989.
22. Macey, M. G. and Newland, A. C. Modulation of T and B cell subpopulations during the high-dose intravenous immunoglobulin therapy. *Plasma Ther. Transf. Technol.* **9**: 139; 1988.
23. Abe, T. and Matsuda, J. Effects of immunoglobulin on cellular and humoral immunity of haemophiliacs with reversed T4/T8 ratio of lymphocytes. *In* "Clinical Use of Intravenous Immunoglobulins" (Eds Morell, A. and Nydegger, U. E.), p. 385. Academic Press, London; 1986.
24. White, W. B., Desbonnet, C. R. and Ballow M. Immunoregulatory effects of intravenous immune serum globulin therapy in common variable hypogammaglobulinemia *Am. J. Med.* **83**: 431; 1987.
25. Tsubakio, T., Kurata, Y., Katagiri, S. *et al.* Alteration of T cell subsets and immunoglobulin synthesis **in vitro** during high-dose gammaglobulin therapy in patients with idiopathic thrombocytopenic purpura. *Clin. Exp. Immunol.* 53: 697; 1983.

Discussion

F. Kanakoudi
Did you observe any exacerbation or recurrence of arthritis in any joint of your patients during the couple of days following the IVIG administration?

We had had such an episode repeatedly in one of our three children with JCA (systemic form) treated with IVIG.

A. Corvetta
No. We have never seen a worsening of the arthritis during IVIG therapy. This was also true for patients affected by connective tissue diseases other than RA (3 SLE and 1 necrotizing vasculitis) we have recently treated by IVIG.

G. Gaedicke
In children there exists a rare disorder that is characterized by recurrent fever, slight splenomegaly and skin rash. In former times this syndrome was called "subsepsis allergica" from Wissler; nowadays it is related to RA. We have treated two such patients with IVIG during recent years and observed a dramatic response concerning the disappearance of fever and a complete remission in one and a long-term remission in the other patient. Three patients with arthritis, however, were rather unresponsive to IVIG. Do you have similar experience?

A. Corvetta
No. High fever and skin rash is uncommon in adult RA. However, from our preliminary experience we got the impression that patients with "systemic" rheumatoid arthritis (high titers of RF, skin nodules, tendency to extra-articular manifestations) are more prone to give a good response to IVIG compared to patients with arthritis alone.

Therapeutic opportunities in systemic vasculitis

C. M. LOCKWOOD

Department of Medicine, Clinical School, Addenbrookes Hospital, Cambridge, UK

Introduction

There is now growing evidence that autoimmune mechanisms play an important role in the systemic vasculitides: their demonstration forms the basis of the first diagnostic laboratory test for this group of diseases and their manipulation constitutes the first advance towards specific immunotherapy for their treatment (1, 2). The systemic vasculitides form a loosely associated group which have as their pathological basis a chronic necrotizing inflammation which affects vessels of varying sizes at varying sites throughout the body. There are primary and secondary forms; primary which involve blood vessels exclusively and which are the subject of this article, and secondary which arise in association with disease elsewhere, for example, vasculitis secondary to Crohn's disease. Some primary forms are associated with granulomata, for example, Takayasu's disease and Wegener's granulomatosis. Because so little is known of their pathogenesis, a morphological approach has been adopted towards their classification (see Table 1). Because of the same uncertainty, the evolution of a treatment strategy has been mainly empirical, driven by the high morbidity and mortality rates if no therapy was given. Thus, until recently, the best evidence that

Immunotherapy with Intravenous Immunoglobulins
ISBN 0-12-370725-0

autoimmune processes played an important role in the systemic vasculitides came from evidence that powerful immunosuppressive agents were beneficial (3), and that these might be humoral mechanisms was supported by the finding that additional plasma exchange was useful in the management of severe forms of these diseases (4).

Table 1

	Granulomata	
Vessel size	Present	Absent
Large	Takayasu's[a]	Giant cell arteritis
Medium	Churg-Strauss[a]	Polyarteritis nodosa
Small	Wegener's granulomatosis[a]	Microscopic polyarteritis[a]
		Kawasaki disease[a]
		Henoch-Schönlein purpura[a]

[a] Vasculitides in which anti-neutrophil cytoplasm antibodies have been reported.

In 1982 Davies *et al.* reported that patients with polyarteritis and renal vasculitis had circulating autoantibodies which reacted with the cytoplasm of normal granulocytes (5). A similar report in 1985 by van der Woude *et al.* documented the same phenomenon occurring in patients with Wegener's granulomatosis (6). These autoantibodies were detected by indirect immunofluorescence techniques which were subjective and relatively insensitive. The development of solid-phase immunoradiometric assays obviated both problems and showed that detection of autoantibodies to neutrophil cytoplasm antigens (ANCA) by these techniques provided both sensitive and specific means for diagnosis of the common primary vasculitides (7). That these autoimmune mechanisms operate in systemic vasculitis has led to new strategies for treatment as detailed below.

ANCA and disease activity

The close association of ANCA with the development of certain vasculitides indicated that serial measurements might reflect disease activity which could be useful not only in managing treatment, but also in predicting disease relapse. Van der Woude showed that by indirect immunofluorescence assays ANCA levels correlated with disease activity (6) and we also used this test in a retrospective study of patients' progress after discharge from hospital. We monitored 18 patients over a period of 3 years. Eight had become ANCA-negative during their initial in-patient treatment but 10 still had detectable ANCA at the beginning of the study. No relapses occurred in the ANCA-negative group, but eight relapses occurred in the ANCA-positive group. In six of the eight who relapsed, relapses seemed to occur in relation to reductions in immunosuppressive therapy. This underlined the connection between ANCA and active disease. However, there were some patients who remained ANCA-positive without symptomatology. In such patients further studies showed the importance of other factors in promoting disease expression, for example, ANCA isotype (see below).

This early experience led us to adopt a treatment strategy aimed at inducing both clinical and serological remission. We then tested the assay's predictive performance in a prospective fashion by assessing patients' progress at regular intervals both clinically and serologically. We have now studied 20 patients who were in clinical and serological remission at the beginning of the study, for a mean of 48 patient weeks. The patients were assessed clinically at monthly intervals. ANCA seroconversion was taken to indicate serological relapse and the CRP level was used as a non-specific indicator either of this or other inflammatory events (such as intercurrent infection). We observed 11 relapses in 9 patients. A rise in ANCA preceded relapse in eight and occurred at the same time in two; no seroconversion could be detected in one relapse. On two occasions ANCA tests became positive, but disease did not follow. Only on one occasion did a rise in CRP precede relapse. Thus, although a rise in CRP was not a good predictive test, ANCA seroconversion was useful. Furthermore, since the mean time to relapse after seroconversion was one month, this raised the prospect that monthly patient follow-up might be carried out remote from specialist centers, with recall if ANCA titers rose.

Class and subclass of ANCA

In Wegener's disease and microscopic polyarteritis ANCA are usually of IgG isotype. Rarely patients with a polyarteritis pulmonary–renal syndrome have been identified where ANCA are restricted to IgM isotype (8). These patients have severe disease, readily responsive to plasma exchange, an appropriate treatment since IgM is predominantly confined to the intravascular compartment. With treatment a late isotype switch (to IgG) has been documented in three patients as the disease remitted, and ANCA of both IgM and IgG isotypes have been eluted from the kidneys of one patient at autopsy. This suggested that the IgM autoantibody might not only have determined the pattern of organ involvement, but also the severity of disease activity. A similar relationship of disease to isotype has been reported for Henoch-Schönlein purpura in adults (who have IgA ANCA) (9).

We have also studied the ANCA IgG subclass in patients at presentation and again in remission (yet still ANCA-positive). Initially there was a predominance of ANCA of IgG_3 isotype, but this later switched to IgG_2 (10). This is interesting since IgG_3 antibodies can fix complement and engage macrophages through receptors which IgG_2 antibodies lack (complement and macrophages can substantially augment the inflammatory response once activated). Thus these findings might explain why some patients in remission continue to have raised ANCA levels yet little disease activity.

Incidence of ANCA-positive systemic vasculitis

For the first time ANCA assays have provided a powerful diagnostic tool for the systemic vasculitides which is not dependent on clinical interpretation. Our laboratory acts as a reference center for the population of East Anglia and this has allowed the incidence of ANCA-positive disease to be estimated at 1:2000, a level greater than for SLE and as high as rheumatoid arthritis. No doubt the tendency for vasculitis to present under any medical discipline, and the lack of a diagnostic laboratory test, has served to diminish estimates of its incidence.

Pathophysiological role of ANCA

Whether ANCA fulfil a pathogenetic role is yet undecided. Levels of ANCA correlate with disease activity (6) and ANCA immunoglobulin can be eluted from vasculitic lesions and will bind to appropriate cells cultured *in vitro* (8, 11). Attempts to transfer disease to an experimental model have been frustrated by lack of a suitable recipient species (cross-reactive antigens are present only in baboons) and by the short time available since serum sickness lesions, themselves vasculitic, develop from day 7 on. In a pilot study in baboons we did find a striking neutropenia in recipients given ANCA-rich immunoglobulin (C. M. Lockwood and C. B. Wilson, unpublished). This turned attention to *in vitro* effects of ANCA on neutrophil function, and on signal transduction in particular. We found that preincubation with ANCA markedly inhibited neutrophil activation brought about by agents such as phorbol myristate acetate (PMA), probably because ANCA can lead to sustained activation of polymorphs (12). This is particularly interesting since systemic vasculitis is hallmarked histologically by evidence of chronic polymorph activation, and argues for a direct role of ANCA in the disease process.

ANCA and network control of immune responses

If autoantibodies in patients with systemic vasculitis can mediate disease, then study of the regulation of these autoimmune responses may help to guide new strategies for treatment. The best understood immunological regulatory mechanisms involve control by way of a "network" of idiotypic anti-idiotypic reactions predicted by the "network theory" (13). Idiotypic determinants have been characterized on autoantibodies occurring in different autoimmune diseases, and heterologous anti-idiotypic antibodies to those have been shown to have a regulatory effect *in vitro* (14). The possibility that natural homeostatic mechanisms operate within the network framework has been supported by the finding that "normal" B cells possess the necessary genetic information to manufacture autoantibodies (15) and, that within the population of normal immunoglobulins, there exist a range of "natural" anti-idiotypic antibodies (16). This has been exploited therapeutically for the treatment of a number of autoimmune diseases, best exemplified by spontaneous anti-factor VIII disease, where control of autoantibody formation has been shown to be explainable by idiotypic anti-idiotypic regulation (17). It is of note that the treatment of choice for Kawasaki disease, an ANCA-positive childhood vasculitis, is the administration of pooled normal immunoglobulin intravenously (18).

This has led us to study the properties of pooled immunoglobulins on ANCA reactions (19). We have shown that $F(ab)_2$ of normal pooled immunoglobulin can inhibit binding of ANCA *in vitro*. The degree of inhibition ranged from 0 to 100%, with up to 75% of a panel of 21 pretreatment ANCA-positive sera being substantially inhibited by a single $F(ab)_2$ preparation of pooled immunoglobulin. Inhibitory reactivity was also found in remission sera, which were ANCA-negative, including sera from patients whose remission occurred spontaneously. That this inhibition of binding fulfilled the criteria of idiotypic anti-idiotypic reactions was demonstrated by showing that the $F(ab)_2$ of affinity-purified immunoglobulin reacted with, and was inhibited in its specific binding by, IgG from normal immunoglobulin. These experimental data have encouraged pilot studies of the use of pooled immunoglobulin for treatment of certain patients with systemic vasculitis.

Treatment of systemic vasculitis with intravenous immunoglobulin (IVIG)

We have treated four patients with pooled normal immunoglobulin given by intravenous infusion (Sandoglobulin®). All had ANCA-positive vasculitis: for two this was the only treatment given, for the other two IVIG was given after failure of conventional immunosuppressive drugs. The four patients were observed for a mean of 3 months before and 6 months after therapy. Clinical disease activity was recorded using a 2, 1, 0 scale (2 = active disease requiring hospital or home care; 1 = still symptomatic but institutionally independent; 0 = remission); levels of ANCA (by radioimmunoassay) and C-reactive protein (CRP) were measured serially. The potential efficacy of the Sandoglobulin® was assessed by an *in vitro* test of inhibition of ANCA-binding activity. The clinical and laboratory data are shown in Table 2 and the sequential ANCA levels are shown in Fig. 1.

Table 2
Clinical and laboratory features of four patients treated with IVIG

Patient no.	Age	Sex	Diagnosis	Other treatment	Disease activity pre/post	CRP mg/100 ml pre/post	Follow-up (months)
1	62	F	WG	CP	2/0	148/10	6
2	57	M	WG	—	1/0	18/N	4
3	73	M	MP	—	1/0	N/N	11
4	61	M	MP	CP	1/0	N/N	5

C = cyclophosphamide; P = prednisolone; N = normal (<6 mg/100 ml); WG = Wegener's granulomatosis; MP = microscopic polyarteritis.

Clinical improvement was seen in all four patients, including the two resistant to standard therapy. After the IVIG ANCA levels rose initially in all four patients, but in three then fell to levels substantially lower than pretreatment values, becoming undetectable in the fourth.

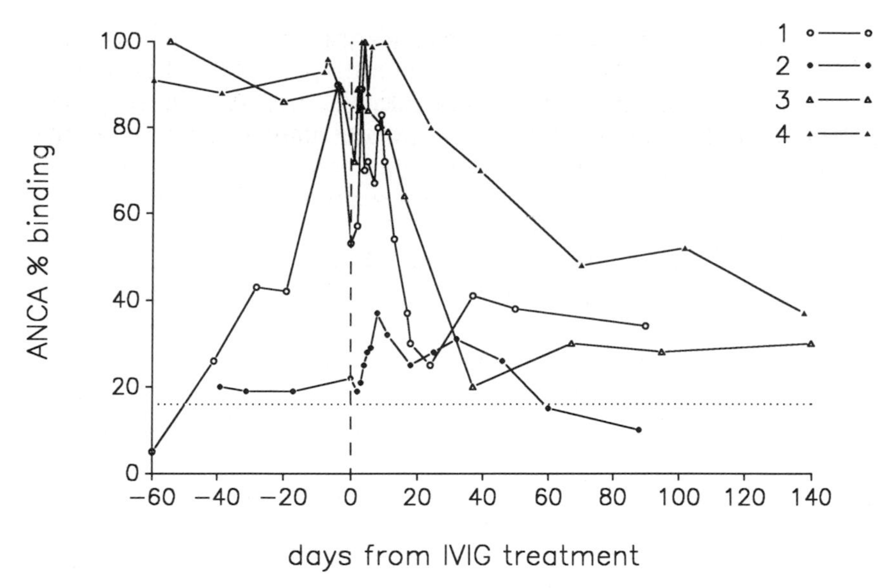

Figure 1. Sequential ANCA binding and IVIG in four patients.

Low levels of ANCA continued to be detectable, without overt evidence of disease, during follow-up in these three patients.

The numbers of patients studied so far is small but some points of interest emerge already. First, clinical improvement occurred in all the patients treated and was maintained for periods of follow-up ranging from 4 to 11 months (mean, 6). Second, after the IVIG infusion ANCA levels rose transiently in all the patients, and remained detectable in three, without deleterious effect on the clinical outcome. The initial rise may have been due to displacement of ANCA from tissue-bound sites, since competitive inhibition of binding was demonstrated between the IVIG ($F(ab)_2$ preparations) and the autoantibodies in each of the patients treated. It is equally possible that the persisting ANCA were from populations of autoantibodies bearing idiotypes not recognized by the normal pooled IgG and possibly not pathogenetically important. Third, in the two untreated patients *in vitro* tests of ANCA producing B-cell activity indicated that in both patients this was abrogated after IVIG infusion, suggesting an immediate down-regulation of autoantibody synthesis had been achieved (Mathieson *et al.* in preparation).

A role for plasma exchange?

The balance of idiotypic and anti-idiotypic reactions appears symmetrical, but if ascendancy of one component could be promoted, then new strategies for therapy could be encouraged. Recently we have found that there is a difference in the isotype of the anti-idiotypic antibodies: a substantial proportion are IgM (16). IgM synthesis rates are markedly faster than IgG. Thus depletion of all circulatory immunoglobulins by plasmapheresis might allow this desired alteration in homeostasis by virtue of the greater synthetic rate of IgM. In this context it is of interest that plasmapheresis has been shown to have an intrinsic benefit in treatment of patients with severe renal and systemic vasculitis (as tested in a randomized prospective controlled trial) (4).

Conclusions

It is now evident that autoimmune mechanisms may play an important role in systemic vasculitis, and their identification is useful for diagnosis and management of these disorders. Their further study may allow an understanding of the pathogenesis of these disorders and open up the prospects of new strategies for treatment. At the present time one such strategy we are exploring involves a combination of treatment by plasma exchange followed by IVIG infusion therapy.

Summary

Serological and clinical parameters have been used to monitor treatment of four patients with systemic vasculitis characterized by the presence of anti-neutrophil cytoplasm antibodies (ANCA). Intravenous immunoglobulin was used alone in two untreated patients and in two patients who had failed conventional cytotoxic and steroid therapy. All four patients improved clinically but ANCA activity diminished only slowly. Evidence is discussed which supports the postulate that these effects may have been produced by perturbation of immunoregulatory mechanisms governed by the "network" theory.

References

1. Savage, C. O. S. and Lockwood, C. M. Autoantibodies in primary systemic vasculitis. *In* "Advances in internal Medicine" (Ed. Stollerman, G. H.), Vol. 35, pp. 73–92. Year Book Medical Publishers, Chicago; 1990.
2. Van der Woude, F. J., Daha, M. R. and Van Es, L. A. The current status of neutrophil cytoplasmic antibodies. *Clin. Exp. Immunol.* 78: 143–148; 1989.
3. Katz, P. and Fauci, A. S. Treatment of immune complex mediated diseases: corticosteroids and cytotoxic agents. *In* "Clinics in Immunology" (Ed. Fauci, A. S.), pp. 415–431. Saunders, Eastbourne; 1981.
4. Pusey, C. D. and Lockwood, C. M. Plasma exchange for glomerular disease. *In* "Nephrology" (Ed. Robinson, R. R.), pp. 1474–1486. Springer Verlag, New York; 1985.
5. Davies, D. J., Moran, J. E., Niall, J. F. and Ryan, G. B. Segmental necrotising glomerulonephritis with antineutrophil antibody: possible arbovirus aetiology? *Br. Med. J.* 285: 606; 1982.
6. Van der Woude, F. J., Rasmussen, N., Lobatto, S., Wiik, A., Permin, H., Van Es, L. A., Van der Giessen, M., Van der Hem, G. K. and The, T. H. Autoantibodies against neutrophils and monocytes: tool for diagnosis and marker for disease activity in Wegener's granulomatosis. *Lancet* i: 425–429; 1985.
7. Savage, C. O. S., Winearls, C. G., Jones, S., Marshall, P. D. and Lockwood, C. M. Prospective study of radioimmunoassay for antibodies against neutrophil cytoplasm in diagnosis of systemic vasculitis. *Lancet* i: 1389–1393; 1987.
8. Jayne, D. R. W., Jones, S. J., Severn, A., Shaumack, S., Murphy, J. and Lockwood, C. M. (1989). Severe pulmonary haemorrhage and systemic vasculitis in association with circulating anti-neutrophil antibodies of IgM class only. *Clin. Nephrol.* 32: 101–106; 1989.
9. Van den Wall Bake, A. W. L., Lobatto, S., Jonges, L., Daha, M. R. and Van Es, L. A. IgA antibodies directed against cytoplasmic antigens of polymorphonuclear leucocytes in patients with Henoch-Schonlein purpura. *In* "Recent Advances in Mucosal Immunity: Part B" (Eds Mestecky, J. *et al.*), p. 1593. Plenum, London; 1987.
10. Jayne, D. R. W. and Lockwood, C. M. Subclass specificity of autoantibodies to neutrophil cytoplasm antigens in systemic vasculitis. (Submitted).
11. Abbott, F., Jones, S. J., Lockwood, C. M. and Rees, A. J. Autoantibodies to glomerular antigens in patients with Wegener's granulomatosis. *Nephrol. Dial. Transpl.* 4: 1–8; 1989.
12. Lai, K. N. and Lockwood, C. M. Down-regulation of signal transduction in human neutrophils by anti-neutrophil cytoplasm antibodies. (Submitted.)

13. Jerne, N. K. Towards a network theory of the immune response. *Ann. Immunol. (Inst. Pasteur)* 125c: 373–389; 1974.
14. Lockwood, C. M. and Pye, R. J. Basic mechanisms in autoimmunity "Advances in Dermatology" (Eds Champion, R. H. and Pye, R. J.) Vol. 8, pp. 71–84. Churchill Livingstone, Edinburgh; 1990.
15. Painter, C., Monestier, M., Bonin, B. and Bing, C. A. Functional and molecular studies of V genes expressed in autoantibodies. *Immunol. Rev.* 94; 75–98; 1986.
16. Rossi, F., Jayne, D. R. W., Lockwood, C. M. and Kazatchkine, M. D. Anti-idiotypes against anti-neutrophil cytoplasmic antigen (ANCA) autoantibodies in normal human polyspecific IgG for therapeutic use and in the remission sera of patients with systemic vasculitis. *Clin. Exp. Immunol.* (In press).
17. Sultan, Y., Rossi, F. and Kazatchkine, M. D. Recovery from anti-VIII:C (anti-haemophilic factor) autoimmune disease dependent on generation of anti-idiotypes against anti-VIII:C autoantibodies. *Proc. Natl. Acad. Sci. USA,* 84: 828–830; 1987.
18. Leung, D. Y. M., Burns, J. C., Neuburger, M. and Geha, R. S. Reversal of lymphocyte activation in vivo in the Kawasaki syndrome by intravenous gamma globulin. *J. Clin. Invest.* 79: 468–472; 1987.

Acknowledgement

Dr C. M. Lockwood is supported by the Wellcome Trust.

Discussion

R. Seger
One obvious question is, of course, what happens to ANCA levels in Kawasaki syndrome upon IVIG treatment? Did you follow these levels?

C. Lockwood
No. The only samples we had were from stored sera from children with Kawasaki disease studied at our children's hospital (Great Ormond Street) who did not receive IVIG. As we published (Savage, C. O. S., Tizard, J., Jayne. D. and Lockwood, C. M. Antineutrophil cytoplasm antibodies in Kawasaki disease. *Arch. Dis. Childh.* 64: 360–363; 1989) both IgM and IgG ANCA raised at presentation fell during follow-up.

Ageing and autoimmunity: lessons learnt from the presence of autoantibodies in patients with malignant conditions

YEHUDA SHOENFELD

Research Unit of Autoimmune Diseases and Department of Medicine 'B', Sheba Medical Center, Tel-Hashomer, Israel

The immune system is dynamic and undergoes continuous morphological and functional changes with age. The immune response reaches its peak value (maximal humoral and cellular reactions against exogenous antigens) at approximately the time of puberty, subsequently declining with advancing age. It is generally agreed that immune functions decline progressively as the effects of senescence of both cellular and humoral immune mechanisms become increasingly apparent. This process has been reported in both elderly experimental animals and people. Furthermore, the production of autoantibodies increases with age. The decreased immune responsiveness and increased autoimmunity that accompany ageing indicate that these are end-results of perturbation in the regulatory mechanisms of the immune system.

Before summarizing the various defects reported in the immune system with ageing, let me emphasize the fact that autoimmune diseases are more prevalent at the second and third decades rather than in the elderly. The age predilection seems to be related in part to

Immunotherapy with Intravenous Immunoglobulins
ISBN 0–12–370725–0

hormonal factors (1), but also in part to intrinsic immune defects (2). Yet, an increased production of autoantibodies can be seen with ageing. To demonstrate this dichotomy, I will summarize some of our recent data concerning autoantibodies, malignancy and ageing (3–5).

Autoantibodies in cancer: are they tumor-related or age-related?

An increased incidence of malignancy was observed among patients with autoimmune diseases (6), and vice versa, a high incidence of autoimmune conditions was recognized in malignancies, especially in lymphoproliferative disorders (7). Moreover, a large number of studies reported an increased incidence of autoantibodies (mainly ANF and RF) in a variety of malignancies (8, 9). Autoantibody production in malignancy may be due to; (1) host immune reaction to tumor-associated antigens, (2) antigenic stimulation as a result of therapy. However, autoantibodies and malignancy may both be associated with another condition rather than each other (e.g. immune deficiency, environmental factors, ageing). Indeed, an association between ageing and autoimmunity has been established (for reviews see references 2 and 10). Therefore, we have decided to evaluate whether or not the association between neoplasia and autoimmunity results from increased incidence of both conditions in old age.

We tested 139 patients (55 of them aged 60 years and younger and 84 older than 60 years) suffering from a variety of malignant tumors, for ANA, RF and anti-erythrocyte antibodies (Coombs's test) (see Table 1). There was no significant difference between the incidences of ANA and RF in the young patients and in the young controls ($X^2 = 1.47$ and 1.05 respectively). Our results suggest that the high incidence of ANA and RF in cancer patients is a result of the old age of these individuals rather than the tumor itself. On the other hand, the incidence of positive Coombs's test in the whole patient group was significantly greater than that reported in the general population—1.5:10 000 (using the binomial test $P < 0.0001$). Therefore, it seems that a positive Coombs' test is a direct result of the tumor itself, in contrast to the case of ANA and RF (4).

Autoantibodies in neoplasia: an unresolved enigma (5)

Based on the above data we have decided to extend our knowledge on the association of antibodies with cancer to a prospective study in

Table 1
Frequency of autoantibodies detected among 164 cancer patients versus 68 age-adjusted normal controls

Autoantibody to	Patients with carcinoma (*n* = 164)	Normal controls (*n* = 68)
ssDNA	8 (4.9%)	3 (4.4%)
dsDNA	5 (3%)	5 (7.4%)
Poly(I)	6 (3.7%)	4 (5.9%)
Poly(G)	7 (4.3%)	5 (7.4%)
Cardiolipin	7 (4.3%)	3 (4.4%)
Histones	12 (7.3%)	3 (4.4%)
RNP	1 (0.6%)	1 (1.5%)
Sm	10 (7.9%)	2 (2.9%)
Ro (SSA)	13 (7.9%)	0 (0%)
La (SSB)	16 (9.8%)	3 (4.4%)

which we have examined 164 sera of patients with solid tumors and 84 sera of patients with lymphomas. We looked for the presence of increased titers of a series of antinuclear antibodies by ELISA, and tried to correlate the presence of autoantibodies with the histological type of the tumor. But the main question we asked ourselves was whether the autoantibodies in these patients with malignancies are tumor-related or age-related. Therefore, a careful sex- and age-matching of the controls to the patients was carried out.

Patients' sera

Sera were obtained from 164 patients with carcinomatous diseases; 102 were females and 62 were males. The group was subdivided according to the origin of the malignancy as follows: 71 with breast cancer (68 females, 3 males); 30 with carcinoma of the colon (18 males, 12 females); 16 with cancer of the prostate gland; 11 with lung cancer; 9 with melanoma, 5 each with carcinomas of the pancreas, gall bladder and multiple primary carcinomas; 3 with carcinoma of the stomach; 2 with carcinoma of the kidney and thyroid; 1 with carcinoma of the ovary and another with seminoma; 3 with sarcoma; and 1 patient with carcinoma of unknown origin. The age distribution was as follows: 0–20 years, 2 patients; 21–40 years, 11 patients; 41–60 years, 59 patients; 61–80 years, 85 patients; and older than 85 years, 7 patients.

The antibodies examined entailed; ssDNA, dsDNA, poly(I), poly(G), cardiolipin, histones, RNP, Sm, Ro and La. For details of the methods used to determine the antibodies the reader is referred to reference 4.

In general, screening for the presence of autoantibodies in sera did not reveal any significant difference between patients with carcinoma and healthy age-adjusted normal controls (Table 1). The results were repeated when subjects were subdivided according to their ages (younger and older than 50 years). A tendency, yet not statistically significant, to a higher incidence of anti-Ro (SSA) and anti-La (SSB) autoantibodies among patients with malignant disorders, was noted.

Furthermore, no distinction could be drawn between the incidence of antinuclear autoantibodies in older carcinomatous patients and younger patients, as well as between elderly and younger controls. Among female patients with carcinoma of the colon, autoantibodies were detected more frequently than in male patients, yet this tendency was not statistically significant.

No excessive autoantibodies were observed in patients with carcinoma of the prostate as well. These results imply that the often observed coexistence between autoimmunity and neoplasia is not manifested serologically by the markers we assessed. This finding remained valid after separation of subjects by origin of tumor, sex and age.

This study concentrated on solid tumors and, in particular, on carcinomas. Meanwhile, we have completed an additional survey in which an identical analysis was carried out on 84 sera of patients with Hodgkin's (29 patients) and non-Hodgkin's lymphomas (55 patients)

Table 2
Frequency of autoantibodies detected among 84 patients with lymphoma versus 46 age-adjusted normal controls

Autoantibody to	Patients with lymphoma (n = 84)	Normal controls (n = 46)	(P-value)
ssDNA	20 (23.8%)	2 (4.3%)	<0.01
dsDNA	6 (7.1%)	4 (8.7%)	NS
Poly (I)	4 (4.8%)	4 (8.7%)	NS
Poly(G)	8 (9.5%)	4 (8.7%)	NS
Sm	14 (16.7%)	1 (2.2%)	<0.05
RNP	16 (19.5%)	2 (4.3%)	<0.05
SS/A	7 (8.3%)	5 (10.9%)	NS
SS/B	12 (14.3%)	3 (6.5%)	NS
Cardiolipin	5 (6%)	3 (6.5%)	NS
Histones	1 (1.2%)	3 (6.5%)	NS
16/6 Id	0 (0%)	1 (2.2%)	NS

(6). Interestingly, the overall calculation pointed to a significantly increased incidence of several autoantibodies in these patients, e.g. anti-ssDNA (27%), anti-Sm (20%) anti-RNP (22%) versus controls 4.5%, 2.2% and 4.5%, respectively (Tables 2 and 3).

Segregating the patients to those with Hodgkin's and non-Hodgkin's lymphoma showed that relatively higher numbers of patients with autoantibodies belonged to the non-Hodgkin's lymphoma (Table 4).

Table 3
Frequency of antibodies detected among 29 patients with Hodgkin's disease versus 46 normal controls

Autoantibody to	Hodgkin's disease	Normal control	(*P*-value)
ssDNA	4 (13.8%)	2 (4.3%)	NS
dsDNA	0 (0%)	4 (8.7%)	NS
Poly(I)	0 (0%)	4 (8.7%)	NS
Poly(G)	2 (6.9%)	4 (8.7%)	NS
Sm	6 (20.7%)	1 (2.2%)	<0.01
RNP	6 (20.7%)	2 (4.3%)	<0.05
SS/A	4 (13.8%)	5 (10.9%)	NS
SS/B	5 (17.2%)	3 (6.5%)	NS
Cardiolipin	2 (6.9%)	3 (6.5%)	NS
Histones	0 (0%)	3 (6.5%)	NS
16/6 Id	0 (0%)	1 (2.2%)	NS

Table 4
Frequency of antibodies detected among 55 patients with non-Hodgkin's lymphoma versus 29 patients with Hodgkin's disease

Autoantibody to	Non-Hodgkin's lymphoma	Hodgkin's disease	(*P*-value)
ssDNA	16 (29.1%)	4 (13.8%)	NS
dsDNA	6 (10.9%)	0 (0%)	<0.1
Poly(I)	4 (7.3%)	0 (0%)	NS
Poly(G)	3 (10.9%)	2 (6.9%)	NS
Sm	8 (14.5%)	6 (20.7%)	NS
RNP	10 (18.2%)	6 (20.7%)	NS
SS/A	3 (5.5%)	4 (13.8%)	NS
SS/B	7 (12.7%)	5 (17.4%)	NS
Cardiolipin	3 (5.5%)	2 (6.9%)	NS
Histones	1 (1.8%)	0 (0%)	NS
16/6 Id	0 (0%)	0 (0%)	NS

This is not surprising as many of the lymphomas are of B-lymphocyte origin, thus resembling the results reported previously on the presence of autoantibody activity in patients with myeloma and macroglobulinemia (13).

In conclusion, we can see that the common belief that cancer is associated with increased incidence of autoantibodies is misleading. By and large they are age-related, and due to the fact that most tumors are more prevalent among elders.

Immune dysfunctions recorded with ageing

Tables 5 and 6 briefly summarize the various defects in both the humoral and the cellular immune systems. For details the reader is referred to reference 2.

Table 5
T-cell defects found in the elderly

	Defects
1	Decrease in the number of Ts cells (OKT 8/Leu-2u)
2	Decrease in the number of Ts cells
3	Decrease in both Ts and T
4	Increase in "null" cells (non-T, non-B-lymphocytes)
5	Progressive decline of mitogen-induced lymphocyte response from birth to old age
6	Cells from old donors enter the G_4 or complete S-phase of the cell cycle to a lesser extent compared with young individuals
7	Deficit of both production of growing factors and expression of specific receptors (exogenous 11–2) can enhance the proliferative response of aged lymphocytes

Table 6
B-cell findings in ageing

1	Number of B lymphocytes is unaffected
2	Increased polyclonal immunoglobulin response to pokeweed mitogen
3	Reduction of both antigen-specific and polyclonal responses with advancing age
4	Intrinsic defect of B-cell maturation in the elderly. II-1 and II-2 are able to enhance B-cell response

Mechanisms of antibody production in the elderly

A considerable controversy surrounds the mechanisms responsible for the increased autoimmunity of ageing. It is well known that many blood components become elevated in elderly persons with no underlying pathological basis. Therefore, Landahl *et al.* (14) have set higher normal limits for any blood components in people 70 years of age and older. Similarly, it is possible that elderly people have higher normal limits for natural autoantibodies, and their increased levels may not represent an impairment of immunological functions.

Many workers claim that the high frequency of autoantibodies observed in elderly people is at least partly associated with undiagnosed diseases appearing with age. The findings of Moulias *et al.* (15) support this view. They found that anti-thyroglobulin antibodies were more frequent in elderly patients (aged 70–90 years) with chronic diseases, but were not elevated in very old healthy subjects (aged 90 years or more) when compared with young controls. The increased levels of thyroid autoantibodies in elderly patients may indicate undiagnosed and asymptomatic autoimmune thyroiditis. Routine autopsy data showing a 2–3-fold increased prevalence of focal thyroiditis in older adults (2) support this concept.

The higher incidence of autoantibodies in the elderly may be a result of unrecognized environmental factors such as intercurrent viral infections. Wilkens and co-workers (16) determined the prevalence of ANF in elderly subjects (aged 59 years and older), and retested these individuals for the same autoantibody 10 months later (16). The prevalence of ANF was 11% in the older persons, compared with 2.5% in the younger control group. Ten months later some individuals showed changes from positive to negative and vice versa. These variations during a 10-month period can be due to unrecognized environmental influences.

Autoantibodies may have a protective role against certain infections that are more prevalent in older people. For example, some workers suggest that IgM-RF is involved in the enhancement of binding of low-affinity IgG antibodies against their antigen (17). Therefore, it is possible that the production of IgM-RF represents a first line of defense against bacterial or viral infections until specific antibody production is activated. Supporting this view are data from Gordon and Rosenthal (18), suggesting that the autoreactive clones accumulating with age are of restricted specificity.

Some workers believe that autoreactive clones of lymphocytes exist in the spleens of young animals, but under normal circumstances produce little autoantibody. With ageing a deregulation of these clones occurs, perhaps as a result of deficient suppressor T-cell function (19). Thoman and Weigel (20) demonstrated that spleens of older animals are less capable of producing suppressor T cells when cultured *in vitro* and that this deficiency can be corrected by adding interleukin-2 (20). Their data suggest that aged animals possess suppressor T cells, but their function cannot be expressed as a result of the inability of older animals to produce interleukin-2. Other workers think that the expansion of autoreactive lymphoid clones is unrelated to suppressor cell activity, and is caused by the normal exposure of the immune system to self-antigen (21). They claim that prolonged exposure to self-antigens and/or alternations of self-antigens resulting from normal catabolic processes can give rise to autoreactive lymphoid clones.

The increased autoimmunity of ageing may represent intrinsic biochemical alternations in lymphoid cells (20). It was found that with age the ratio of cAMP to cGMP in the splenic T cells of mice is five times lower than in youth. Similar changes in cyclic nucleotides were found in human peripheral T cells (22). The shift in the cyclic nucleotide ratio can result from changes in intrinsic T-cell properties that may account for the increased production of autoantibodies in older animals. Supporting this view are the findings that in SLE patients the cyclic nucleotides are maintained at levels characteristic of older populations (22). The alternations in cAMP and cGMP levels can be explained by the free radical theory of ageing: the excess of free radicals occurring in older mammals leads to activation of guanylate cyclase and an increase in cGMP, which in turn activates phosphodiesterase and induces a decrease in cAMP. Another important finding that can explain the age-related changes in intrinsic T-cell properties was reported by Trail and co-workers (24). They found that membrane fluidity of peripheral blood lymphocytes is decreased in old subjects. The decreased fluidity of the cell membrane could result in disruption of ionic channels leading to changes in intracellular ionic composition. This in turn can lead to changes in cellular activity resulting in overproduction of autoantibodies (24).

Another common explanation of the age-dependent increased production of autoantibodies is increased somatic mutations (25). Age-dependent increase in the rate of somatic mutations can give rise to cellular clones producing autoantibodies.

In summary, as can be seen, ageing is associated with increased production of autoantibodies. It can also explain the increased generation of autoantibodies with solid tumors. Yet, these phenomena are not associated with overt autoimmune diseases.

Summary

Ageing is associated with increased production of a variety of autoantibodies. This phenomenon is represented by the author in a large group of patients with solid tumors (carcinoma). In contrast to a common belief, patients with carcinomas generate more anti-nuclear autoantibodies because of their older age rather than because of the tumor itself. Yet, a true higher incidence of autoantibodies was noted among patients with lymphomas.

The increased autoimmunity of ageing is the end result of the combination of immune defects (e.g. Ts cell dysfunction), with an increased exposure to environmental agents. The increased autoimmunity with ageing usually is not associated with overt autoimmune diseases.

Acknowledgement

We would like to thank Ms Shira Lancry for excellent secretarial assistance.

References

1. El-Roeiy, A. and Shoenfeld, Y. Autoimmune diseases in pregnancy. *Am. J. Repnoa. Immunol.* **9**: 28–32; 1985.
2. Tomer, Y. and Shoenfeld, Y. Ageing and autoimmunity. *Autoimmunity* **1**: 141–149; 1988.
3. Swissa, M., Amital-Teplizki, H., Haim, N., Cohen, Y. and Shoenfeld, Y. Autoantibodies in neoplasia. An unresolved enigma. *Cancer* **65**: 2554–2558; 1990.
4. Huminer, D., Tomer, Y., Potlick, S. and Shoenfeld, Y. Autoantibodies in cancer patients: are they tumor related or age related? *Autoimmunity* **5**: 232–233; 1990.
5. Swissa, M., Cohen, Y. and Shoenfeld, Y. Autoantibodies in lymphoma. (Submitted.)
6. Albin, R. J. Malignancy associated with antinuclear antibodies. *Lancet* **2**: 1253–1254; 1972.
7. McCarty, G. A. Autoimmunity and malignancy. *Med. Clin. North Am.* **69**: 599–615; 1985.
8. Burnham, T. K. Antinuclear antibodies in patients with malignancies. *Lancet* **2**: 426–427; 1972.
9. Albin, R. J. Antibodies in malignant diseases. *Br. Med. J.* **2**: 767; 1972.

10. Kay, N. E. and Anderson, K. Direct antiglobulin Coombs' test. *N. Y. State J. Med.* **78**: 1244; 1978.
11. Wortman, J., Rosse, W. and Logue, G. Cold agglutinin autoimmune hemolytic anemia in non-hematologic malignancies. *Am. J. Hematol.* **6**: 275–276; 1975.
12. Tatal, N., and Bunin, J. J. Development of malignant lymphoma in the course of Sjogren's syndrome. *Am. J. Med.* **36**: 529–540; 1969.
13. Abu-Shakra, M., Krupp, M., Agrov, S., Buskila, D., Slor, H. and Shoenfeld, Y. The detection of anti-Sm-RNP antibodies in sera of patients with monoclonal gammaptthies. *Clin. Exp. Immunol.* **76**: 349–353; 1989.
14. Landahl, S., Jagenbuerg, R. and Svanborg, A. Blood components in a 70 year old population. *Clin. Chim. Acta* **112**: 301–304; 1981.
15. Moulias, R., Proust, J. and Wang, A. Age related increase in autoantibodies. *Lancet* **1**: 1128–1129; 1984.
16. Wilkens, R. F., Whitaker, R. R., Anderson, R. V. and Berven, D. Significance of antinuclear factors in older persons. *Ann. Rheum, Dis.* **26**: 306–309; 1967.
17. Silverstris, F., Anderson, W., Goodwin, J. S. and Williams Jr, R. C. Discrepancy in the expression of autoantibodies in healthy aged individuals. *Clin. Immunol. Immunopathol.* **35**: 234–244; 1985.
18. Gordon, J. and Rosenthal, M. Failure to detect age-related increase of non-pathological autoantibodies. *Lancet* **1**: 231–234; 1984.
19. Skias, D., Reder, A. T., Bania, M. B. and Antel, J. P. Age related changes in mechanism accounting for low levels of polyclonally induced immunoglobulin secretion in humans. *Clin. Immunol. Immunopathol.* **35**: 191–199; 1985.
20. Thoman, L. M. and Weigel, W. O. Deficiency in suppressor T cell activity in aged animals. Reconstitution of this activity by interleukin-2. *J. Exp. Med.* **157**: 2184–2192; 1983.
21. Goidl, E. A., Michelis, M. A., Siskind, G. W. and Weksler, M. E. Effect of age on the induction of autoantibodies. *Clin. Exp. Immunol.* **44**: 24–30; 1981.
22. Walford, R. L. Immunology and ageing. *Am. J. Clin. Pathol.* **74**: 247–253; 1980.
23. Antel, J. P., Oger, J. F. J., Dropcho, E., Richman, D. P., Kuo, H. H. and Arnason, B. G. W. Reduced T-lymphocyte cell reactivity and function of human ageing. *Cell Immunol.* **54**: 184–192; 1980.
24. Trail, K. N., Schonitzer, D., Jurgens, G., Bock, G., Pfeilschifter, R., Hilchenbach, M., Holasek, A., Forster, O. and Wick, G. Age-related changes in lymphocyte subset proportions, surface differentiation antigen density and plasma membrane fluidity: application of the Europe Senieur protocol admission criteria. *Mech. Ageing Dev.* **33**: 39–66; 1985.
25. Heimer, R., Levin, F. M. and Rudd, E. Globulins resembling rheumatoid factor in serum of the aged. *Am. J. Med.* **35**: 175–181; 1963.

Part V
New/prospective indications

New concepts in the pathogenesis of allergies and asthma

GARY L. LARSEN, BRUCE D. MAZER and ERWIN W. GELFAND

Department of Pediatrics,
National Jewish Center for Immunology & Respiratory Medicine,
University of Colorado School of Medicine,
Denver, Colorado, USA

Introduction

Insight into the pathogenesis of common allergic disorders including atopic asthma has come from recent studies of antigen-induced late phase responses (LPRs). These reactions have been observed in the skin (1) as well as the upper (2) and lower airways (3) of man. While LPRs have been known to exist for some time, only recently has the potential clinical significance of these responses received emphasis (4). For example, in contrast to the immediate asthmatic response, the late asthmatic response (LAR) persists for hours or days instead of minutes, may be prevented by corticosteroids but not adrenergic agents, and is associated with more frequent and severe asthma as well as increases in airways responsiveness (3). All these features are characteristics of the chronic asthmatic state. In addition, atopic asthmatics with LARs may develop a vicious cycle in which heightened airways responsiveness allows enhanced reactions to allergens as

Immunotherapy with Intravenous Immunoglobulins
ISBN 0–12–370725–0

well as non-immunologic stimuli such as irritants and exercise (5), leading to more persistent symptoms and greater morbidity from the disease. These features of late responses in general, and the LAR in particular, have spurred new interest in the pathogenesis of these disorders.

The purpose of this brief review is to present current thoughts regarding the pathogenesis of LPRs. The immunology and pathology of these responses will be presented. In addition, factors that either protect or predispose to LPRs will be reviewed. Newer therapeutic regimens used to treat chronic asthma based on the inflammatory nature of this disease will be noted. While the major focus will be on atopic asthma and the antigen-induced LAR, studies of LPRs in the skin (late cutaneous response) and the upper airways (late nasal response) that provide insight into LPRs in general will be cited. Observations from both clinical investigations and studies employing animal models will be reviewed. To put the findings in the models in the proper context, studies utilizing animals will be compared to observations in man when possible.

The immunology of late phase responses

While antigen-induced LPRs have been recognized for decades, only recently have their immunologic bases been examined. The observations of Pepys *et al.* (6) in patients with allergic bronchopulmonary aspergillosis and late reactions in skin and lung led to the hypothesis that LPRs were Arthus phenomena, the type III response of Coombs and Gell. However, recent studies of cutaneous late phase reactions have suggested that responses with this time course are not necessarily representative of the Arthus phenomenon. For example, Solley and associates (1) found heating of atopic human serum before passive sensitization greatly reduced the capacity to transfer both immediate and late cutaneous responses. In addition, removal of IgE by passing the serum over an anti-IgE immunoabsorbent abolished the ability to transfer the reactions while IgE recovered from the immunoabsorbent restored the responses. Therefore, in human skin, the evidence is strong that late responses to antigen may be IgE-dependent.

The hypothesis that the antigen-induced LAR may also be dependent on IgE has been difficult to approach in man. A report by Kirby *et al.* (7) found that inhalation of sheep anti-human IgE led to an LAR in one atopic asthmatic. With use of a rabbit model of the LAR, the importance of antigen-specific IgE to this pattern of airways obstruction has also been addressed (8, 9). In a study involving neonatal immunization to *Alternaria tenuis*, rabbits with predominantly or only antigen-specific IgE to this mold developed both early and late airways obstruction (8). In rabbits passively sensitized with intravenous infusions of sera containing anti-*Alternaria* IgE, late responses were again noted after antigen challenge (8, 9). In both actively and passively sensitized rabbits, the presence of antigen-specific IgG was associated with blunting of the LAR. Immunoglobulin and complement deposition within the rabbit airways was not found (9, 10). Thus, as in human skin, LPRs within the airways of both man and rabbits have been associated with the presence of antigen-specific IgE. As recently reviewed (11), animal models of the LAR have now been developed in six species of animals. While the relative importance of antigen-specific IgE and IgG to these responses has not been examined in detail in most species, reports from two separate groups employing guinea-pig models have also suggested antigen-specific IgE may be more important than antigen-specific IgG in producing LARs in this species (12, 13). However, in one model in rats passively sensitized with a monoclonal IgE antibody, immediate but not late changes in airway mechanics were produced by antigen challenge, suggesting additional immunologic and/or physiologic factors may be necessary to produce LARs in this species (14).

While suppression of the LAR has been associated with antigen-specific lgG in the rabbit, no comparable observations have been made in human asthma. However, in subjects treated with ragweed immunotherapy, Pienkowski *et al.* (15) noted suppression of ragweed-induced late cutaneous responses was related to the level of antigen-specific IgG in sera. Fling *et al.* (16) found that the late cutaneous response in mountain cedar-sensitive patients was suppressed by immunotherapy to this antigen with the suppression strongly correlated with mountain cedar-specific lgG_4.

A recent general-population study by Burrows *et al.* (17) concluded that the prevalence of asthma was closely related to the serum IgE level standardized for age and sex. The authors concluded that asthma is almost always associated with some type of IgE-related reaction, challenging the concept that there are basic differences between allergic ("extrinsic") and non-allergic ("intrinsic") forms of the disease. These observations highlight the potential importance of IgE-related mechanisms in asthma.

The pathology of late phase reactions

Late phase reactions in both the upper and lower airways as well as the skin of man and/or animal models have been associated with inflammation within the involved tissue. For example, in human skin, Solley and associates (1) noted the late cutaneous response was characterized by edema and a mixed cellular infiltrate. A recent study by Frew and Kay (18) noted a significant association between the numbers of CD4+ cells and activated eosinophils in human late phase allergic skin reactions 24 h after antigen exposure. In man, bronchoalveolar lavage performed after antigen challenge that led to an LAR has also shown accumulation of inflammatory cells. For example, de Monchy *et al.* (19) found the LAR was associated with the accumulation of eosinophils in the lung while Metzger *et al.* (20) found lavage fluids contained both neutrophils and eosinophils during the late time period. In actively immunized rabbits with IgE to *Alternaria tenuis*, simultaneous challenge of the skin and lungs led to interstitial edema and vessel dilation in the skin and airways within 15—30 min of exposure while the period of the LAR (6 h) was characterized by edema and a mixed cellular infiltrate of polymorphonuclear leukocytes and mononuclear cells (10). Within the lung, these abnormalities were found in both the large and small airways, but not within alveoli. Forty-eight hours after antigen challenge, the edema had subsided, and the cellular infiltrate was more mononuclear in character. By 7 days, the histology of both the skin and airways was normal.

In man and various animal models, the LAR and accumulation of granulocytes within the airways have been temporally related. However, this temporal association does not necessarily mean accumulation of cells and release of mediators are responsible for the late response or subsequent increase in airways responsiveness. However, from work in an animal model of the late cutaneous reaction, there are suggestions that granulocytes play an important role in late phase reactions. Lemanske *et al.* (21) depleted rats of neutrophils with vinblastine, and found the late cutaneous response induced by either anti-IgE or mast cell granules was significantly attenuated. In addition, these investigators partially reconstituted the late cutaneous reaction by administering exogenous neutrophils to the granulocytopenic animals at the time of challenge. In terms of the LAR in man, the mechanistic importance of the inflammatory cells is difficult to address. However, the importance of granulocytes to the antigen-induced LAR in rabbits has also been approached through depletion and partial repletion of these cells (22). In immune rabbits made neutropenic with the administration of nitrogen mustard, subsequent antigen challenge led to an immediate asthmatic response but no LAR or increase in airways responsiveness. When granulocytopenic ragweed-immune and granulocytopenic ragweed non-immune rabbits were transfused with a neutrophil-rich population of white cells at the time of ragweed exposure, control (non-ragweed immune) rabbits had neither immediate nor late asthmatic responses after exposure to this antigen while ragweed-immune rabbits had early and late decreases in lung function. In addition, marked increases in airways reactivity to histamine were noted in the ragweed-immune group. These observations suggest that the granulocytic series of cells is important in the production of the LAR and the subsequent increase in airways reactivity in this model.

Potential mediators of late phase responses

Mediators of inflammation and immediate hypersensitivity that may be important in LPRs have been most extensively studied in the sheep model of the LAR where several lines of evidence have suggested lipoxygenase products are important in producing a LAR (23). However, at this time, the role of eicosanoids in the pathogenesis of LARs in man has primarily been suggested by their relevant *in vitro* activities, their production by lung tissue after appropriate stimulation *in vitro*, and their pharmacologic effects after *in vivo* administration in humans (24). A recent report by Britton and co-workers (25) found that while an oral leukotriene D_4 antagonist led to a small reduction in the immediate asthmatic response after antigen challenge of atopic asthmatics, it had no significant effect on the LAR. Thus, the potential importance of lipoxygenase products of arachidonic acid metabolism in human LARs remains to be explored in more detail.

Other mediators have also been associated with late phase reactions. For example, Dorsch and co-workers performed studies that suggest that thromboxanes may be involved in late cutaneous reactions in man (26). In the upper airways, Naclerio and associates (2) found histamine, TAME-esterase, kinin, and prostaglandin D_2 were all released during the immediate response to antigen while only the first three were released during late responses. This led to speculation that basophils were the cellular source of the mediators during the late response.

Another mediator that has attracted much attention in terms of LPRs has been platelet activating factor (PAF). However, administration of PAF to humans led only to immediate and not late airways obstruction (27). These investigators did note PAF caused an increase in airways reactivity in man, and as noted earlier, this may be one of the most important consequences of antigen exposure.

To summarize, there is currently much confusion about the relative importance of various mediators in terms of late phase reactions. Realistically, one mediator is unlikely to be responsible for all the manifestations of this disorder. Rather, a series of cell-to-cell interactions mediated through the products they release are likely to be responsible for the pathologic and physiologic features of the disease (24).

Factors that may modulate late phase responses

In all likelihood, several factors interact to determine if an allergic reaction subsides after an immediate response or progresses to a LPR. These factors are listed in Table 1. The first factor that may be of importance is the antigen load. While information in the lung is minimal, observations in the skin of atopic subjects suggest that by increasing the dose of antigen, most atopic subjects will develop a late cutaneous response (15). A second modulating factor is the level of antigen-specific IgE present within the host. In studies that have looked at the determinants of the LAR, higher levels of IgE have generally correlated with the development of these responses (28, 29). Conversely, as discussed previously, antigen-specific IgG may protect against these reactions (8, 9, 15, 16). Another potentially important factor is the level of airways reactivity in that asthmatics with more reactive airways are more likely to develop late phase responses (28, 29).

Table 1
Factors that may modulate late phase responses

Factor	References
Antigen load	15
Antigen-specific IgE	28,29
Antigen-specific IgG	8,9,15,16
Airways responsiveness	28,29
T lymphocytes	18,30
Histamine releasing factors	31
Endogenous corticosteroids	32
Viral respiratory infections	33
Time of day	34

Other factors have also been identified that may separate early responders from those that have a late response. Studies by Gonzalez and associates (30) found that in atopic asthmatics with only an immediate asthmatic response, there was a significant increase in the percentage and absolute number of T suppressor cells (OKT8) in bronchoalveolar lavage, raising the possibility that mobilization of T suppressor cells into the lung is associated with prevention of a subsequent LAR. In addition, histamine releasing factors, factors derived from mononuclear cells and other sources and which may be found in late phase reactions *in vivo*, may be important for the development of LPRs (31). Observations in a canine model of the late asthmatic response have suggested that endogenous glucocorticosteroids may also determine if an LAR will occur (32). Other factors such as co-existent or recent viral respiratory infections may also predispose to LARs (33). The time of day when antigen exposure occurs also appears to be an important variable (34).

The relative importance of the factors listed in Table 1 in terms of their ability to modulate LPRs is unknown. However, this list presents several variables that probably interact to determine the outcome of antigen exposure.

New approaches to therapy of allergic asthma

The concept that late allergic airway responses more closely resemble severe asthma together with the demonstration that LARs are associated with an inflammatory reaction within the airways has led to new approaches to the therapy of chronic asthma. Thus, therapy in the milder asthma patient with episodic wheezing is more likely to include drugs with anti-inflammatory actions such as corticosteroids and sodium cromoglycate at an earlier stage in the disease. In addition, in the difficult to control steroid-dependent asthma patient, drugs with anti-inflammatory actions such as cytotoxic drugs (35) or macrolide antibiotics (36) are used in attempts to achieve clinical stability while reducing the need for corticosteroids.

The possible benefit of therapy with agents that have anti-inflammatory and/or immunomodulatory effects has also led to the use of intravenous immunoglobulin (IVIG) in patients with asthma (37–39). The efficacy of IVIG in decreasing the symptoms of asthma in immunodeficient children was suggested by the study of Page *et al.* (38). In a more comprehensive study of eight immunocompetent children with steroid-dependent asthma, Mazer *et al.* (39) demonstrated significant clinical benefit as defined by improved lung function and symptom scores when the children received 2 g/k of IVIG over two consecutive days every month for 6 months. In addition, the patients were able to tolerate significantly less oral corticosteroids without deterioration in lung function while receiving this therapy. In the seven subjects who exhibited positive skin tests prior to treatment, a highly significant decrease in prick skin test reactivity to a battery of aeroallergens was demonstrated. The mechanisms through which this improvement was achieved are undefined.

Summary

Late phase responses in the skin, upper airways and lungs of atopic individuals represent important clinical problems in many of their features. Studies in human skin and the lower airways in man and animal models have suggested that antigen-induced late phase responses are initiated by an IgE-mediated reaction. When late phase responses develop, they have been associated with an influx of inflammatory cells. Several mediators, including an increasing array of cytokines released by both resident and infiltrating cells, may contribute to late phase reactions and their sequelae. Factors that determine if an allergic reaction subsides after an immediate response or progresses to include a late phase reaction probably include the magnitude of antigen exposure, levels of antigen-specific IgE and IgG, 'responsiveness' of the target tissue, the number and type of T lymphocytes in the area of the response, histamine releasing factors, and endogenous levels of corticosteroids, as well as recent viral infections and time of antigen exposure. Within the lung, recognition of the inflammatory nature of late phase responses has supported the use of therapeutic regimens with anti-inflammatory and/or immunomodulatory potential including macrolide antibiotics, methotrexate, and intravenous immunoglobulin. In terms of the latter therapy, one study of immunocompetent children with steroid-dependent asthma suggested that a beneficial clinical response together with a steroid sparing effect may be seen with monthly high dose immunoglobulin infusions. Continued study of late phase responses should provide additional insight into the mechanisms responsible for and the best therapeutic approaches to difficult clinical problems such as steroid-dependent asthma.

Acknowledgement

This work was supported in part by Grants No. HL-27063, HL-31376, HL-36577, and AI-26490 from the National Institutes of Health. Dr Mazer is a fellow of the Medical Research Council of Canada. Dr Gelfand is a Scholar of the Raymond and Beverly Sackler Foundation.

References

1. Solley, G. O., Gleich, G. J., Jordon, R. E. and Schroeter, A. L. The late phase of the immediate wheal and flare skin reaction: its dependence upon IgE antibodies. *J. Clin. Invest.* 58: 408; 1976.
2. Naclerio, R. M., Proud, D., Togias, A. G., Adkinson, N. F. Jr., Meyers, D. A., Kagey-Sobotka, A., Plaut, M., Norman, P. S. and Lichtenstein, L. M. Inflammatory mediators in late antigen-induced rhinitis. *N. Engl. J. Med.* **313**: 65; 1985.
3. O'Byrne, P. M., Dolovich, J. and Hargreave, F. E. State of art: late asthmatic responses. *Am. Rev. Respir. Dis.* **136**: 740; 1987.
4. Gleich, G. J. The late phase of the immunoglobulin E-mediated reaction: a link between anaphylaxis and common allergic disease? *J. Allergy Clin. Immunol.* **70**: 160; 1982.
5. Cockcroft, D. W. Mechanisms of perennial allergic asthma. *Lancet* **2**: 253; 1983.
6. Pepys, J., Turner-Warwick, M., Dawson, P. L. and Hinson, K. F. W. Arthus (type III) skin reactions in man. Clinical and immunopathological features. *In* "Allergology, Proceedings of the Sixth Congress of the International Association of Allergology" (Eds Rose, B., Richter, M., Sehon, A. and Frankland, A. W.), pp. 221–235. Excerpta Medica International Congress Series, Amsterdam; 1968.
7. Kirby, J. G., Robertson, D. G., Hargreave, F. E. and Dolovich, J. Asthmatic responses to inhalation of anti-human lgE. *Clin. Allergy* **16**: 191; 1986.
8. Shampain, M. P., Behrens, B. L., Larsen, G. L. and Henson, P. M. An animal model of late pulmonary responses to *Alternaria* challenge. *Am. Rev. Respir. Dis.* **126**: 493; 1982.
9. Behrens, B. L., Clark, R. A. F., Marsh, W. and Larsen, G. L. Modulation of the late asthmatic response by antigen specific immunoglobulin G in an animal model. *Am. Rev. Respir. Dis.* **130**: 1134; 1984.
10. Behrens, B. L., Clark, R. A. F., Presley, D. M., Graves, J. P., Feldsien, D. C. and Larsen, G. L. Comparison of the evolving histopathology of early and late cutaneous and asthmatic responses in rabbits after a single antigen challenge. *Lab. Invest.* **56**: 101; 1987.

11. Larsen, G. L. Animal models of the late asthmatic response. *In* "The Allergic Basis of Asthma" (Ed. Kay, A. B.), pp. 91–109. W. B. Saunders, London; 1988.
12. Brattsand, R., Andersson, P., Wieslander, E., Linden, M., Axelsson, B. and Paulsson, I. Pathophysiological characteristics of a guinea pig model for dual bronchial obstruction. *In* "Glucocorticoids, Inflammation and Bronchial Reactivity" (Eds Hogg, J. C., Ellul-Micallef, R. and Brattsand, R.), pp. 51–66. Excerpta Medica, Amsterdam; 1985.
13. Iijima, H., Ishii, M., Yamauchi, K., Chao, C-L., Kimura, K., Shimura, S., Shindoh, Y., Inoue, H., Mue, S. and Takishima T. Bronchoalveolar lavage and histologic characterization of late asthmatic response in guinea pigs. *Am. Rev. Respir. Dis.* **136**: 922; 1987.
14. Sorkness, R., Blythe, S. and Lemanske, R. F. Jr. Pulmonary antigen challenge in rats passively sensitized with a monoclonal IgE antibody induces immediate but not late changes in airway mechanics. *Am. Rev. Respir. Dis.* **138**: 1152; 1988.
15. Pienkowski, M. M., Norman, P. S. and Lichtenstein, L. M. Suppression of late-phase skin reactions by immunotherapy with ragweed extract. *J. Allergy Clin. Immunol.* **76**: 729; 1985.
16. Fling, J. A., Ruff, M. E., Parker, W. A., Whisman, B. A., Martin, M. E., Moss, R. B. and Reid, M. J. Suppression of the late cutaneous response by immunotherapy. *J. Allergy Clin. Immunol.* **83**: 101; 1989.
17. Burrows, B., Martinez, F. D., Halonen, M., Barbee, R. A. and Cline, M. G. Association of asthma with serum IgE levels and skin-test reactivity to allergens. *N. Engl. J. Med.* **320**: 271; 1989.
18. Frew, A. J. and Kay, A. B. The relationship between infiltrating CD4+ lymphocytes, activated eosinophils, and the magnitude of the allergen-induced late phase cutaneous reaction in man. *J. Immunol.* **141**: 4158; 1988.
19. de Monchy, J. G. R., Kauffman, H. F., Venge, P., Koeter, G. H., Jansen, H. M., Sluiter, H. J. and deVries, K. Bronchoalveolar eosinophilia during allergen-induced late asthmatic reactions. *Am. Rev. Respir. Dis.* **131**: 373; 1985.
20. Metzger, W. J., Zavala, D., Richerson, H. B., Moseley, P., Iwamota, P., Monick, M., Sjoerdsma, K. and Hunninghake, G. W. Local allergen challenge and bronchoalveolar lavage of allergic asthmatic lungs. Description of the model and local airway inflammation. *Am. Rev. Respir. Dis.* **135**: 433; 1987.
21. Lemanske, R. F., Guthman, D. A., Oertel, H., Barr, L. and Kaliner, M. The biologic activity of mast cell granules. VI. The effect of vinblastine-induced neutropenia on rat cutaneous late phase reactions. *J. Immunol.* **130**: 2837; 1983.
22. Murphy, K. R., Wilson, M. C., Irvin, C. G., Glezen, L. S., Marsh, W. R., Haslett, C., Henson, P. M. and Larsen, G. L. The requirement

for polymorphonuclear leukocytes in the late asthmatic response and heightened airways reactivity in an animal model. *Am. Rev. Respir. Dis.* **134**: 62; 1986.

23. Abraham, W. M. The importance of lipoxygenase products of arachidonic acid in allergen-induced late responses. *Am. Rev. Respir. Dis.* **135**: S49; 1987.
24. Smith, H. R. and Henson, P. M. Mediators of asthma. *Sem. Respir. Med.* **8**: 287; 1987.
25. Britton, J. R., Hanley, S. P. and Tattersfield, A. E. The effect of an oral leukotriene D_4 antagonist L-649,923 on the response to inhaled antigen in asthma. *J. Allergy Clin. Immunol.* **79**: 811; 1987.
26. Dorsch, W., Ring, J. and Melzer, H. A selective inhibitor of thromboxane biosynthesis enhances immediate and inhibits late cutaneous allergic reactions in man. *J. Allergy Clin. Immunol.* **72**: 168; 1983.
27. Cuss, F. M., Dixon, C. M. S. and Barnes, P. J., Effects of inhaled platelet activating factor on pulmonary function and bronchial responsiveness in man. *Lancet* **2**: 189; 1986.
28. Boulet, L. P., Roberts, R. S., Dolovich, J. and Hargreave, F. E. Prediction of late asthmatic responses to inhaled allergen. *Clin. Allergy* **14**: 379; 1984.
29. Crimi, E., Brusasco, V., Losurdo, E. and Crimi, P. Predictive accuracy of late asthmatic reaction to *Dermatophagoides pteronyssinus*. *J. Allergy Clin. Immunol.* **78**: 908; 1986.
30. Gonzalez, M. C., Diaz, P., Galleguillos, F. R., Ancic, P., Cromwell, O., and Kay, A. B. Allergen-induced recruitment of bronchoalveolar helper (OKT4) and suppressor (OKT8) T-cells in asthma: relative increases in OKT8 cells in single early responders compared with those in late-phase responders. *Am. Rev. Respir. Dis.* **136**: 600; 1987.
31. MacDonald, S. M., Naclerio, R. M., Plaut, M., Warner, J., Kagey-Sobotka, A. and Lichtenstein, L. M. Human late-phase reactions. *In* "Allergy and Inflammation" (Ed. Kay, A. B.), pp. 293–305. Academic Press, London; 1987.
32. Sasaki, H., Yanai, M., Shimura, S., Okayama, H., Aikawa, T., Sasaki, T. and Takishima, T. Late asthmatic response to *Ascaris* antigen challenge in dogs treated with metyrapone. *Am. Rev. Respir. Dis.* **136**: 1459; 1987.
33. Lemanske, R. F. Jr., Dick, E. C., Swenson, C. A., Vrtis, R. F. and Busse, W. W. Rhinovirus upper respiratory infection increases airway hyperreactivity and late asthmatic reactions. *J. Clin. Invest.* **83**: 1; 1989.
34. Mohiuddin, A. A. and Martin, R. J. Circadian basis of the late asthmatic response. *Am. Rev. Respir. Dis.* **139**: A67; 1989.
35. Mullarkey, M. F., Blumenstein, B. A., Andrade, W. P., Bailey, G. A., Olason, I. and Wetzel, C. E. Methotrexate in the treatment of corticosteroid-dependent asthma. *N. Engl. J. Med.* **318**: 603; 1988.

36. Wald, J. A., Friedman, B. F. and Farr, R. S. An improved protocol for the use of troleandomycin (TAO) in the treatment of steroid-requiring asthma. *J. Allergy Clin. Immunol.* 78: 36; 1986.
37. Smith, T. F., Muldoon, M. F., Bain, R. P., Wells, E. L., Tiller, T. L., Kutner, M. H., Schiffman, G. and Pandey, J. P. Clinical results of a prospective, double-blind, placebo-controlled trial of intravenous γ-globulin in children with chronic chest symptoms. *Monogr. Allergy* 23: 168; 1988.
38. Page, R., Friday, G., Stillwagon, P., Skoner, D., Caliguiri, L. and Fireman, P. Asthma and selective immunoglobulin subclass deficiency: improvement of asthma after immunoglobulin replacement therapy. *J. Pediatr.* 112: 127; 1988.
39. Mazer, B. D., Giclas, P. C. and Gelfand, E. W. Immunomodulatory effects of intravenous immunoglobulin in severe steroid-dependent asthma. *Clin. Immunol. Immunopathol.* 53(2): S156; 1989.

Discussion

F. De Baets
Have you looked for IgG subclass deficiencies in your asthmatic children treated by IVIG?

G. L. Larsen
In the study, Drs Mazer and Gelfand looked at both absolute levels of IgG subclasses and the response of the children to immunization with specific antigens. They found no evidence of a subclass deficiency in any of the children included in their study.

A. Reshef
B. Kay's group has suggested a role for low-affinity IgE receptors (FcRII/CD32) on inflammatory cells other than mast cells in LPR.

Do you think that IVIG down-regulates such receptor expression on the LPR sites?

G. L. Larsen
To my knowledge, this important question has not yet been addressed.

C. Diener
Could you tell us something about the individual allergic sensitization of the asthmatic patients receiving IVIG?

G. L. Larsen

Seven of the 8 children had evidence of allergic sensitization as reflected by at least one positive immediate hypersensitivity skin test to a standard panel of common Colorado antigens. The antigens to which this group was sensitive included a wide range of antigens (trees, grasses, weeds, etc.). While some of the children may have had some seasonal increases in symptoms, they also had severe perennial symptoms that required large doses of steroids to maintain clinical stability.

H. D. Ochs

This is the devil's advocate question: Did the intense medical attention these children received during the trial and the possible "urge" to decrease the steroid dose (or other drugs) change the clinical presentation of these children? Did the subjects receive comparable medical care during the 6 months prior to the trial?

G. L. Larsen

Because of the severity of disease in these children, they all had received considerable medical attention in the 6 months prior to this study. However, it would be misleading to imply this was comparable to the attention they received while subjects of this study. To role out a significant placebo effect independent of an effect of IVIG, Dr Mazer and Dr Gelfand's preliminary study should be followed by a double-blind, placebo-controlled study of steroid-dependent asthmatics. Ideally, the study should also incorporate a cross-over design and involve several centers with expertise in immunology and pulmonology.

Induction of immune tolerance in hemophiliacs with inhibitors, by combined treatment with IVIG, cyclophosphamide and factor VIII or IX—the Malmö model

INGA MARIE NILSSON and ERIK BERNTORP

Department for Coagulation Disorders, University of Lund, Malmö General Hospital, Malmö, Sweden

Introduction

A most serious complication, both in hemophilia A and B, following substitution therapy, is the development of antibodies to factor VIII or factor IX. It occurs in 8–20% of patients with severe hemophilia A, and in 2.5–16% of patients with hemophilia B. The inhibitors are antibodies of IgG class, and usually of subclass 4 (1, 2). Clinically, patients with inhibitors can be divided into "high responders", who have a strong anamnestic response after exposure to factor VIII or factor IX, and "low responders", who have little or no anamnestic response. There are two main goals in the treatment of patients with inhibitors. The first is to control severe acute bleeding episodes, and the second is the induction of tolerance, thus rendering the patient available to regular substitution therapy as given to ordinary hemophiliacs without inhibitors. From our center a new method has been reported for the temporary removal of high-titer antibodies in patients

Immunotherapy with Intravenous Immunoglobulins
ISBN 0–12–370725–0

with hemophilia A and B by extracorporeal adsorption to protein A (3). We recently described a new approach to the problem of inducing tolerance in high-responding patients with hemophilia A and B by giving high-dose intravenous IgG in combination with cyclophosphamide and factor VIII or factor IX (Malmö treatment model) (4–7).

Here we report our experience with removal of coagulation inhibitory antibodies by extracorporeal protein A adsorption, and with the induction of immune tolerance in hemophilia A and B patients with inhibitors to factor VIII or IX according to the Malmö treatment model.

Methods

Factor VIII assays

Factor VIII coagulant activity (VIII:C) was determined both with a one-stage assay (8) and with a chromogenic assay (Coatest, KabiVitrum). Factor VIII antigen (VIII:Ag) was measured with two different methods: (1) a two-site solid-phase IRMA with a hemophilic antibody as solid phase and ^{125}I-labeled monoclonal antibody as tracer, both these antibodies being directed against the factor VIII heavy chain; (2) an ELISA based on monoclonal antibodies against factor VIII light chain (7). The results were expressed in international units (IU).

Factor IX assays

Factor IX coagulant activity (IX:C) was measured with a one-stage assay, and IX antigen (IX:Ag) with an IRMA using both polyclonal and monoclonal factor IX antibodies (9).

Factor VIII and IX inhibitor

A neutralization assay was used (10). The inhibitory activity of the plasma is expressed as the number of units of factor VIII or factor IX inactivated by 1 ml of the plasma, with one Malmö inhibitor unit (MIU) corresponding to 3 Bethesda inhibitor units (BIU) per ml of plasma (11).

Computer-controlled extracorporeal protein A adsorption for removal of factor VIII and IX inhibitors

The clinical set-up consists of two monitors, the first being a plasma separator and the second a computerized adsorption system (Fig. 1). Plasma is obtained using an ordinary cell centrifuge. Venous blood is drawn with a flow rate of up to 50 ml/min, and immediately citrated. The citrate is added both as an anticoagulant and to prevent complement activation in the plasma separator and in the gel. After separation in the cell separator, the plasma is pumped over on-line to the plasma treatment monitor (Citem 10, Excorim, Lund) at a rate of 10–25 ml/min. The adsorption unit includes two columns each containing 62 ml sterile protein A–Sepharose (Immunosorba, Excorim, Lund). Protein A binds to the Fc portion of IgG antibodies of subclasses 1, 2 and 4; the binding capacity is 20 mg IgG/ml. The plasma is passed over the first column until this column is saturated with IgG; it is then switched over to the second column while the first is rinsed and the IgG eluted with a pH gradient from pH 7.0 to pH 2.2. The column is neutralized before new plasma is applied. The eluting fluids from the column are controlled by continuous pH and ultraviolet detectors, the data from which aid computer identification

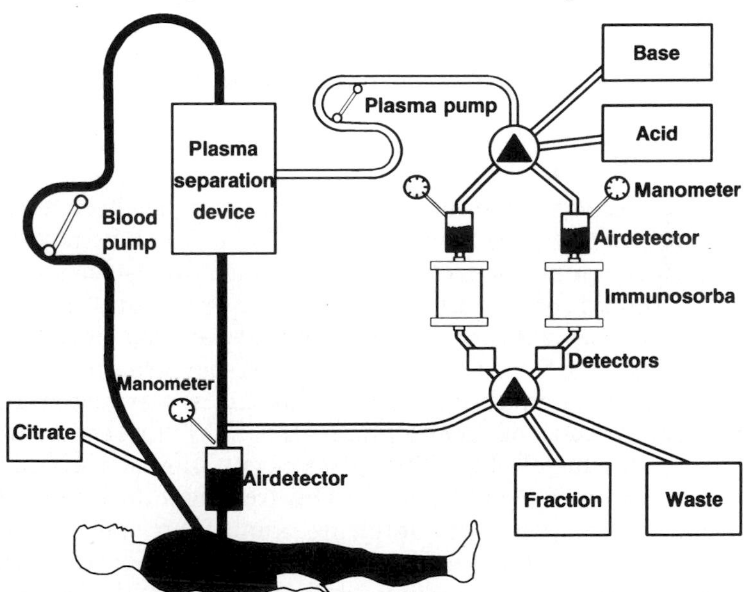

Figure 1. The procedure for removal of antibodies from plasma by adsorption to protein A–Sepharose (Citem 10, Excorim, Lund).

of plasma, waste and fraction. A series of sorting valves guide the fluids in the right direction. The treated plasma containing no antibodies is then reinfused with the blood cells to the patient. The same columns can be used on repeated treatments.

The Malmö treatment model

When the factor VIII/IX inhibitor concentration is initially high (>3 MIU/dl), the antibodies are first removed by extracorporeal adsorption to protein A. Cyclophosphamide is given from the first day of treatment, first i.v. at daily doses of 12–15 mg/kg body weight for 2 days, and then orally, at daily doses of 12–15 mg/kg for 8–10 days. The initial dose of factor VIII/IX is varied as necessary to raise VIII:C/IX:C to a concentration of 40–100 IU/dl. Factor VIII/IX is then given at intervals of 8 – 12 h to maintain VIII:C/IX:C at a level of 30–80 IU/dl. When the VIII:C/IX:C concentration decreases, the total daily dose of factor VIII/IX is increased. Beginning on day 4 of treatment, IgG is given at daily doses of 0.4 g/kg for 5 days. After disappearance of the coagulation inhibitor, regular factor VIII/IX treatment (30 IU/kg) is given 2–3 times a week.

Results and comments

Removal of inhibitors by extracorporeal protein A adsorption

So far, high-titer antibodies have been almost completely removed on 21 occasions in 11 patients (4 with hemophilia A, 3 with hemophilia B, and 4 non-hemophilic patients with antibodies against factor VIII). The time required for a course of treatment depends on the inhibitor titer and the IgG level. Six to twelve hours is the average time required for the processing of 5–12 l. For high titers, a 2-day session including a night's rest for the equilibration of intra- and extravascular IgG is the best choice. In the hemophiliacs, the inhibitor concentration decreased to low levels, and the IgG concentration was reduced to 5–40% of its original level (Table 1). This treatment does not prevent the anamnestic response on antigenic stimulation, but it enables hemostasis to be controlled in situations of severe bleeding or surgical operation. In the four non-hemophilic patients with factor VIII antibodies, admitted for this treatment because of severe bleeding episodes, it was not possible to reduce the inhibitors as efficiently as in

Table 1
Extracorporeal adsorption to protein A for removal of antibodies against factor VIII/IX

Patient	Diagnosis	Episode	Inhibitor titer BIU/ml[a] Before	After	Reduction of IgG (%)
1	Hem A	1	129	5.7	78
		2	14.1	5.4	72
		3	17	3.3	84
		4	3	0	
2	Hem A	1	1.2	0	66
3	Hem A	1	4200	10	95
		2	30	3	
4	Hem A	1	20	0	
		2	18	0	
5	Hem B	1	18	3.6	80
		2	12.6	1.7	67
6	Hem B	1	16	1.8	61
		2	16.5	1.6	74
7	Hem B	1	27	2	

[a] 1 MIU = 3 BIU.

the other hemophilic patients, probably owing to the extremely high levels of inhibitors and the presence of complexes between factor VIII and inhibitor. In these patients 10–50 l of plasma were processed.

Induction of immune tolerance according to the Malmö treatment model

The main goal in treatment of hemophiliacs with inhibitors is the induction of tolerance to factor VIII or IX therapy. Tolerance is defined as the elimination of the inhibitors, the normalization of the half-life of infused factor VIII or IX, and the absence of anamnestic response.

In 1980, we reported a patient with severe hemophilia B and inhibitor of high-responding type (12). Preceding a surgical operation, his antibodies were removed by protein A adsorption. He was given cyclophosphamide and factor IX. After 7 days his antibodies reappeared in high titer. When 2 years later he had to be treated once more, the patient was given the same treatment as in 1980, but with the addition of intravenous immunoglobulin (given as prophylaxis against infection). This time there was no anamnestic response (4).

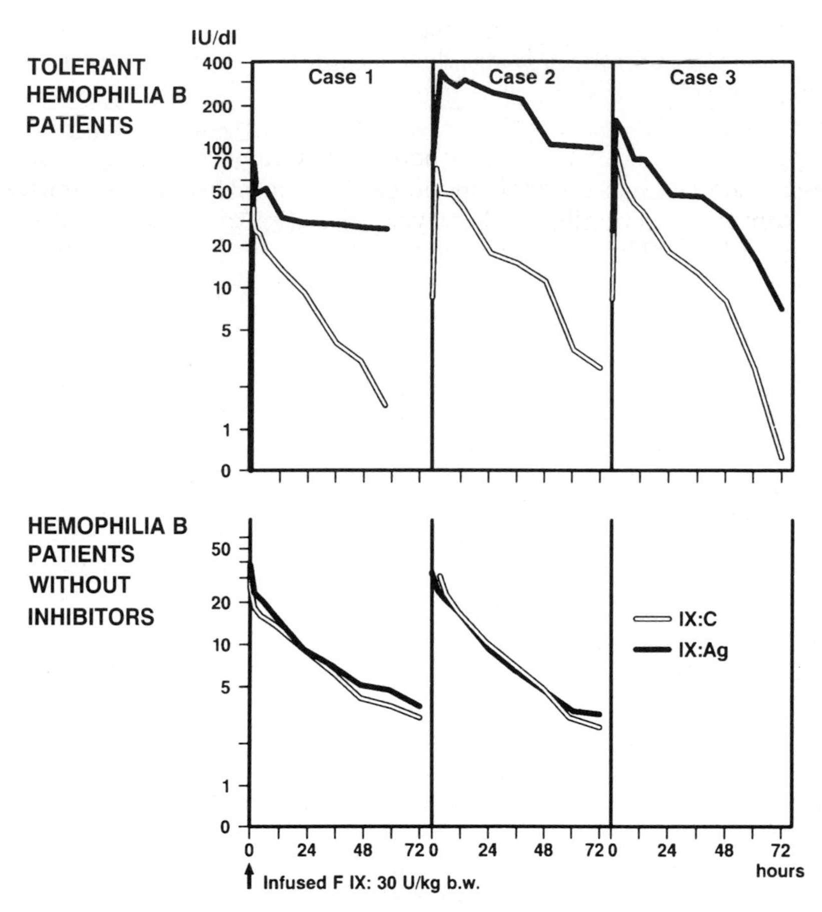

Figure 2. In vivo *disappearance curves for IX:C* ( ) *and IX:Ag* ( ) *in cases 1, 2 and 3 with hemophilia B and inhibitors after induction of tolerance, and in two patients with hemophilia B without inhibitors. The dose of factor IX was 30 U/kg body weight. Blood samples were collected before injection, 10 min afterwards, and then at various intervals.*

This treatment protocol (Malmö model) has now been successfully tried in three more patients with hemophilia B, and it has also been applied in 11 hemophilia A patients, in nine of whom it resulted in the elimination of the factor VIII clotting inhibitory antibodies.

Hemophilia B

The four patients with hemophilia B had all high-responding antibodies of IgG_4 type against factor IX (5). Earlier treatment with factor

IX alone or with factor IX and cyclophosphamide, or with factor IX and IgG, had given rise to a marked anamnestic response. When the combined treatment was given, the secondary antibody response was suppressed; and after 2–3 weeks' treatment the coagulant antibodies disappeared. The *in vivo* recovery and half-life of IX:C was the same in these patients as in ordinary hemophilia B patients (Fig. 2). In contrast to ordinary hemophiliacs, however, the IX:Ag in our patients remained high. Thus, even when the patients only received factor IX twice a week, IX:Ag material was constantly found in their plasma. It has been shown that the IX:Ag material is not an anti-idiotypic antibody (13). The IX:Ag material could be completely adsorbed to protein A, indicating that the IX:Ag circulates in complex with IgG. With the immunoblotting technique, the complexes were found to consist of factor IX and an IgG_4 antibody without IX:C inhibitory activity. The original IX:C inhibitors were also of the IgG_4 subclass. The "new" non-coagulation inhibitory antibodies are believed to recognize other epitopes of factor IX than the original IX:C inhibitory antibodies. Circulating persisting IX:Ag complexes were only observed during treatment with the cyclophosphamide, factor IX, and IgG combination; tolerance induction was only successful when such complexes were produced (5). It is known that modified antigen may act as a tolerogen. It is tempting to speculate that the circulating factor IX antigen and IgG complexes have a tolerance inducing effect.

In one of the hemophilia B patients, the antibodies reappeared after 6 months, but in the others the tolerant state appears to be stable, the first patient treated having now been tolerant for 8 years.

Hemophilia A

The Malmö Model has been applied in 11 patients with hemophilia A and inhibitors (Table 2). All the coagulation inhibitory alloantibodies had been found to be of IgG_4 class. Case 6 was classed as an intermediate responder, and case 8 as a low responder. In all the other cases earlier treatment with factor VIII alone, or with factor VIII and cyclophosphamide or with factor VIII and IgG had given rise to a marked anamnestic response. In cases 9, 10 and 11, protein A adsorption was first performed to reduce the inhibitor level below 3 MIU/ml. In seven cases the anamnestic response was suppressed after only one course of the combined treatment. In cases 5 and 10, two courses of the combined treatment were required to eradicate the inhibitor. One patient, case 9, has been treated three times; the anamnestic response decreased after each treatment, and he now behaves like a low responder and is on regular treatment. In case 11,

Table 2
Results of treatment in 11 patients with hemophilia A and inhibitors

Case (age in years)	Maximal antibody concentration after treatment (MIU/ml[a])				No. of treatments
		F VIII + Cy	F VIII + IgG	(Malmö protocol) F VIII + Cy + IgG	
1 (17)		15–20		0	(1)
2 (16)		7–16		0	(1)
3 (56)		~30		0	(1)
4 (18)		9		0	(1)
5 (15)	4			1	(2)
				0	
6 (46)	2			0	(1)
7 (5)	95			0	(1)
8 (3)	1			0	(1)
9 (5)	35			33	(3)
				7 (PA)	
				1–2 (PA)	
10 (21)		>100	111	10 (PA)	(2)
				0–0.6 (PA)	
11 (29)	>1000			1000–13 000 (PA)	(2)
				10 (PA)	

[a] 1 MIU = 3 BIU.
PA = protein A adsorption.

where the inhibitor concentration was extremely high, the protocol failed.

After induction of tolerance the patients continued with regular prophylaxis consisting of about 30 IU factor VIII/kg, 2–3 times a week. The *in vivo* recovery and half-life of infused VIII:C was the same in the tolerant patients as in ordinary hemophiliacs.

The hemophilia A patients have now been tolerant for periods varying between 3 and 7 years, and in none of them has the inhibitor reappeared.

We have recently found that, like hemophilia B patients, the tolerant hemophilia A patients also develop circulating immunocomplexes (7). For demonstration of complexes between factor VIII and an IgG antibody, we collected plasma samples from the tolerant patients 3 h after infusion of a factor VIII concentrate, or added a purified factor VIII concentrate to the plasma. As controls, similar samples were collected from non-inhibitor hemophiliacs. The plasma samples were gel filtered in AcA 34. The void fractions containing factor VIII/vWF complexes were pooled and incubated with protein A–Sepharose. To detect factor VIII and IgG subclass adsorbed to protein A, radiolabeled $F(ab')_2$ fragments from a monoclonal factor VIII antibody and radiolabeled $F(ab')_2$ fragments from monoclonals against the individual IgG subclasses were used. The tolerant plasma samples all gave strong signals with the radiolabeled antifactor VIII monoclonal antibody, indicating that the samples contained complexes between IgG and factor VIII. The tolerant plasma samples had no detectable IgG_1, IgG_2 and IgG_3 bound to protein A, but high counts for IgG_4. These findings indicate that, despite having no demonstrable VIII:C inhibitory activity, the tolerant patients have IgG_4 antibodies capable of forming complexes with factor VIII both *in vivo* and *in vitro*. After factor VIII infusion all factor VIII in the tolerant patients circulated in complex with the IgG_4 antibody.

From another type of experiment we have obtained supporting evidence of the presence *in vivo* of immunocomplexes between factor VIII and a "new" antibody without VIII:C inhibitory activity. Figure 3 shows the disappearance rates of VIII:C and of VIII:Ag, after

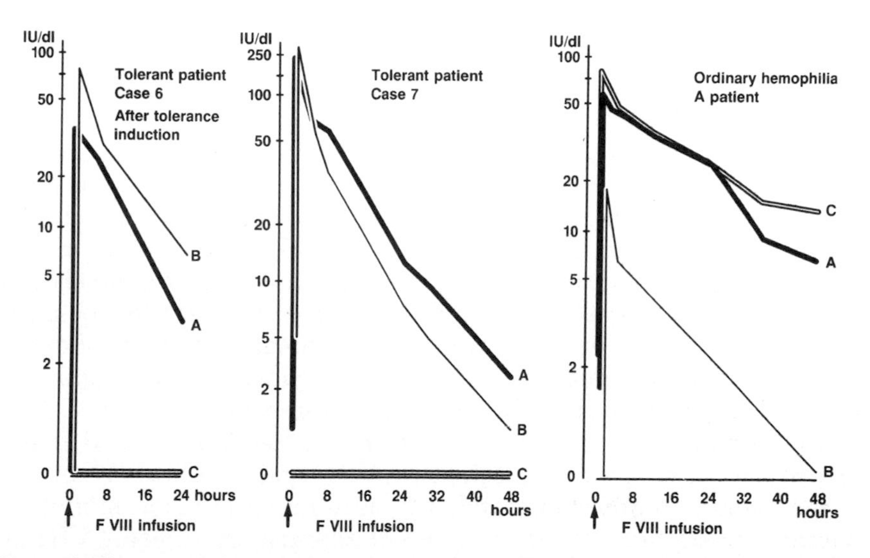

Figure 3. The rate of elimination of infused factor VIII in two patients with hemophilia and inhibitors after induction of tolerance and in one patient with severe hemophilia A without inhibitors. The dose of factor VIII (Monoclate, Armour) was 30 IU/kg body weight. Samples were drawn at intervals, and factor VIII was measured with (A) a functional assay VIII:C (▬); (B) VIII:Ag IRMA (——), and (C) VIII:Ag ELISA (▭).

infusion of factor VIII concentrate to two tolerant patients (case 6 and 7) and to one ordinary hemophilia A patient. The tolerant patients had a normal disappearance rate of VIII:C and of VIII:Ag, as determined with an IRMA specific for the factor VIII heavy chain. Surprisingly, the ELISA specific for factor VIII light chain gave zero values. Similar results were seen in one further patient (case 10). In ordinary hemophiliacs, VIII:C and ELISA results parallel each other. In further *in vitro* experiments the "ELISA inhibitor" was identified as an IgG_4 antibody blocking the interaction between factor VIII light chain and at least one of the monoclonals in the ELISA, but lacking any coagulation inhibitory activity. The antibodies blocking the factor VIII reaction in the ELISA could be demonstrated in final dilutions of 1:6 to 1:24 of the tolerant plasma samples. Thus, the amount of antibody present in the tolerant state suffices to complex all factor VIII given in substitution therapy.

Using radiolabeled factor VIII heavy chain (kindly provided by Dr O. Nordfang, Copenhagen) it was possible to show that some patients had a coagulation inhibitor against the heavy chain before the induction of tolerance, but not in their tolerant plasma which ELISA showed to contain an inhibitor against the light chain. These findings provide further evidence that the antibodies seen before and after the induction of tolerance are different.

In conclusion, the "Malmö model" comprising cyclophosphamide, antigen (factor VIII or IX) and high-dose IVIG is mostly successful in eliminating previously established coagulation inhibitory antibodies against factor VIII or IX. All components of the treatment appear to be necessary. The modification of the immune response has been found to persist during prophylactic factor VIII and IX treatment. In Bonn, Brackmann (14) has shown that it is possible to suppress antibodies to factor VIII by giving prolonged infusions of very large quantities of factor VIII over a period of 1–2 years. The advantages with the Malmö model are that the inhibitors can be eliminated within weeks and that success is possible even with high-responding patients.

After induction of tolerance according to the Malmö model, the patients still have circulating IgG_4 antibodies against factor VIII or IX. These antibodies differ in specificity, have no coagulation inhibitory activity and do not enhance the rate of elimination of factor VIII or IX. The tolerant antibodies are directed against other epitopes of factor VIII or IX, than are the pretolerance coagulation inhibitory antibodies. The soluble circulating immunocomplexes containing antibodies with secondary specificity are believed to be involved in the modification of the immune response.

It is important to discover the mechanism responsible for the tolerance-inducing effect. Not only would this pave the way for refinements of the method, but also add to our basic knowledge of immunological tolerance in general. Treatment with cyclophosphamide, antigen and high-dose unspecific IgG may even prove to be an effective means of suppressing established antibody production in other disease conditions.

Summary

A serious complication in hemophilia A and B is the development of antibodies to factor VIII or factor IX. A new treatment model has been evolved for inducing tolerance in such patients by giving cyclophosphamide, factor VIII/IX and high-dose IVIG, followed by regular factor VIII/IX treatment; when the initial antibody concentration exceeds 10 BIU/ml, treatment is preceded by extracorporeal antibody adsorption to protein A. This protocol has been applied in 15 hemophiliacs (11 A; 4 B), all with IgG_4 antibodies, in 13 of whom it resulted in the elimination of the factor VIII/IX clotting inhibitory antibodies. After the induction of tolerance, the patients still have circulating IgG_4 antibodies against factor VIII/IX, though these antibodies differ in specificity, have no coagulation inhibitory activity and do not enhance the rate of elimination of factor VIII/IX.

Acknowledgement

The investigation was supported by grants from the Swedish Medical Research Council (19X–00087).

References

1. Shapiro, S. S. Antibodies to blood coagulation factors. *Clin. Haematol.* **8**: 207–214; 1979.
2. Hoyer, L. W., Gawryl, M. S. and de la Fuente, B. Immunochemical characterization of factor VIII inhibitors. *Progr. Clin. Biol. Res.* **150**: 73–85; 1984.

3. Nilsson, I. M., Sundqvist, S.-B. and Freiburghaus, C. Extracorporeal protein A Sepharose and specific affinity chromatography for removal of antibodies. *Progr. Clin. Biol. Res.* **150**: 225–241; 1984.
4. Nilsson, I. M. and Sundqvist, S.-B. Suppression of secondary antibody response by intravenous immunoglobulin and development of tolerance in a patient with haemophilia B antibodies. *Scand. J. Haematol.* **33** (Suppl. 40): 203–206; 1984.
5. Nilsson, I. M., Berntorp, E. and Zettervall, O. Induction of split tolerance and clinical cure in high-responding hemophiliacs with factor IX antibodies. *Proc. Natl. Acad. Sci. USA* **83**: 9169–9173; 1986.
6. Nilsson, I. M., Berntorp, E. and Zettervall, O. Induction of immune tolerance in patients with hemophilia and antibodies to factor VIII by combined treatment with intravenous IgG, cyclophosphamide, and factor VIII. *N. Engl. J. Med.* **318**: 947–950; 1988.
7. Nilsson, I. M., Berntorp, E., Zettervall, O. and Dahlbäck, O. Non-coagulation inhibitory factor VIII antibodies after induction of tolerance to factor VIII in hemophilia A patients. *Blood* **75**: 378–383; 1990.
8. Nilsson, I. M., Kirkwood, T. B. L. and Barrowcliffe, T. W. In vivo recovery of factor VIII: A comparison of one-stage and two-stage methods. *Thromb. Haemost.* **42**: 1230–1239; 1979.
9. Wallmark, A., Ljung, R., Nilsson, I. M., Holmberg, L., Hedner, U., Lindvall, M. and Sjögren, H. O. Polymorphism of normal factor IX detected by mouse monoclonal antibodies. *Proc. Natl. Acad. Sci. USA* **82**: 3839–3843; 1985.
10. Nilsson, I. M. and Hedner, U. Immunosuppressive treatment in haemophiliacs with inhibitors to factor VIII and factor IX. *Scand. J. Haematol.* **16**: 369–382; 1976.
11. Kasper, C. K., Aledort, L. M., Counts, R. B., Edson, J. R., Fratantoni, J., Green, D., Hampton, J. W., Hilgartner, M. W., Lazerson, J., Levine, P. H., McMillan, C. W., Pool, J. G., Shapiro, S. S., Shulman, N. R. and von Eys, J. A more uniform measurement of factor VIII inhibitors. *Thromb. Diath. Haemorrh.* **34**: 869–871; 1975.
12. Nilsson, I. M., Jonsson, S., Sundqvist, S.-B., Ahlberg, Å. and Bergentz, S.-E. A procedure for removing high titer antibodies by extracorporeal protein A–Sepharose adsorption in hemophilia B and antibodies. *Blood* **58**: 38–44; 1981.
13. Zettervall, O., Sundqvist, S.-B. and Nilsson, I. M. Characterisation of the tolerant state in a patient with haemophilia B after removal of high-titer factor IX antibodies. *Scand. J. Haematol.* **34**: 446–454; 1985.
14. Brackmann, H.-H. induced immunotolerance in factor VIII inhibitor patients. *Progr. Clin. Biol. Res.* **150**: 181–185; 1984.

Combined use of plasmapheresis and intravenous gammaglobulin in the treatment of HIV-positive and HIV-negative autoimmune syndromes

RAPHAEL B. STRICKER and DOBRI D. KIPROV

San Francisco Children's Hospital, San Francisco, California, USA

Therapeutic apheresis and intravenous gammaglobulin (IVIG) have both been used in the treatment of various autoimmune disorders. The goal of our pilot study was to investigate the synchronous use of plasma exchange and IVIG in immune neurologic, hematologic and myopathic diseases. In addition, we wished to determine the optimal treatment regimen for combined plasmapheresis + IVIG. Finally, we wanted to assess the immunologic alterations that occur during this therapy.

Twenty-nine patients were included in our study. Twelve were positive for the human immunodeficiency virus (HIV), and 17 were HIV-negative. The diseases of these patients are listed in Table 1. Eleven patients had peripheral neuropathy, and seven patients had polymyositis. Ten of the HIV-positive patients had AIDS-related complex, and two had overt AIDS. All patients were on stable doses of medication during the study.

Although we did not test every possible combination, we found that the optimal treatment regimen appeared to be one plasma volume

Immunotherapy with Intravenous Immunoglobulins
ISBN 0-12-370725-0

Table 1
Diseases of patients in study

	Number of patients
1. HIV-Positive	
Peripheral neuropathy	5
Polymyositis	3
Immune thrombocytopenic purpura	4
Total	12
2. HIV-Negative	
Peripheral neuropathy	6
Polymyositis	2
Myasthenia gravis	5
Multiple sclerosis	2
Thrombotic thrombocytopenic purpura	2
Total	17

Table 2
Response criteria used in study

1. Clinical improvement

— Subjective improvement
— Physical examination
— Karnofsky performance status

2. Objective criteria

— Laboratory parameters
(Platelets, CPK/LDH, acetylcholine receptor antibody)
— Specialized tests
(EMG, muscle/nerve biopsy)
— Immunologic alterations
(Lymphocyte subsets, circulating immune complexes, beta-2-microglobulin)

exchange (with 5% albumin replacement) combined with 0.2–0.3 g/kg of IVIG per treatment. This combination was used twice weekly for 3–4 weeks. The optimal follow-up regimen has not been established, but it appears to be a similar combination given once every 3–4 weeks.

The response criteria used in the study are shown in Table 2. Clinical improvement was assessed by patient reporting of subjective improvement, physical examination, and Karnofsky performance status. Objective improvement was assessed by laboratory tests, such as platelet count, enzyme levels and antibody titers. Patients with myopathy or neuropathy also had muscle or nerve biopsies and electromyographic (EMG) testing. Finally, immunologic alterations in the HIV-positive patients were studied using assays of lymphocyte subsets, immune complexes and beta-2-microglobulin.

The response of HIV-positive patients with peripheral neuropathy, polymyositis or immune thrombocytopenic purpura (ITP) to combined plasmapheresis and IVIG is shown in Table 3. Nine of the 12 patients responded to combined treatment. In the case of patients with neuropathy or myopathy, response to treatment was often characterized by significant improvement in the patient's functional status. Improvement has persisted for 6 months or more in many patients on maintenance treatment.

Table 3
Response of HIV-positive patients to combined plasmapheresis and IVIG

Diagnosis	Number	Response
Peripheral neuropathy	5	3
Polymyositis	3	2
ITP	4	4
Total	12	9

The response of one HIV-positive patient with ITP is shown in Fig. 1. The patient had suffered two serious bleeding episodes with platelet counts less than 10 000/μl. With combined plasmapheresis + IVIG treatment, his platelet count rose from 6000/μl to a high of 48 000/μl. He was switched to IVIG treatment alone and his platelet count dipped to 28 000/μl. Subsequently he was restarted on combined therapy, and his platelet count has remained at 44 000–50 000/μl over 6 months with biweekly treatments. He has had no further bleeding on this regimen.

Muscle and nerve biopsies were obtained from several HIV-positive patients. Sural nerve biopsies showed intense IgG staining of myelin. After combined treatment with plasma exchange and IVIG, the antibody deposits disappeared on follow-up nerve biopsy. Muscle biopsy prior to treatment in patients with myopathy revealed diffuse lymphocytic infiltrates and intense myofibrillar vacuolization. After treatment, repeat muscle biopsy showed that the muscle fibers had

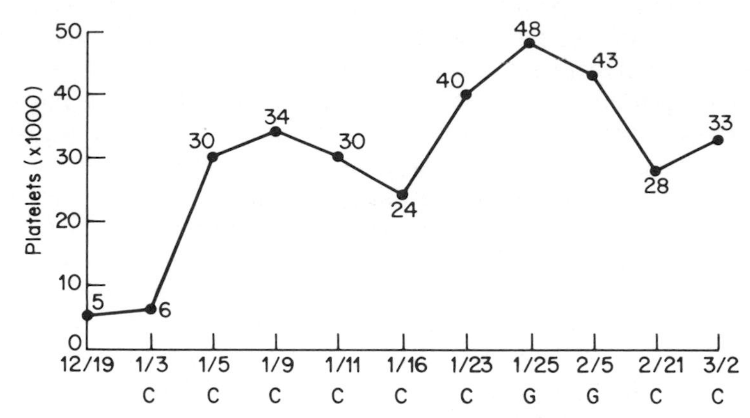

Figure 1. Response of an HIV-positive patient with immune thrombocytopenic purpura to combined plasmapheresis and IVIG treatment (C) and IVIG treatment alone (G).

become normal. This improvement correlated with clinical resolution of myopathy, which was not related to zidovudine (AZT) in any of our patients.

The response of HIV-negative patients to combined plasma exchange + IVIG is shown in Table 4. Ten of 17 patients responded to combined therapy. All seven patients with polymyositis or myasthenia gravis improved with treatment. None of the patients with multiple sclerosis or thrombotic thrombocytopenic purpura (TTP) improved on this regimen, although the TTP patients improved with intensive plasmapheresis and fresh frozen plasma replacement.

Three of six neuropathy patients improved on the combined regimen. The response of these patients appeared to correlate with the presence of a serum paraprotein, as shown in Table 5. Four of the neuropathy

Table 4
Response of HIV-negative patients to combined plasma exchange + IVIG

Diagnosis	Number	Response
Peripheral neuropathy	6	3
Polymyositis	2	2
Myasthenia gravis	5	5
Multiple sclerosis	2	0
TTP	2	0
Total	17	10

patients had an associated IgM or IgG paraprotein. Three of these patients responded to combined treatment. In contrast, two patients did not have a paraprotein, and these patients did not respond to the combined regimen. The antigen specificity of the paraprotein was not determined in these patients.

Table 5
Response of HIV-negative peripheral neuropathy patients to combined regimen

Associated finding	Number	Response
Paraprotein (+)	4	3
Paraprotein (−)	2	0

We conclude that combined therapy with plasmapheresis + IVIG appears to be especially effective for patients with HIV-associated syndromes in whom immunosuppressive or cytotoxic therapy is contraindicated. Plasmapheresis + IVIG is also effective for HIV-negative patients with polymyositis or myasthenia gravis. Combined plasma exchange + IVIG does not appear to be effective for patients with multiple sclerosis or TTP, based on our small sample. In HIV-negative patients with peripheral neuropathies, the presence of a monoclonal gammopathy may be an indication for combined therapy with plasmapheresis + IVIG. The results of this pilot study are now being evaluated in larger controlled trials.

Summary

We used a combination of therapeutic plasmapheresis plus intravenous gammaglobulin (IVIG) to treat various autoimmune diseases. Twenty-nine patients were included in our study. Twelve patients were infected with the human immunodeficiency virus (HIV), while 17 patients were HIV-negative. Nine of 12 HIV-infected patients with peripheral neuropathy, myopathy or immune thrombocytopenia responded to combination treatment with plasmapheresis + IVIG. Ten of 13 HIV-negative patients with neuropathy, myopathy or myasthenia gravis also responded to combination therapy. In contrast, patients with multiple sclerosis or thrombotic thrombocytopenic purpura failed to improve on this regimen. The optimal combination appeared to be one plasma volume per exchange plus 0.2–0.3 g/kg IVIG per treatment. We conclude that combined plasmapheresis + IVIG appears to be effective for HIV-positive and HIV-negative patients with various autoimmune neurologic, myopathic and hematologic diseases.

IVIG treatment in chronic inflammatory demyelinating polyneuropathy

M. VERMEULEN[1], P. A. van DOORN[1], I. LUNDKVIST[2], and A. BRAND[2]

[1] *Department of Neurology, University Hospital Dijkzigt, Rotterdam, The Netherlands*

[2] *Department of Immunohematology and Bloodbank, University Hospital Leiden, The Netherlands*

Definition of CIDP

Chronic inflammatory demyelinating polyneuropathy (CIDP) (1) is the chronic form of the Guillain-Barré syndrome (GBS) (2); the main difference is the course and the prognosis. In GBS the onset of symptoms is subacute with initially mild tingling of the toes and fingers followed by advancing symmetrical weakness of the legs and arms. In approximately two-thirds of the patients the symptoms were preceded by an upper respiratory or gastrointestinal infection. Evolution of weakness is complete after 2 weeks in 50% of the patients and after 4 weeks in 90%. The progressing phase is followed by a plateau phase varying from one day to many weeks, before recovery starts. After 4–6 months, approximately 80% of the patients have made a satisfactory recovery. On neurological examination in patients with GBS, weakness appears to predominate over sensory loss and most patients have areflexia. After one week of symptoms, the CSF protein

Immunotherapy with Intravenous Immunoglobulins
ISBN 0–12–370725–0

is elevated without pleocytosis. Neurophysiological studies show conduction blocks in the acute phase and later on slowed nerve conduction velocities are more clearly noticeable.

Signs and symptoms of CIDP are similar to GBS but there are some differences; CIDP patients have more often sensory loss but less frequently respiratory involvement. The main difference is the progression of weakness and sensory symptoms which takes in CIDP several months. Moreover, CIDP may have a recurrent course. Another difference is the prognosis which is worse in CIDP; the majority of patients have no tendency for a spontaneous good recovery.

In many studies, CIDP has been defined as a peripheral nerve disorder of the demyelinating type in the absence of another disease. Recently, it has been emphasized that clinical and laboratory features indistinguishable from CIDP may occur in patients with thyrotoxicosis, chronic active hepatitis, inflammatory bowel disease, HIV infection, Hodgkin's disease and monoclonal gammopathy (3). CIDP may also occur in association with hereditary neuropathy and has been reported in patients with central nervous system demyelination.

Nerve biopsies may show inflammatory cell infiltrates predominantly in the endoneurium; direct immunofluorescence assays demonstrated IgG or IgM deposits. In sera of CIDP patients antibodies against whole peripheral nerve myelin, Schwann cells and other neural constituents have been demonstrated (4–6). Lymphocyte transformation tests showed proliferation in the presence of peripheral nerve extracts in a large proportion of patients with inflammatory demyelinating neuropathies in contrast to tests in patients with other neuropathies (7).

Treatment modalities in CIDP

Prednisone

In a placebo-controlled clinical trial, prednisone was shown to cause a small but statistical significant improvement assessed by a neurological disability scale (8). Patients with CIDP are usually treated with prednisone. The recommended dosage is 100 mg daily. After an initial 4 weeks of therapy, this dosage is tapered over 10 weeks to a 100 mg single-dose, alternate-day schedule by gradually reducing an alternate off-day by 10 mg per week. The alternate day dose is thereafter gradually reduced (9). In this treatment program, patients are on rather high doses of prednisone for more than one year. However, meanwhile some patients may have reached a spontaneous remission. We have observed patients, who had deteriorated over 4–7 months and who rapidly improved on placebo treatment. If these patients had been treated with prednisone, improvement would certainly have been attributed to treatment and high-dose prednisone treatment would have been continued.

Prednisone treatment is not safe; side effects are aseptic necrosis of hip or shoulders, osteoporosis, cataract, infection, gastric ulcer, psychosis, hyperglycemia, hypertension, altered appearance and weight gain.

Plasma exchange

A study comparing plasma exchange with sham exchange showed no difference in the neurological disability scores between the two groups, but it was concluded that plasma exchange had a beneficial effect on some manifestations of the disease (10). Plasma exchange has only few side effects, especially when plasma substitutes instead of citrate plasma are infused. However, this therapy is rather inconvenient if regular treatment is necessary and may be impossible due to problems in vascular access. An alternative could be treatment with IVIG (11).

IVIG treatment

Several uncontrolled studies have described improvement in CIDP patients after treatment with IVIG (11–15). The effect of IVIG in CIDP was studied in a placebo-controlled cross-over study (16). IVIG treatment was discontinued in seven patients with CIDP who had previously been judged to have responded to IVIG and who needed this treatment at regular intervals to prevent relapse. The first trial treatment, albumin or IVIG, was given when the patient's condition had deteriorated, and the second trial treatment when on day 8 after the onset of the first treatment, the clinical condition had further deteriorated. If the patient's clinical condition had not changed, the second treatment was postponed until further deterioration occurred. If the patient's condition had improved after the first treatment, the second treatment started when the patient's condition again deteriorated.

All patients received one placebo (albumin) treatment and one IVIG. The two treatments could not be distinguished. Treatment consisted of 0.4 g/kg body weight/day for 5 consecutive days or the same amount of albumin. The treatment responses were assessed with a clinical disability score. After IVIG, all 7 patients had improved on day 8 after the onset of treatment. After placebo, none of the patients had improved, the condition had deteriorated in 2 and was unchanged in 5. Three of these 5 patients further deteriorated after 1 week and 2 after 3 weeks. The time lapses since day 8 of the trial treatment until deterioration were significantly different between the two groups. The mean of the time lapses were 6.4 weeks after IVIG and 1.3 weeks after placebo (Table 1).

Table 1
Time lapse in weeks after trial treatment until clinical deterioration

Patient	After IVIG	After placebo
1	3	1
2	4	0
3	4	0
4	6	1
5	8	3
6	9	3
7	11	1
Mean	6.4	1.3

The mean of the nerve conduction velocity of the median motor nerve slightly increased in the IVIG treatment group and did not change in the placebo group. The mean of the compound muscle action potential (CMAP) of the abductor pollicis brevis after stimulation of the median nerve at the wrist increased and decreased in the placebo group. The mean CMAP after stimulation of the elbow increased more in the IVIG group than in the placebo group. These physiological changes did not reach statistical significance.

The results of this study show that CIDP patients may respond to IVIG, but the study did not address the question whether IVIG is effective treatment for all patients judged to have CIDP. This was investigated in a recently completed clinical trial in which patients with the clinical diagnosis CIDP, and who had not been treated with IVIG, were randomized to IVIG or placebo. The treatment was the same as in the cross-over trial. None of the patients were on corticosteroids or other immunosuppressive drugs. The total number of patients randomized was 28 which is approximately the same number of patients analyzed in the controlled studies on the effectiveness of prednisone and of plasma exchange. Treatment responses were assessed after 16 days with a disability scale and with the MRC muscle strength score of six muscle groups.

The results showed no differences between the treatment and placebo groups. In the treatment group 4 of 15 patients improved and in the placebo group 3 of 13 patients. The 4 patients who improved in the treatment group did not improve more than the 3 patients in the placebo group.

Two features stand out in the results of this study; first, the low proportion of patients, approximately 25%, who responded to treatment and second, the remarkable feature that patients may improve spontaneously at a rate faster than that of deterioration, which is in contrast to what we expected in CIDP patients with spontaneous recovery. A possible explanation for the low proportion of patients who responded to treatment is that this treatment is effective in few patients with CIDP; another explanation is that some of these patients had a neuropathy different from CIDP.

Retrospective evaluation of a group of 52 CIDP patients, including many patients of the two trials, who were treated with IVIG showed that in at least 10 of the 52 patients the subsequent course showed that another diagnosis was more likely. The most important other neuropathies to consider are: first, chronic axonal neuropathy as described by McLeod *et al.* (17) (if these patients are seen late in the course of the disease, they may have slowed nerve conduction velocities and increased CSF protein in the absence of another disease and this makes distinction from CIDP very difficult), second, vasculitic neuropathy confined to the peripheral nervous system (18), third, multifocal motor neuropathy (19), and fourth, multifocal demyelinating neuropathy (20). In the study in 52 patients judged to have CIDP, five factors appeared to be related to improvement after IVIG; these factors are shown in Table 2. The probability of improvement if all these factors are present is 93%.

The results of the cross-over trial showed that patients with CIDP do respond to IVIG but this could not be confirmed in a trial in which

Table 2

Clinical factors associated with improvement in descending order of importance

— Progression of weakness until treatment
— Absence of discrepancy in weakness between arms and legs
— Disease duration less than one year
— Areflexia arms
— Nerve conduction velocity median motor nerve less than 80% of normal

patients judged to have CIDP were randomized. Therefore, the selection of patients who are treated with IVIG should be improved. Prospective randomized studies are needed to investigate if the five factors of Table 2 are useful in this selection. The design of these studies should also take account of the fact that CIDP patients may have rapid spontaneous improvements.

Summary

Several uncontrolled studies described improvement of chronic inflammatory demyelinating polyneuropathy (CIDP) after IVIG. A beneficial treatment response to IVIG was confirmed in a cross-over trial in a selected series of patients who were judged to be dependent on regular IVIG treatment. However, a beneficial treatment effect could not be confirmed in a randomized clinical trial in patients with the diagnosis CIDP. Explanations for the different results of these two trials are firstly that the diagnosis CIDP is difficult and that patients judged to have CIDP may in fact have another neuropathy and secondly that patients with CIDP may have a fast spontaneous improvement. Analysis of patients treated with IVIG showed that five simple factors were related to treatment response. Prospective studies are needed to investigate if these factors are useful in selecting CIDP patients for treatment with IVIG.

References

1. Dyck, P. J., Lais, A. C., Ohta, M. *et al.* Chronic inflammatory polyradiculoneuropathy. *Mayo Clin. Proc.* **50**: 621; 1975.
2. Asbury, A. K., Arnason, B. G. W., Karp, H. R. and McFarlane, D. E. Criteria for diagnosis of Guillain-Barré syndrome. *Ann. Neurol.* **3**: 565; 1978.
3. Barohn, R. J., Kissel, J. T., Warmolts, J. R. and Mendell, J. R. Chronic inflammatory demyelinating polyradiculoneuropathy, clinical characteristics, course and recommendations for diagnostic criteria. *Arch. Neurol.* **14**: 878; 1989.
4. Melnick, S. C. Thirty-eight cases of the Guillain-Barré syndrome: an immunological study. *Br. Med. J.* **1**: 368; 1963.
5. Koski, C. L., Humphrey, R. and Shin, M. L. Anti-peripheral myelin antibody in patients with demyelinating neuropathy: quantitative and kinetic determination of serum antibody by complement component 1 fixation. *Proc. Natl. Acad. Sci. USA* **82**: 905; 1985.

6. Van Doorn, P. A., Brand, A. and Vermeulen, M. Anti-neuroblastoma cell line antibodies in inflammatory demyelinating polyneuropathy: inhibition in vitro and in vivo by IV immunoglobulin. *Neurology* **38**: 1592; 1988.
7. Korn-Lubetzki, I. and Abramsky, O. Acute and chronic demyelinating inflammatory polyradiculoneuropathy. Association with autoimmune diseases and lymphocyte response to human neuritogenic protein. *Arch. Neurol.* **43**: 604; 1986.
8. Dyck, P. J., O'Brien, P. C., Oviatt, K. F. *et al.* Prednisone improves chronic inflammatory demyelinating polyradiculoneuropathy more than no treatment. *Ann. Neurol.* 11: 136; 1982.
9. Dalakas, M. C. and Engel, W. K. Chronic relapsing (dysimmune) polyneuropathy: pathogenesis and treatment. *Ann. Neurol.* **9**: 134; 1981.
10. Dyck, P. J., Daube, J., O'Brien, P. *et al.* Plasma exchange in chronic inflammatory demyelinating polyradiculoneuropathy. *N. Engl. J. Med.* **314**: 461; 1986.
11. Vermeulen, M., van der Meché, F. G. A., Speelman, J. D., Weber, A. and Busch, H. F. M. Plasma and gamma-globulin infusion in chronic inflammatory polyneuropathy. *J. Neurol. Sci.* **70**: 317; 1985.
12. Cook, J. D., Delgrado, M. R. and Soutter-Glass, D. Treatment of childhood autoimmune polyneuropathy: IV gammaglobulin. *Neurology* 37(Suppl. 1): 253; 1987.
13. Albama, M., McNamara, M. E., Sokol, M. and Wijshock, E. Improvement of neurologic function in chronic inflammatory demyelinating polyradiculoneuropathy following intravenous gammaglobulin infusion. *Arch. Neurol.* **44**: 248; 1987.
14. Curro Dossi, B. and Tezzon, F. High-dose intravenous gammaglobulin for chronic inflammatory demyelinating polyneuropathy. *Ital. J. Neurol. Sci.* **8**: 321; 1987.
15. Fead, J. M., Day, B., Pollock, M. *et al.* High-dose intravenous human immunoglobulin in chronic inflammatory demyelinating polyneuropathy. *Neurology* **39**: 422; 1989.
16. Van Doorn, P. A., Brand, A., Strengers, P. F. W., Meulstee, J. and Vermeulen, M. High-dose intravenous immunoglobulin treatment in chronic inflammatory demyelinating polyneuropathy: A double blind placebo controlled cross-over study. *Neurology* **40**: 209; 1990.
17. McLeod, J. G., Tuck, R. R., Pollard, J. D., Cameron, J. and Walsh, J. C. Chronic polyneuropathy of undetermined cause. *J. Neurol. Neurosurg. Psychiatry* **47**: 530; 1984.
18. Dyck, P. J., Benstead, T. J., Conn, C. L., Stevens, J. C., Windebank, A. J. and Low, P. A. Nonsystemic vasculitic neuropathy. *Brain* **110**: 843; 1987.
19. Pestronk, A., Cornblath, D. R., Ilyas, A. A. *et al.* A treatable multifocal motor neuropathy with antibodies to GM1 ganglioside. *Ann. Neurol.* **24**: 73; 1988.

20. Lewis, R. A., Sunner, A. J., Brown, M. J. and Asbury, A. K. Multifocal demyelinating neuropathy with persistent conduction block. *Neurology* 32: 958; 1982.

Discussion

J. A. Schifferli
A small subgroup of your patients responded to IVIG and from the literature we know that a small group of patients responds to plasma exchange. You had a patient who responded to both, and we have made a similar observation in a young girl. Do you think it is the same group of patients who responds to both forms of treatment?

M. Vermeulen
The patients with CIDP who had plasma exchange and IVIG responded to both with one exception. This was a patient who initially had a slight improvement after IVIG but repeated infusions had no effect. Thereafter this patient had repeatedly a beneficial response to plasma exchange.

Intravenous immunoglobulin in idiopathic inflammatory bowel disease: results of an open-label therapeutic trial

HANS D. OCHS[1], SUSANNA H. FISCHER[1], DENNIS L. CHRISTIE[1], RODGER C. HAGGITT[2] and DOUGLAS S. LEVINE[3]

[1]Department of Pediatrics, [2]Department of Pathology and [3]Department of Medicine, University of Washington School of Medicine, Seattle, Washington, USA

Introduction

Idiopathic inflammatory bowel disease (IIBD) affecting the large intestine can be divided into two major entities: ulcerative colitis (UC) and Crohn's colitis (1). Although these two disorders share many clinical, pathologic and epidemiologic features, there are usually sufficient differences to allow their separation as distinct clinical entities. In approximately 10—20% of patients with IIBD, a distinction between the two disorders may not be possible. The etiology of both types of IIBD is unknown.

Two main theories have been proposed for the cause of IIBD.

1. The immunologic hypothesis proposes that the immune system is reacting abnormally or inappropriately against one or more antigens (e.g. intestinal bacterial or viral agents) to which everyone is commonly exposed.
2. The infectious hypothesis proposes that a yet undiscovered

Immunotherapy with Intravenous Immunoglobulins
ISBN 0–12–370725–0

pathogen is causing the disease and that the immune system is simply responding appropriately to it.

The immune system has long been suspected of playing a major role in IIBD. This hypothesis is based on the pathology of the lesions, the response of the disease to immunosuppressive drugs, the systemic complications such as circulating immune complexes, arthritis and uveitis, and a variety of laboratory observations of immune abnormalities. In UC, the most common histologic abnormalities include inflammation limited to the colonic mucosa with infiltrating neutrophils, eosinophils, plasma cells and lymphocytes within the epithelium and lamina propria. In Crohn's colitis the entire thickness of the bowel wall may be infiltrated with inflammatory cells accompanied by lymphangiectasia, lymphedema, lymph node hyperplasia and granulomas. Attempts have been made to characterize the immune defect(s) associated with IIBD. The T-cell subset recognized by the monoclonal antibody HNK-1 has been reported to be increased in patients with active Crohn's disease and its number correlated with the *in vitro* suppression of pokeweed mitogen-induced immunoglobulin synthesis (2). Patients with IIBD are also found to have an increase in circulating "activated T cells" which are positive for CD 71 identified by the monoclonal antibody OKT9 recognizing the transferrin receptor (3). Another activation antigen (4F2) has also been reported to be increased in peripheral blood T cells of patients with Crohn's disease (4). Serum immunoglobulin concentrations have been reported to be normal in the majority of patients with IIBD. Studies using radiolabeled immunoglobulin suggest an increased catabolic and synthetic rate for IgG. Abnormal metabolism of IgG correlates directly with disease activity (5). Antibodies to colonic epithelial cells have been consistently identified in patients with IIBD (1, 6). A high prevalence of antibodies to intestinal epithelial antigens in patients with IIBD and their relatives has been described by Fiocchi *et al.* (6). The majority of patients with IIBD have normal proliferative responses to mitogens; a subset of patients with Crohn's disease may have decreased proliferative responses to PHA. Little is known about lymphokine production by peripheral blood lymphocytes from IIBD patients. Elevated levels of circulating interferon have been demonstrated in the blood of some patients with IIBD (7, 8).

Case reports have appeared in the literature suggesting a beneficial effect of intravenous immunoglobulin (IVIG) infusions in IIBD (9, 10). However, these observations may have represented spontaneous remissions of IIBD; the number of study patients was small, no controls were included, and the degree of refractoriness to standard therapies in the responders was not always described.

To obtain more experience with IVIG in IIBD, we treated 12 medically refractory patients with active and extensive idiopathic ulcerative and Crohn's colitis.

Material and methods

Patients

Twelve patients, including eight females and four males who had a history of IIBD for at least 6 months, were enrolled in the study (Table 1). Patients were selected for IVIG therapy if they were medically refractory or dependent on large doses of corticosteroids to prevent their symptoms of colitis. Clinical and laboratory examination, colonoscopic findings, and histologic examination of mucosal biopsies supported the diagnosis of ulcerative colitis (UC) in nine and of Crohn's colitis in three patients. At enrolment all patients were symptomatic except patient 12, who denied symptoms but was steroid-dependent. Colonoscopic examination showed moderate to severe mucosal inflammation to at least the splenic flexure in all 12 patients despite the use of multiple standard prescription medications including corticosteroids. Nine of the 12 patients were previously hospitalized for treatment of severe colitis.

Laboratory evaluation

Standard laboratory tests obtained at the beginning of the study included CBC, WBC and differential, sedimentation rate, serum immunoglobulin levels, IgG subclass concentrations, liver enzymes and a battery of blood chemistry determinations. None of the patients had abnormal liver enzymes or abnormal blood chemistries. In six of the patients one or more IgG subclasses were below the normal range of age-matched controls. Two patients had elevated total serum IgG and IgG_1 levels. White blood cell counts, sedimentation rates and hemoglobin concentrations were abnormal in some but not in all patients (Table 2).

Immunoglobulin therapy

Two lots of Sandoglobulin® (No. 73712710 and No. 8371310) were used throughout the study. During induction (phase A) a total of 2 g/kg was infused either over a 2-day period (1 g/kg per day) or over a

Table 1
Status of patients enrolled in the study

Patient Age (years) Sex Dx	Duration, extent of symptoms	Other medical problems	Medication at enrolment	Clinical status and symptoms at study entry	Extent of disease at study entry
1. LMC 16 F UC	GI symptoms at 8 years of age and relapse at 15 years of age; good initial response to therapy; symptoms of 4 weeks duration requiring hospitalization	—	Prednisone 40 mg/day, sulfasalazine, trimethoprim and sulfamethoxazole	Cushingoid, malnourished, nausea, vomiting, bloody diarrhea >10 stools/day	Up to transverse colon: severe (E)[a]; moderate—severe (H)[b]
2. MLK 20 F Crohn's	First GI symptoms at 19 years; good initial response to therapy; symptoms of 6-months duration at enrolment	Allergies including severe asthma	Prednisone 25 mg/day, corticosteroid enemas	Cushingoid, over-weight, 2–4 liquid stools/day, abdominal cramping	Pancolitis: moderate (E); mild (H)
3. JLE 66 M UC	For 3.3 years, persistent moderate—severe bloody diarrhea not responding to therapy	Ankylosing spondylitis	Prednisone 40 mg/day, sulfasalazine, corticosteroid enemas	5–10 liquid bloody stools/day, explosive at times	Up to hepatic flexure: severe (E); proximal mild, distal severe (H)
4. KAL 23 F UC	For 1.5 years, severe bloody diarrhea not responding to therapy; previously hospitalized	Juvenile diabetes since age 9, brittle; severe retinopathy; osteoporosis	Prednisone 20 mg/day, sulfasalazine	Cushingoid, malnourished, 9–15 bloody liquid stools/day	Pancolitis: proximal mild, distal moderate (E); proximal mild, distal severe (H)

5. BDR 17 M UC	GI symptoms for 6 months requiring hospitalization 10 days prior to enrolment	Allergies	Methylprednisolone 60 mg/day, sulfasalazine, metronidazole, TPN	Cushingoid, weight loss, 3–10 bloody liquid stools/day, cramping	Pancolitis: proximal moderate, distal severe (E); mild–moderate (H)
6. JIF 7 M UC	GI symptoms at 4 years of age; 3 relapses requiring hospitalization; relapse 3 weeks prior to enrolment.	—	Methylprednisolone 40 mg/day	Anexoria, weight loss, 5–8 bloody liquid stools/day, cramping	Previous documentation of colitis to transverse colon of severe degree
7. KCM 42 F Crohn's	GI symptoms (pain) and arthritis for 10 years, diarrhea for 1 year; hospitalized for 2 weeks prior to enrolment	Thyroidectomy	Methylprednisolone 40 mg/day, TPN, ibuprofen	Cushingoid, overweight, 4–5 loose to watery stools/day, cramping	Pancolitis: proximal moderate—severe, distal mild (E); proximal severe, distal mild (H)
8. AKH 29 F Crohn's	Perirectal, rectovaginal fistulae for 10 years; previous hospitalization for right hemi-colectomy; I&D for rectal abscesses	—	Methylprednisolone 200 mg/day, tobra-, clindamycin, TPN	Draining perirectal abscess	Rectal disease only
9. MEH 51 M UC	Uncontrollable bloody diarrhea of 8.5 years duration unresponsive to therapy	Coronary bypass surgery	Prednisone 60 mg/day sulfasalazine, corticosteroid enemas	Cushingoid, overweight, liquid bloody diarrhea	Pancolitis: proximal mild, distal severe (E); proximal mild–moderate, distal severe (H)
10. RMH 17 F UC	GI symptoms at age 15; relapse 10 days prior to enrolment requiring hospitalization	Hepatitis age 6	Methylprednisolone 60 mg/day metronidazole, TPN	Severe bloody diarrhea, malnourished	Up to splenic flexure (limit of exam): severe (E) and (H)

Table 1 Continued

Patient Age (years) Sex Dx	Duration, extent of symptoms	Other medical problems	Medication at enrolment	Clinical status and symptoms at study entry	Extent of disease at study entry
11. JM 10 F UC	Recurrent GI symptoms since age 6; two previous hospitalizations; admitted 5 days prior to enrolment with severe symptoms	—	Methylprednisolone 48 mg/day, metronidazole, TPN	Bloody diarrhea, hepatomegaly, clubbing, malnourished	To transverse colon (limit of exam): severe (E), moderate (H)
12. HAN 17 F UC	GI symptoms for 6 months; 4 previous hospitalizations	Azathioprine-induced pancreatitis, allergies including asthma	Prednisone 20 mg/day	Cushingoid, asymptomatic but steroid dependent	Pancolitis: proximal mild, distal moderate (E); mild (H)

[a] E = endoscopic examination.
[b] H = histologic evaluation of bx.

Table 2

Laboratory evaluation of patients

Patient	IVIG therapy	IgG at study entry (mg/dl)	Laboratory values WBC (× 1000) Sedimentation rate (mm/h) HGb (g/dl) pre/post	Status at termination of study		Extent of disease on follow-up
				Medication	Clinical status	
1. LMC	Phase A[a] × 2 Phase B[b] 200 mg/kg every 2 weeks × 6	Total IgG= 574(low) IgG_1= 544 IgG_2= 62 (low) IgG_3= 15 (low) IgG_4= 2 (low)	14.1/4.6 29/7 11/14	None	Asymptomatic	No endoscopic or histologic follow-up at 3 or 6 months (refused follow-up colonoscopy)
2. MLK	Phase A × 1 Phase B: 400 mg/kg every 2 weeks × 6	Total IgG= 1040 IgG_1= 471 IgG_2= 413 IgG_3= 43 IgG_4= 21	7.9/6.2 15/27 13.8/12.8	None	Asymptomatic	*3 months*—pancolitis mild (E); mild (H) *6 months*—pancolitis, mild with rectal sparing (E); no inflammation (H)
3. JLE	Phase A × 1 Phase B: 400 mg/kg every 2 weeks × 6	Total IgG= 1288 IgG_1= 1064 IgG_2= 5(low) IgG_3= 29(low) IgG_4= 10	7.9/6.2 30/60 11.5/11.0	Topical steroid enemas, sulfasalazine	Markedly improved	*3 months*—up to transverse colon: proximal mild, distal severe (E); mild, focally severe (H) *6 months*—left-sided colitis: moderate (E); mild (H)
4. KAL	Phase A × 1 Phase B: 400 mg/kg every 2 weeks ×6	Total IgG= 864 IgG_1= 491 IgG_2= 77(low) IgG_3= 37(low) IgG_4= 37	7.3/5.7 31/32 12.2/12.0	Prednisone 10 mg every other day	Unchanged	*3 months*—up to hepatic flexure: mild (E); mild, focally severe (H) *6 months*—pancolitis: endoscopic assessment not possible; mild, moderate and severe (H)

Table 2 Continued

Patient	IVIG therapy	IgG at study entry (mg/dl)	Laboratory values WBC (× 1000) Sedimentation rate (mm/h) HGb (g/dl) pre/post	Status at termination of study		Extent of disease on follow-up
				Medication	Clinical status	
5. BDR	Phase A × 1 Phase B: 400 mg/kg every 2 weeks × 12	Total IgG= 699 IgG_1= 507 IgG_2= 88(low) IgG_3= 14(low) IgG_4= 18	19.6/6.4 11/4 7.8/13.6	None	Asymptomatic	*3 months*—no colitis: no inflammation (E, H) *6 months*—no colitis: no inflammation (E, H); mild proctitis (H)
6. JIF	Phase A × 1 Phase B: 400 mg/kg every 2 weeks × 12	Total IgG= 699 IgG_1= 462 IgG_2= 309 IgG_3= 23 IgG_4= 48	16.4/8.0 48/3 13.4/13.3	Prednisone 12.5 mg every other day	Markedly improved	*8 months*—up to splenic flexure: moderate (E); moderate inflammation (H)
7. KCM	Phase A × 1 Phase B: 200 mg/kg × 1 colectomy	Total IgG= 679 IgG_1= 233(low) IgG_2= 159 IgG_3= 34 IgG_4= <3(low)	7.3/10.3 30/41 10.5/9.3	Prednisone 60 mg/day	Unchanged	Study incomplete
8. AKH	Phase A × 1 Phase B: 200 mg/kg every 2 weeks × 2 colectomy	Total IgG= 1282 IgG_1= 586 IgG_2= 497 IgG_3= 97 IgG_4= 49	10.2/4.1 133/18 11.4/9.6	TPN	Unchanged	Study incomplete
9. MEH	Phase A × 1 Phase B: 400 mg/kg × 1 colectomy	Total IgG= 806 IgG_1= 372(low) IgG_2= 136 IgG_3= 54 IgG_4= 15	6.5/5.8 23/57 12.8/12.2	Prednisone 20 mg/day, corticosteroid enema	Unchanged	Study incomplete

Patient	Treatment	IgG		Other therapy	Response	Outcome
10. RMH	Phase A × 2 colectomy	Total IgG= 1810(high) IgG_1= 1526(high) IgG_2= 106 IgG_3= 80 IgG_4= 5	10.9/11.5 29/97 11.6/9.7	Prednisone 40 mg/day, metronidazole	Markedly improved	Study incomplete
11. JM	Phase A × 2 colectomy	Total IgG= 1700(high) IgG_1= 1534(high) IgG_2× 129 IgG_3= 67 IgG_4= 29	24.8/28.4 not done 10.2	Prednisone 40 mg/day, metronidazole	Markedly improved	Study incomplete
12. HAN	Phase A = 1 Phase B: 400 mg/kg every 2 weeks × 3 colectomy	Total IgG= 1097 IgG_1= 530 IgG_2= 226 IgG_3= 41 IgG_4= 70	7.6/5.4 7/10 12.0/12.5	Prednisone 11 mg/day	Tolerated reduction of steroids by 50%	Study incomplete

[a] Induction phase.
[b] Follow-up treatment phase.
E = endoscopic examination.
H = histologic evaluation of bx.

5-day period (400 mg/kg per day). The material was prepared as a 6% solution and infused at a rate of 1 ml/kg/h (60 mg/kg/h) during the first 15 min of the infusion and subsequently at a rate of 3 ml/kg/h. Three patients (1, 10 and 11) required a second induction phase to achieve significant improvement. In six of the 12 patients, long-term therapy (phase B) was started 1–2 weeks following the induction phase and consisted of 200–400 mg/kg IgG infused every 2 weeks for a total of 12 weeks (four patients) or 24 weeks (two patients). The remaining six patients dropped out of the study either before starting or before completing phase B (see Table 2).

Results

Safety

All patients tolerated the IVIG infusions well and only mild side effects (headache, chills, chest tightness) were experienced by three patients during a small proportion of the infusions; the side effects resolved upon reduction of the rate of infusion.

Patient participation

Patients 1–6 completed the study. The other six (patients 7–12) dropped out before completion of the protocol: two patients required urgent surgical intervention and four patients electively discontinued their participation in the study protocol to undergo surgery. Patient 7, who had severe Crohn's colitis of more than 10 years duration, failed to respond to IVIG and required emergency colectomy due to a limited perforation 4 weeks after initiating IVIG. Patient 8 had Crohn's colitis of 10 years duration with extensive perirectal abscesses at the time of enrolment and required a diverting ileostomy during early phase B, 7 weeks after initiating IVIG. Patient 9 with UC of 9 years duration elected to have a colectomy after the induction phase just 3 weeks after initiating IVIG. Patient 10 had UC of 2 years duration, responded to two induction courses but then elected to have colectomy 3 weeks after initiating IVIG. Patient 11, with a 4-year history of UC, became asymptomatic after the induction phase but her parents decided to withdraw from the study prior to phase B with ultimate colectomy in mind. Patient 12 had a 6-month history of UC and was steroid-dependent at the time of enrolment. Despite success in reducing her steroid dose she elected to have colectomy during phase B, 11 weeks after initiating IVIG.

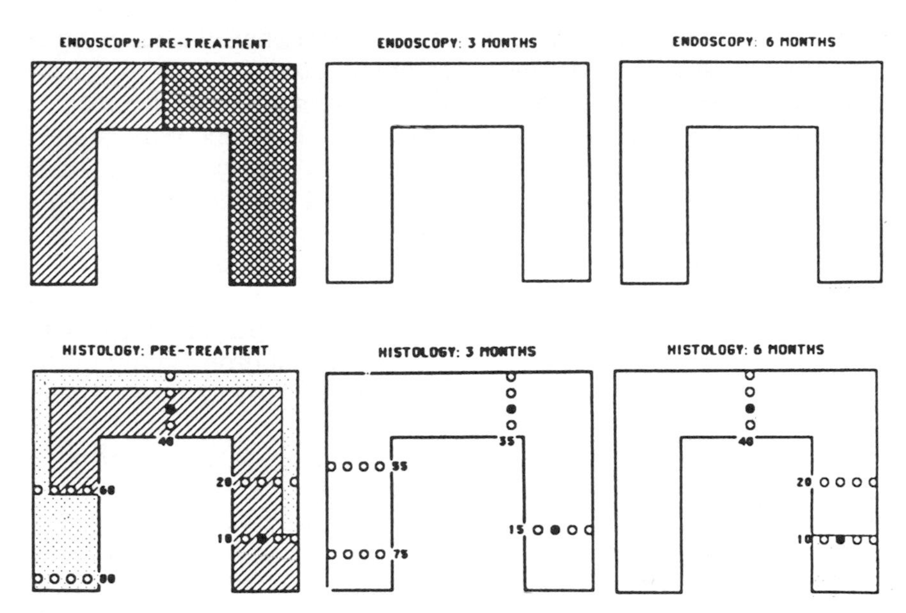

Figure 1. Distributions of inflammatory change in the colonic mucosa of patient 5 (BDR) before and during a 6-month course of treatment with intravenous immunoglobulin (IVIG) for chronic ulcerative colitis. Corresponding endoscopic and histologic examinations demonstrate elimination of inflammation following therapy and recurrence of mild rectal inflammation 6 months after initiating IVIG. Key: The degree of inflammatory change was assessed independently by direct visualization of the mucosa during total colonoscopy and by histologic examination of coded colonoscopic biopsies. Pretreatment endoscopic and histologic evaluations were completed within 1 week of initiating IVIG, and the follow-up evaluations were completed 3 and 6 months after initiating IVIG. These schematic diagrams depict the ascending colon and more proximal regions on the left, and the descending colon and more distal regions on the right. Circles represent biopsy sites (4-quadrant locations at each level), and numbers represent the level of these biopsies in centimetres from the anus. Darkened circles (at 40 cm and 10 cm in this case) represent biopsies that were photographed and illustrated in Fig. 2. Intensity of inflammation is depicted in affected areas of colonic mucosa as follows: double hatching, *severe;* single hatching, *moderate;* stippled, *mild;* blank, *no inflammation. Endoscopic inflammatory change was scored as follows:* severe, *multiple erosions and ulcers, exudate, and spontaneous hemorrhage;* moderate, *mucosal friability and erosions;* mild, *edema and loss of normal vascular pattern;* no inflammation, *intact mucosa with retained normal vascular pattern. Histologic inflammatory change was scored as follows:* severe, *ulcerated mucosa and granulation tissue;* moderate, *numerous crypt abscesses;* mild, *scattered crypt abscesses, cryptitis, or increased inflammatory cell content in the lamina propria;* no inflammation, *uninflamed mucosa and abnormalities of crypt architecture consistent with quiescent chronic ulcerative colitis.*

General response to therapy

Response to therapy was monitored by standard clinical assessment at regular intervals and evaluations of symptom diaries completed by the patients. Of the six patients who completed the study, four (patients 1, 2, 3 and 5) became asymptomatic or had significant reduction in symptoms during phase B and were tapered off systemic steroids completely (Tables 1 and 2). Patient 6 showed marked improvement during phase B and substantially reduced his steroid dose. Patient 4 had brittle, insulin dependent diabetes mellitus; her clinical improvement was equivocal, although her steroid doses were reduced without significant worsening of her diarrheal symptoms, a part of which could be ascribed to the diabetes. Of those patients who dropped out of the study project, two (patients 10 and 11) showed a marked improvement following phase A.

All patients showed a marked increase in serum IgG concentration during IVIG therapy. The mean IgG level of 1079 (± 391 = 1 SD) mg/dl observed before initiation of therapy increased to 3378 (± 578) mg/dl at the completion of phase A. The trough and peak IgG concentrations at the last dose of IVIG during phase B were 1390 (± 396) mg/dl and 1850 (± 397) mg/dl, respectively. After completion of phase B, white blood cell counts of most patients had normalized. Improvement of sedimentation rate and hemoglobin concentration was less prevalent (Table 2).

Endoscopic and histologic observations

Results of colonoscopies performed before initiating IVIG, at the completion of phase B, and at the end of the 12-week observation phase are summarized in Tables 1 and 2. Four (patients 1, 2, 3 and 5) of the six patients who completed the study protocol had objective improvement based on direct visualization of the colonic mucosa and histologic evaluation of numerous endoscopic biopsy samples (12–28 per patient) taken during each colonoscopic procedure. Patient 1 refused to have follow-up colonoscopy. Patient 4 with brittle diabetes mellitus showed no improvement on colonoscopy. Examples of distribution and severity of inflammatory change before, during and after IVIG therapy are illustrated in Figs 1 and 2.

Discussion

The "stubborn problem of inflammatory bowel disease" (11) continues to resist efforts to identify the pathologic mechanisms and to effectively

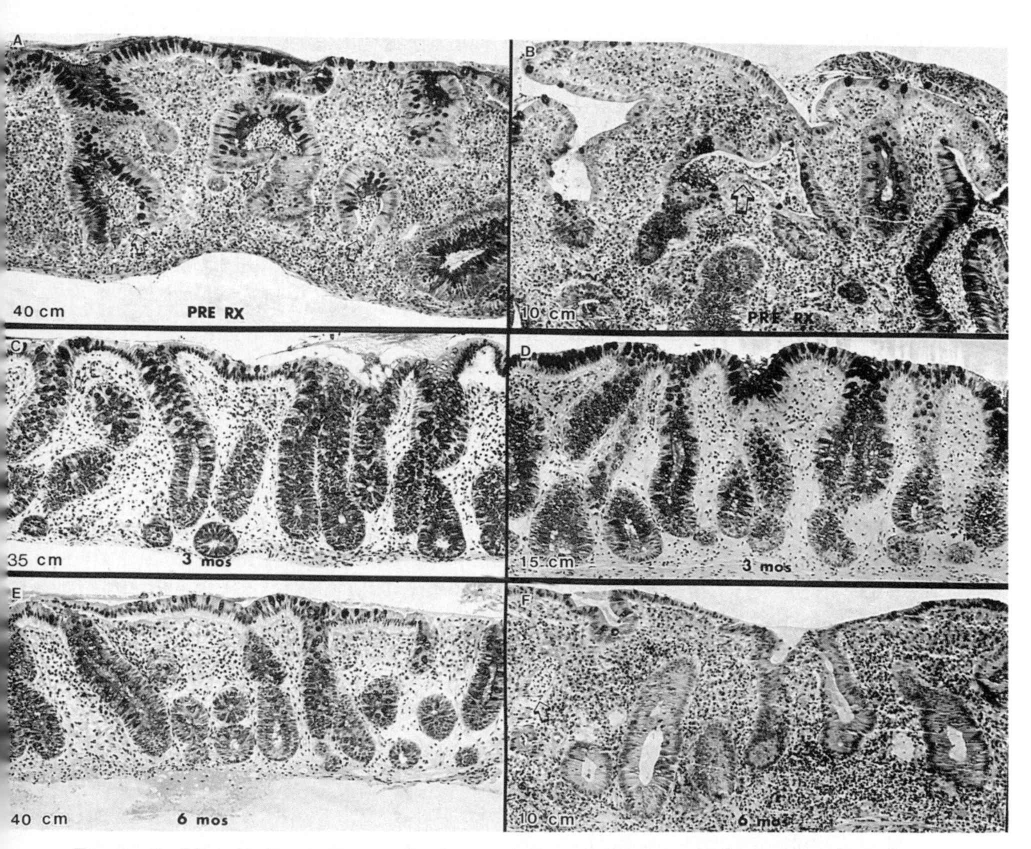

Figure 2. Histologic sections of representative colonoscopic biopsies taken from patient 5 (BDR) (see Fig. 1) before treatment with IVIG (A,B), 3 months after initiating IVIG (C, D), and 6 months after initiating IVIG (E,F) at comparable sites in the colon (35–40 cm from anus: A,C,E; 10–15 cm from anus: B,D,F). (A) Pre-IVIG treatment biopsy at 40 cm shows moderate inflammation with increased lamina propria inflammatory cells and numerous crypt abscesses (arrows). (B) Pre-IVIG treatment biopsy at 10 cm shows moderate inflammation with numerous crypt abscesses (arrow) and architectural distortion with a villiform configuration of the mucosal surface. (C) Biopsy at 35 cm obtained 3 months after initiating IVIG shows no inflammation. (D) Biopsy at 15 cm obtained 3 months after initiating IVIG shows no inflammation. (E) Biopsy at 40 cm obtained 6 months after initiating IVIG shows no inflammation. (F) Biopsy at 10 cm obtained 6 months after initiating IVIG shows mild inflammation with increased lamina propria inflammatory cells, epithelial mucin depletion, and occasional crypt destruction (arrow). (All biopsies were fixed in Hollandes, processed, step-serially sectioned at 4 μm thickness, and stained with hematoxylin, eosin, saffron, and Alcian blue at pH 2.5. Magnification × 200; photographically reduced to 50%, A–F.)

treat all afflicted patients. The variable clinical course of IIBD and the diversity of its pattern of remissions and exacerbations can make it difficult to assess treatment success. In some patients, IIBD becomes chronic and may ultimately result in complications necessitating surgical intervention. Morbidity may be considerable and often interferes with day to day activities of afflicted patients. The long-term outcome is uncertain. Many patients are dependent on intermittent or continued use of systemic corticosteroids, azathioprine, or 6-mercaptopurine. More recently, other potent immunosuppressive drugs have been evaluated and were found to be partially effective in IIBD, including methotrexate (12) and cyclosporine A (11, 13). However, these drugs are toxic and may be associated with long-term adverse effects. The ultimate immunosuppressive therapy, removal of lymphocytes by leukapheresis, is associated with considerable morbidity and is not practical as a long-term treatment strategy (14). The rationale for using IVIG in the treatment of UC and Crohn's colitis is based on the hypothesis that IIBD is caused either by an abnormal immune response to gut-associated antigens or directly by an infectious agent. It has been shown that in addition to neutralizing antibodies, IVIG contains anti-idiotypic antibody that may be directly responsible for its immunomodulating properties (15).

In view of the limited experience with IVIG in the treatment of IIBD, we decided to carry out an open-label study designed to address safety, efficacy and optimal dosing of IVIG. Of the 12 patients enrolled, three developed mild adverse effects, two during a single infusion and one on several occasions. In most patients, 2 g of IgG/kg given either over a 2-day or a 5-day period (induction phase) successfully induced remission. In three patients, the induction phase had to be repeated. The lack of reliable and easy-to-perform laboratory parameters to assess the activity of extensive IIBD made it difficult to adjust the dose to the need of individual patients. Of the six patients completing 3 or 6 months of therapy with biweekly infusion of 400 mg of IgG/kg, five showed either remission or significant improvement. The patient (patient 4) who did not respond to IVIG therapy had severe diabetes mellitus and diarrhea that may have been directly related to diabetes. Most of the responders began to feel better following the first few IVIG infusions, gained weight, had a marked decrease in the number of loose stools per day, and showed objective laboratory changes including a decrease in WBC and sedimentation rate and an increase in hemoglobin concentration. Total colonoscopy with multiple mucosal biopsies and histologic assessment of the colonic distribution and intensity of inflammatory changes was helpful in documenting treatment response.

At present, at least 3 months after completing phase B, patient 1 is off steroids and remains in remission. Two patients require low-dose steroids to remain asymptomatic (patient 5) or to keep symptoms at a minimum (patient 6). Patient 2 was asymptomatic and off steroids for 3 months after completing phase B before she relapsed. Patient 3 relapsed 4 months after his last dose of IVIG and underwent elective colectomy 4 months later. Patient 4 died of complications related to her diabetes 8 months after completing IVIG. In patients 7–12, who did not complete at least 3 months of therapy, IVIG was not promptly effective or could not be evaluated: patients 7 and 8 developed surgical complications within 5–7 weeks of initiating IVIG, patient 9 elected to have a colectomy just 3 weeks after initiating IVIG, and patients 10, 11 and 12 preferred colectomy in spite of clinical improvement following induction with IVIG.

Because the etiology of IIBD remains unknown, it is difficult to speculate as to the mechanism(s) of action of IVIG in UC and Crohn's colitis. IVIG preparations derived from large pools of plasma may contain antibodies to an unknown "etiologic agent". Alternatively, anti-idiotypic antibody present in IVIG may shut off autoantibody synthesis (15). The recent finding that IVIG may interfere with the excess production and excretion of lymphokines (IL-1, interferon-gamma, tumor necrosis factor) in Kawasaki disease (16) may also be of relevance for IIBD. Increased IL-1 production by activated intestinal lamina propria mononuclear cells obtained from patients with IIBD has been recently demonstrated (7). It may be hypothesized that other lymphokines, e.g. tumor necrosis factor, may be produced in excess locally, contributing to the pathophysiology of IIBD. It has been recently suggested that the non-specific inflammatory processes of IIBD are caused by locally generated leukotrienes and prostaglandins (17, 18, 19). It is possible, but not proven, that IVIG interferes with the local production of these potent mediators of inflammation.

The observed results of our open-label therapeutic trial of IVIG, although encouraging, have to be considered preliminary in nature and must be confirmed by a carefully designed placebo-controlled study before IVIG can be recommended as a therapy for patients with IIBD. Furthermore, the duration of disease remission in responders must be evaluated because of the tendency for some patients to relapse following completion of courses of IVIG therapy. Since both antibody-mediated and cellular mechanisms may play a role in the etiology of IIBD, a combination of IVIG and a cytotoxic drug affecting mainly T cells, such as cyclosporine A, may be more effective than each agent alone. The devastating nature of IIBD and the suspected role of the immune system in the pathogenesis of IIBD justifies continued investigation of immunomodulating therapeutic agents for these diseases.

Summary

Two hypotheses have been proposed as etiology for idiopathic inflammatory bowel disease (IIBD): (a) an abnormal or inappropriate immune response to one or more common antigens, and (b) a yet-undiscovered pathogen. For both of these etiologic options, high dose intravenous immunoglobulin (IVIG) may be beneficial. Therefore, we designed a pilot study to explore the effect of IVIG on the clinical manifestation and steroid requirement of IIBD. Twelve patients, nine with ulcerative colitis and three with Crohn's colitis received 2 g/kg body weight during the induction (phase A) and 200–400 mg/kg every 2 weeks for a total of 12–24 weeks (phase B). Patients were observed for an additional 12 weeks while off IVIG (phase C). Of the six patients who completed the study four became asymptomatic and could be taken off systemic steroids completely; one patient showed marked clinical improvement and achieved substantial reduction in the dose of steroids required. In parallel to the clinical responses, objective improvements were observed during colonoscopy and in evaluating the histologic appearance of multiple mucosal biopsies. Of the six patients who failed to complete the study, two showed marked clinical improvement following the initiation phase.

Acknowledgements

This work was supported by a grant from Sandoz Pharmaceuticals and in part conducted through the Clinical Research Center of the University of Washington (RR–37).

References

1. Kirsner, J. B. and Shorter, R. G. (Eds) "Inflammatory Bowel Disease", 3rd edn. Lea and Febiger, Philadelphia; 1988.
2. James, S. P., Neckers, L. M., Graeff, A. S. *et al*. Suppression of immunoglobulin synthesis by lymphocyte subpopulations in patients with Crohn's disease. *Gastroenterology* **86**: 1510–1518; 1984.
3. Raedler, A., Fraenkel, S., Klose, G. *et al*. Involvement of the immune

system in the pathogenesis of Crohn's disease. Expression of the T_9 antigen on peripheral immunocytes correlates with the severity of the disease. *Gastroenterology* **88**: 978–983; 1985.
4. Pallone, F., Montano, S., Fais, S. *et al.* Studies of peripheral blood lymphocytes in Crohn's disease. Circulating activated T cells. *Scand. J. Gastroenterol* **18**: 1003–1008; 1983.
5. Jensen, K. B., Jarnum, S., Koudahl, G. and Kristensen, M. Serum orosomucoid in ulcerative colitis. Its relation to clinical activity, protein loss, and turnover of albumin and IgG. *Scand. J. Gastroenterol.* 11: 177–183; 1976.
6. Fiocchi, C., Roche, J. K. and Michener, W. M. High prevalence of antibodies to intestinal epithelial antigens in patients with inflammatory bowel disease and their relatives. *Ann. Intern. Med.* **110**: 786–794; 1989.
7. Fiocchi, C. Lymphokines and the intestinal immune response. Role in inflammatory bowel disease. *Immunol. Invest.* **18**: 91–102; 1989.
8. Lieberman, B. Y., Fiocchi, C., Youngman, K. R. *et al.* Interferon gamma production by human intestinal mucosal mononuclear cells. Decreased levels in inflammatory bowel disease. *Dig. Dis. Sci.* **33**: 1297–1304; 1988.
9. Rohr, G., Kusterer, K., Schille, M. *et al.* Treatment of Crohn's disease and ulcerative colitis with 7S-immunoglobulin. *Lancet* **1**: 170; 1987 (letter).
10. Cottier, H. and Hässig, A. Immunoglobulin in chronic inflammatory diseases. *Vox Sang.* 51(Suppl.2): 39–43; 1986.
11. Sachar, D. B. Cyclosporine treatment for inflammatory bowel disease. A step backward or a leap forward? *N. Engl. J. Med.* **321**: 894–896; 1989.
12. Kozarek, R. A., Patterson, D. J., Gelfand, M. D. *et al.* Methotrexate induces clinical and histologic remission in patients with refractory inflammatory bowel disease. *Ann. Intern. Med.* **110**: 353–356; 1989.
13. Brynskov, J., Freund, L., Rasmussen, S. N. *et al.* A placebo-controlled, double-blind, randomized trial of cyclosporine therapy in active chronic Crohn's disease. *N. Engl. J. Med.* **321**: 845–850; 1989.
14. Bicks, R. O. and Groshart, K. D. The current status of T-lymphocyte apheresis (TLA) treatment of Crohn's disease. *J. Clin. Gastroenterol.* 11: 136–138; 1989.
15. Nydegger, U. E., Sultan, Y. and Kazatchkine, M. D. The concept of anti-idiotypic regulation of selected autoimmune diseases by intravenous immunoglobulin. *Clin. Immunol. Immunopathol.* **53**: S72–S82; 1989.
16. Leung, D. Y. M., Cotran, R. S. and Kurt-Jones, E. *et al.* Endothelial cell activation and high interleukin-1 secretion in the pathogenesis of acute Kawasaki disease. *Lancet* ii: 1298–1302; 1989.
17. Sharon, P. and Stenson, W. F. Enhanced synthesis of leukotriene B_4 by colonic mucosa in inflammatory bowel disease. *Gastroenterology* **86**: 453–460; 1984.

18. Lauritsen, K., Laursen, L. S., Bukhave, K. *et al.* Effects of topical 5-aminosalicylic acid and prednisolone on prostaglandin E_2 and leukotriene B_4 levels determined by equilibrium *in vivo* dialysis of rectum in relapsing ulcerative colitis. *Gastroenterology* 91: 837–844; 1986.
19. Laursen, L. S., Naesdal, J., Bukhave, K. *et al.* Selective 5-lipoxygenase inhibition in ulcerative colitis. *Lancet* 335: 683–685; 1990.

The response of patients with chronic fatigue syndrome to intravenously administered gammaglobulin

J. M. DWYER, A. R. LLOYD, I. B. HICKIE, D. WAKEFIELD and C. R. BOUGHTON

Departments of Immunology and Infectious Diseases, Division of Medicine; and the Mood Disorders Unit, Division of Psychiatry, Prince Henry Hospital, University of New South Wales, Sydney, Australia

Introduction

The chronic fatigue syndrome (CFS) is a condition of unknown etiology, characterized by extreme fatigue exacerbated by minimal physical activity, and neuropsychiatric symptoms such as difficulties with concentration and short-term memory (1). Patients may have an insidious onset of the syndrome, but frequently its development is preceded by an episode of what appears to be an infectious disease. Viral infections, including Epstein-Barr virus (2), a number of enteroviruses, and Ross River virus (3) may represent potent triggering stimuli. Non-viral infections (including *Toxoplasma gondii*) have also been reported to trigger the onset of CFS (1).

Disordered cell-mediated immunity (CMI) is a common feature of patients with CFS, as is IgG subclass deficiency (4,5). We believe the immunological disturbances may be central to the pathogenesis of the

Immunotherapy with Intravenous Immunoglobulins
ISBN 0–12–370725–0

syndrome. We have hypothesized that in CFS disordered immunoregulation allows antigen stimulation to be followed by the production of excessive amounts of cytokines over a prolonged period, which may produce the symptomatology. Cytokines such as alpha-interferon commonly produce a CFS-like syndrome when used therapeutically (6).

Because of this hypothesis supported by a CD8 lymphopenia and anergy in many patients, we examined the efficacy of immunomodulatory therapy with high-dose intravenous immunoglobulin (IVIG), previously shown to be beneficial in a number of diseases featuring disordered immunoregulation. Following an uncontrolled trial in which 67% of patients had a favorable response, we undertook a randomized double-blind, placebo-controlled trial of IVIG therapy for CFS.

Methods

Subjects

For a diagnosis of CFS we required: (1) a history of marked exercise-aggravated muscle fatigue present for at least 6 months, associated with typical constitutional and neuropsychiatric symptoms (7); (2) a significant degree of morbidity associated with CFS requiring frequent medical consultations, and a substantial reduction in ability to participate in usual daily activities when compared to the subject's premorbid state. Time lost from academic activities or work, an inability to participate in sport, and other similar indicators were documented. To examine a homogenous group of subjects, patients were required to have chronic and persisting symptomatology, though in the community there is a relapsing and remitting course occasionally reported for this syndrome; (3) a physical examination and a standardized investigation protocol to exclude other chronic infectious or immunodeficiency-related disorders, as well as other medical conditions which should be considered in the differential diagnosis of a patient with fatigue and neuropsychiatric disturbances.

Forty-nine adult patients enrolled, who met these criteria and had received no previous immunological therapy. The patients (25 males and 24 females) ranged in age from 16 to 63 years (mean = 36 years) and had been suffering from CFS from 12–180 months (median = 47 months). In only a few of these cases could we document the onset of CFS following a specific infection (Epstein-Barr virus in 4, and *Toxoplasma gondii* in 1).

Subjects were randomly allocated to receive either IVIG (Intragam, Commonwealth Serum Laboratories (CSL), Melbourne, Australia), administered by continuous infusion in a dosage of 2 g IgG/kg or placebo (10% w/v maltose in equivalent volume). Three infusions lasting 24h were administered at monthly intervals.

Monitoring

At a standardized interview, all subjects underwent an assessment of the severity of their symptoms and the degree of disability. Specific details of the degree of involvement at work, academic, leisure, sporting and social activities were recorded. A standardized psychiatric interview was conducted by a psychiatrist prior to treatment. At this interview, psychiatric diagnoses were made according to a standard diagnostic schedule (DSM-IIIR) (8). Effectiveness of therapy was assessed 3 months after the second infusion, at an interview conducted by both a physician and a psychiatrist. Symptomatic and functional improvement was assessed, with neither the patient nor the interviewer being aware of which treatment had been received. Subjects having a major reduction in the severity of symptoms and an improvement in functional capacity (as assessed by the physician) were designated as "responders", providing the patient agreed with this assessment. Patients were only considered to have improved functional capacity if there was a substantial return to involvement in at least two of the three following areas of activity: work, leisure, or social (each assessed in the context of that achieved prior to the onset of CFS). The patients interviewed by the psychiatrist at enrolment were interviewed again to enable the psychiatrist to make a post-infusion evaluation of improvement in psychological morbidity. In addition, the psychiatrist rated each subject before and after treatment using the detailed Hamilton depression scale (9).

Patients were evaluated using self-report measures of physical and psychological symptomatology as well as laboratory measures of immune status. A quality of life (QAL) visual analog scale (modified to include ten aspects of physical and neuropsychiatric symptomatology typical of CFS) was completed by the patients on entry, and at monthly intervals throughout the trial (10). The patients who had been interviewed by the psychiatrist before treatment completed self-report measures of depression (Zung scale) at entry and at monthly intervals throughout the trial.

Cell-mediated immunity was assessed by analysis of peripheral blood T-cell subsets, delayed-type hypersensitivity (DTH) skin testing, and T-cell stimulation with phytohemagglutinen (PHA). IgG subclass levels were assayed at entry by radial immunodiffusion.

Adverse effects were monitored both during and after infusions by a combination of investigator recordings and patient reports of local and constitutional symptoms during and after the infusions. For the purpose of analysis, the changes in the physical, psychological and immunological parameters for each subject were expressed as a percentage of improvement in the entry score of each measure. Any change in DTH score was expressed by subtracting the cumulative diameter measured at entry from that measured at the conclusion of the study (δDTH).

Results

Evaluation at entry

Twenty-three patients received immunoglobulin, and 26 placebo. There was no significant difference in demographic variables, or entry measures of physical or psychological well-being, or indicators of immune function between the treatment groups (*Table 1*). At entry, a reduction in the absolute count of the T-cell subsets equal to or below the lower limit of the normal ranges for our laboratory was found in 21 patients (43%). T-Cell lymphopenia was more marked in the CD8 subset (37% of patients). Reduced DTH responses were demonstrated in 33 patients (67%). Forty of the 49 patients (82%) had abnormal CMI evidenced by reduced DTH responses and/or T-Cell lymphopenia. Sixty-two per cent of the immunoglobulin recipients and 31% of the placebo recipients had IgG subclass deficiencies.

Only 21% of the patients met criteria for a current major depressive episode at entry into the study. None of these met the criteria for the more melancholic subtype, *i.e.* the patients did not have an endogenous depression. Fifty-eight per cent scored above the recommended cut-off point for identifying mild depression in community settings. The pattern and severity of psychiatric morbidity seen in these 33 patients were consistent with that found in general medical settings.

Evaluation of response

Ten of the immunoglobulin recipients (10/23: 43%) and 3 of the placebo recipients (3/26: 11%) had a marked reduction in symptoms

Table 1
Entry data for 49 patients with chronic fatigue syndrome

Entry data	Immunoglobulin recipients (n = 23)	Placebo recipients (n = 26)
Age (years)[a]	39 (10)	33 (12)
Sex – males (%)	9 (39)	15 (58)
Disease duration (months)[a]	73 (53)	61 (43)
Immune measures		
CD4 lymphocyte count[a] (cells × 10^3/mm^3)	0.8 (0.4)	0.9 (0.3)
CD8 lymphocyte count[a] (cells × 10^3/mm^3)	0.3 (0.2)	0.3 (0.1)
PHA response[a] (cpm × 10^3)	69 (30)	89 (36)[c]
IgG subclass analysis[b]	13 (62%)	8 (31%)
DTH response[b]	14 (61%)	19 (73%)
Psychological measures		
Quality of life score[a] (n = 49)	36 (14)	41 (16)
Hamilton score[a] (n = 33)	10.7 (2.8)	10.5 (3.4)
Zung score[a] (n = 33)	42 (8)	38 (11)

[a] Mean (SD) of each group.
[b] Number (per cent) of subjects in each group with values below normal range: mean ± 2 SD;
[c] $P < 0.05$.

Table 2
Physician and psychiatrist (blinded) rating of response to immunoglobulin or placebo infusions in patients with chronic fatigue syndrome

	Immunoglobulin recipients	Placebo recipients
Physician	(n = 23)	(n = 26)
Response	10	3
No response	13	23
		$\chi^2 = 4.85$[a]
Psychiatrist	(n = 16)	(n = 17)
Response	6	2
No response	10	15
		$\chi^2 = 1.72$

[a] $P < 0.05$.

and improvement in functional capacity, fulfilling the criteria for response ($\chi^2 = 4.85$, $P = 0.03$) (Table 2). Six of the 13 patients who responded (6 immunoglobulin recipients) resumed their pre-morbid employment status in full-time occupations or housework. Eleven of the 13 responders (9 immunoglobulin, 2 placebo recipients) resumed improvement in leisure or sporting activities such as tennis, gardening or carpentry.

Psychiatric assessment of psychological morbidity at follow-up determined that six of 16 (38%) of the immunoglobulin recipients, and 2 of 17 (12%) of placebo recipients were significantly improved. The patient-rated QAL score improved by a mean of 41% in the responders in comparison to a mean of −12% in those patients who did not respond. The psychiatrist-rated Hamilton depression score changed by 42% in the responders vs. −12% in the non-responders (Table 3).

The 10 immunoglobulin and 3 placebo recipients who were rated by the physicians as having responded also had a significant improvement in their measures of cell-mediated immunity. These patients had a significantly greater percentage change in the CD4 count (37% vs. −3%), and an increase in DTH skin responses, than the 36 patients designated as having no improvement. This degree of change in the immunological measurements in the 13 responders thus presented a resolution of abnormal values in 7 of 8 patients who had reduced DTH responses at entry, and in 2 of the 5 with reduced CD4 counts at entry (Table 3).

In the 23 immunoglobulin recipients, the percentage change in QAL was positively correlated with the improvement in Hamilton depression score, and the improvement in cell-mediated immunity (measured by CD4 count and DTH). Discriminant function analysis, utilizing the measures of cell-mediated immunity recorded at entry, correctly allocated 87% of the immunoglobulin recipients to the "responder" or "non-responder" categories. CD4 lymphocyte counts made the largest contribution to the discriminant function.

Adverse effects

Phlebitis and constitutional effects, worsening of fatigue and concentration impairment occurred more commonly in the immunoglobulin recipients than in patients receiving placebo. An exacerbation of constitutional symptoms occurred with 53 of the 65 immunoglobulin infusions (82%), and 19 of the 78 placebo infusions (24%). The symptoms in both immunoglobulin and placebo recipients typically developed 12–24 h after the completion of the infusion, and persisted for up to 10 days.

Table 3
Physical, psychological and immunological measures before and after immunoglobulin or placebo infusions in patients with chronic fatigue syndrome

	Before		After[a]	
	Immunoglobulin ($n = 23$)	Placebo ($n = 26$)	Immunoglobulin ($n = 23$)	Placebo ($n = 26$)
Immune measures mean (SD)				
CD4 lymphocytes (cells $\times 10^3/mm^3$)	0.8 (0.4)	0.9 (0.3)	0.9 (0.4)	0.9 (0.3)
PHA response ($\Delta cpm \times 10^3$)	69 (30)[b]	89 (36)[b]	95 (42)	100 (36)
DTH response[c]	14 (61%)	19 (73%)	7 (23%)	14 (56%)
Physical and psychological measures mean (SD)				
Quality of life score	36 (14)	41 (16)	36 (21)	38 (14)
Hamilton score	10.7 (2.8)	10.5 (3.4)	9 (5)	10 (3)
Zung score	42 (8)	38 (11)	41 (11)	40 (12)

[a] 3 months after third infusion.
[b] $P < 0.05$.
[c] Number (per cent) of subjects in each group with responses below normal range: mean ± 2 SD.

Discussion

The results of this study demonstrate that a significant proportion of patients (43%) with very well-characterized severe and long-standing chronic fatigue syndrome responded to high-dose intravenous immunoglobulin therapy. This response was characterized by recommencement of employment, leisure and social activities as well as by a significant reduction in physical and psychological morbidity, and improvement in indicators of immune function. Thus this represents the first report of an effective treatment modality for at least some patients with CFS, evaluated in a double-blind, placebo-controlled trial.

The majority of patients in this study had a long-standing disability from CFS (mean duration = 47 months) with the not unexpected secondary physical and psychological disabilities associated with chronic illness. These secondary factors may have prevented a satisfactory treatment response in some patients. We remain open to the possibility that the dosage regimen used may not be suitable for all patients, and that the underlying pathophysiology in the production of fatigue may not be the same in all subjects.

Response to immunoglobulin therapy was significantly predicted by the immunological measures recorded at entry (particularly, low CD4 lymphocyte count), supporting the concept that cellular immunity is important in both the pathogenesis and response to treatment in patients with CFS. The association between recovery from CFS and resolution in abnormalities in cell-mediated immunity is strengthened by the demonstration of immunological improvement in both the placebo responders tested at follow-up. We are currently engaged in a study to define the dose–response relationship of immunoglobulin/benefit in the treatment of patients with CFS, and are carefully analyzing the time-course and the permanency of beneficial effects noted. While a number of patients have remained well for periods now extending beyond 18 months, some have relapsed, only to improve again following further infusions of gammaglobulin.

Summary

Chronic Fatigue Syndrome (CFS) is a condition of uncertain etiology characterized by profound fatigue, neuropsychiatric dysfunction and frequent abnormalities in indicators of immunological competence. No effective therapy is known. Forty-nine patients participated in a randomized, double-blind placebo-controlled trial to determine the effectiveness in this condition of intravenously administered IgG. The patients received three intravenous infusions of a placebo solution or IgG, at a dose of 2 g/kg per month.

Assessment of the severity of symptoms and associated disabilities (both before and after treatment) was completed at detailed interviews by a physician and psychiatrist unaware of the treatment received by the patients. Changes in physical symptoms and functional capacity were recorded using visual analogue scales, while changes in psychological morbidity were assessed using patient-rated indices of depression. Immunological capacity was evaluated by T cell sub-set analysis, delayed-type hypersensitivity (DTH) skin testing, and by lymphocyte transformation with phytohaemagglutinin (PHA). Three months after the final infusion, 10 of 23 (43%) immunoglobulin recipients, and 3 of 26 (12%) placebo recipients were assessed as having responded, with a substantial reduction in their symptoms, and recommencement of work, leisure and social activities. The patients designated as "responders" had improvement in both physical and psychological measures ($P=<0.01$ for each).

We hypothesise that CFS is associated with an excessive and prolonged release of cytokines, following antigenic stimulation. A disturbance in immunoregulatory function, perhaps induced by exposure to particular antigens in a genetically susceptible individual, may establish the circumstances for such a pathogenesis. Immunomodulatory treatment with IgG is effective in a significant number of patients with CFS, a finding which supports the concept that an immunological disturbance may be important in the pathogenesis of this disorder.

Acknowledgements

The data presented at this meeting were subsequently published in the *American Journal of Medicine* and are reproduced here with the permission of the Editors. (*Am. J. Med.* 89: 561–568; 1990.)

References

1. Lloyd, A., Wakefield, D., Boughton, C. and Dwyer, J. What is myalgic encephalomyelitis? *Lancet* i: 1286–1287; 1988.
2. Straus, S. The chronic mononucleosis syndrome. *J. Infect. Dis.* 157: 405–412; 1988.

3. Behan, P., Behan, W. and Bell, E. The postviral fatigue syndrome – an analysis of the findings in 50 cases. *J. Infect.* 10: 211–222; 1985.
4. Lloyd, A., Wakefield, D., Boughton, C. and Dwyer, J. Immunological abnormalities in the chronic fatigue syndrome. *Med. J. Aust.* 151: 122–124; 1989.
5. Linde, A., Hammarstrom, L. and Smith, C. IγG subclass deficiency and chronic fatigue syndrome. *Lancet* i: 885–886; 1988.
6. McDonald, E., Mann, A. and Thomas, H. Interferons as mediators of psychiatric morbidity. An investigation in a trial of recombinant α-interferon in hepatitis-B carriers. *Lancet* ii: 1175–1177; 1987.
7. Holmes, G., Kaplan, J., Gantz, N. *et al.* Chronic fatigue syndrome: a working case definition. *Ann. Intern. Med.* 108: 387–389; 1988.
8. American Psychiatric Association. "Diagnostic and Statistical Manual of Mental Disorders", 3rd edn revised. APA, Washington, DC; 1987.
9. Hamilton, M. A rating scale for depression. *J. Neurol. Neurosurg. Psychiatry* 23: 56–62; 1960.
10. Gill, W. Monitoring the subjective well-being of chronically ill patients over time. *Community Health Stud.* 8: 288–297; 1984.

Discussion

R. Stiehm

Do you have any evidence of T-cell activation in these disorders?

J. M. Dwyer

One hundred consecutive patients with chronic fatigue syndrome and 100 control subjects were examined for the presence of DR^+ mononuclear cells in peripheral blood. Thirty-nine subjects with chronic fatigue syndrome and 14 control subjects had an increase of DR^+ cells ($P < 0.05$ in chi square).

Intravenously administered IgG for the treatment of thyroid eye disease

J. M. DWYER, ELIZABETH M. BENSON, J. N. CURRIE and J. O'DAY

Department of Clinical Immunology, Prince Henry Hospital, University of New South Wales, Sydney, Australia; and the Department of Medicine, Alfred Hospital, Monash Medical School, Melbourne, Australia

Introduction

Despite a significant improvement in our understanding of how immunological reactions can produce a range of thyroid abnormalities, mechanisms responsible for thyroid eye disease (TED), most often associated with Graves' disease remain unclear (1). Just as autoimmune thyroid disease covers the spectrum from hyper- to hypothyroidism, so too TED manifests itself in many different ways. The ophthalmopathy may occur in patients with Hashimoto's thyroiditis or primary hypothyroidism, and is sometimes found even in the absence of thyroid disease. Patients may have nothing more than an almost unnoticeable lid retraction, to a fulminating malignant proptosis (2). If inadequately managed, permanent damage to vision and ocular movement can result. Patients may be left with such consequences, but have no evidence of active TED. A lack of inflammatory processes and fibrotic change in ocular muscles limit therapeutic options at this stage. It is thus important to distinguish inactive thyroid eye disease to

Immunotherapy with Intravenous Immunoglobulins
ISBN 0–12–370725–0

distinguish it from active TED, where aggressive treatment is called for (3). The four major signs of active TED are: increasing proptosis; eyelid edema; conjunctival edema; and the appearance of papilloedema and visual disturbances. Increased ocular pressure, ophthalmoplegia (with the inferior recti being particularly susceptible), and a loss of color vision are all common.

Previously (2) TED was thought to represent the orbital manifestations of that thyroid abnormality characterized by the presence in the serum of thyroid stimulating immunoglobulins (TSIgG). We now know that these antibodies are not responsible for the orbital disease, but are often co-associated with the responsible immune disturbances (4–6). Cell-mediated immunity to retro-orbital antigens (7, 8) and antibodies to retro-orbital muscle antigens have been described (9). These antigen-specific immunoglobulins do not cross-react with thyroid antibodies, and have not been shown to be pathogenic (10). The pathogenesis of TED is likely to involve both humoral and cell-mediated mechanisms.

At present all of the therapeutic strategies available are less than satisfactory. Active disease features enlarged, indeed swollen, eye muscles (most readily detected on CT scan), severe proptosis, ophthalmoplegia or failing vision. Patients with these symptoms are usually treated with large doses of steroids, often with a good therapeutic response but with serious side effects (11, 12). Irradiation of the orbit may give a transient, or even prolonged relief, but such an approach often induces cataract formation, retinal arteritis and lachrymal gland dysfunction (13). Plasma exchange is not useful as an isolated manoeuvre (14). Recently, a combination of steroids and cyclosporin A has been reported to be beneficial in some patients (15).

In an attempt to modify the course of TED by immuno-manipulation rather than immunosuppression, thus avoiding potentially serious side effects, we have treated eight patients with severe TED with an intravenous preparation of IgG. The results have been encouraging.

Subjects

Eight women (whose ages ranged from 40 to 72 years), all with severe TED, were studied. The details of the cases are summarized in Table 1. Five of the eight had failed to respond to immunosuppressive agents, including in one case cyclosporin A. Other cases featured chronic active TED despite orbital irradiation and surgery. None of the patients studied were thyrotoxic, but all had serum antibodies to

Table 1
Response of thyroid eye disease to intravenous gammaglobulin

Case no.	Sex/ age	Euthyroid	Proptosis	Visual disturbance	Ophthal moplegia	Failed immuno suppressives?	Color vision	Ocular pressure	TSH-R antibody	Satisfactory response
1	F 63	12 years	++++ ↓ +	6/12 ↓ 6/6	++++ ↓ ++	Yes and surgery	Normal	Raised ↓ Normal	Elevated ↓ Reduced	Yes
2	F 43	2 years Angina	++ ↓ -	6/9 ↓ 6/6	++++ ↓ -	Yes Worse	Episodic loss ↓ Normal	Raised ↓ Normal	Elevated ↓ Reduced	Yes
3	F 52	5 years	+ ↓ -	6/12 ↓ 6/6	++ ↓ +	Yes including cyclosporin	Decreased ↓ Normal	High ↓ Improved	Elevated ↓ Reduced	Yes ?Fibrosis
4	F 50	Yes then TED	No	6/24 ↓ 6/9	+++ ↓ +	Yes Plasma exchange	Variable ↓ Improved	High ↓ Improved	Very high ↓ Reduced	Transient Better with Cy A
5	F 51	2 years	+++ ↓ +	6/12 ↓ 6/6	No	Yes Orbital irradiation	Decreased ↓ Improved	Increased ↓ Normal	None detected	Yes
6	F 40	2 months Pre-tibial myxoedema	Peri- orbital edema	6/12 ↓ 6/6	No chemosis	No	Decreased ↓ Improved	Normal	88(0–15) ↓ 44	Yes
7	F 66	TED 3 years then hyperthyroid	+++ ↓ +	No	+++ ↓ +	No	No	Normal	No Thyroid yes	Yes
8	F 72	16 years	+++ ↓ +	Dry eyes No	+++ ↓ +	No Failed surgery	Normal	Increased ↓ Decreased	Thyroid colloid only	Yes

thyroid-related antigens. Proptosis, visual fields and acuity, the degree of ophthalmoplegia, color vision perception, and ocular pressure were measured before and after treatment.

Methods

Therapeutic protocol

All patients received intravenous infusions of IgG using a protocol previously shown to be satisfactory in the control of acute idiopathic thrombocytopenic purpura (ITP), and a number of other autoimmune diseases (16). Doses of 2 g/kg of IVIG (Intragam, Commonwealth Serum Laboratories, Melbourne, Australia) were administered over 2–5 days. At least three infusions were given, one month apart. TSIgG and TSH-R antibodies were measured, using standard assays (17, 18).

Results

Of the eight patients studied, proptosis was a major feature in six, as was a decrease in visual acuity. Five patients reported a loss of normal color vision, and six had an increase in intra-ocular tension. Five patients had detectible and elevated levels of TSIgG and TSH-R antibodies. The serum of one patient contained neither of these antibodies, but did contain antibody to thyroid cytoplasmic antigens. In case 8 (Table 1) antibody to thyroid colloid was detected.

All patients experienced subjective and objective clinical improvement following therapy. In only one case (number 4) was the response less than satisfactory. After each infusion her symptoms improved, but for no longer than 2 or 3 weeks. A fourth infusion was combined with a plasma exchange, and the subsequent administration of cyclosporin A therapy for 2 weeks. Remission (currently lasting 14 months) has resulted. A further case (number 6) also experienced only a transient response, and a fourth and fifth infusion were necessary, with the latter being associated with a 24-day tapering course of prednisone. The patient went into remission at this time, and she is free of symptoms and signs 12 months later. In case 7, severe symptoms of ocular irritation subsided after the first infusion. Her proptosis and diplopia improved markedly but more slowly. Prior to treatment, she had experienced diplopia with 10° of lateral gaze movement to the left. After treatment, diplopia was not induced before 50° of lateral gaze movement. Currently, this improvement has been maintained for 6 months. An 80% improvement in the symptoms and signs occurred in case 8, and the patient was less troubled by TED than at any time in the previous 16 years.

Side effects from the administration of the gammaglobulin were not significant. The authors know of two cases of TED treated by others using the above protocol, where no success was achieved. In both, the poor results may have been related to attempts to treat patients with severe but inactive TED.

Discussion

We are encouraged by our results with intravenously administered IgG for the treatment of TED. A harmless and effective protocol is important, not only for those patients with severe disease, but also for those more common cases where congestive symptoms are troublesome and steroids seem inappropriate. All of our patients had protracted disease. Five patients had serious disease and had failed conventional therapy, and thus had a poor prognosis. The prolonged remissions obtained suggest that immuno-manipulation has in some way reconstituted the regulation of those autoreactive T- and B-cell clones responsible for disease.

Pharmacological doses of IVIG have been shown to induce many changes within the immune system of recipients. In terms of the prolonged benefit seen here, and with many other diseases, perhaps those changes associated with the regulation of autoantibody production and T-cell activity by dimers in the gammaglobulin product consisting of autoantibodies complexed to an antibody to their idiotypic regions (id–anti-id complexes) may be the most important (19). However, the generation of immunological tolerance (20), altered macrophage function (21), enhanced suppressor T-cell function (22), and depression of natural killer cell activity (23) have all been reported, and could be playing a role in our manipulation of TED.

In our cases, autoantibody levels fell in five cases after IVIG. We agree that it is unlikely that any of the antibodies we measured produced the pathology treated, but it is of interest that a subset of TSH-R antibodies have been shown to stimulate collagen synthesis in human fibroblasts. This subset of antibodies correlates well with Graves' ophthalmopathy (24).

Recent studies (19) have demonstrated that the larger the pool of donors contributing to the preparation of a batch of intravenous IgG, the more id–anti-id dimers are likely to be present. Some anti-id antibodies may in fact be able to bind to a large number of $F(ab')_2$ fragments from autoantibodies present in the serum of patients with a number of autoimmune diseases. This suggests that there may be a regulatory anti-idiotypic antibody which exerts a modifying influence over a number of autoreactive B-cell clones. As anti-id complex to $F(ab')_2$ can regulate T-cell function as well *via* a suppressor T-cell mechanism, it is possible that regulatory anti-id molecules in our IVIG preparation suppress both the cellular and humoral attacks on the extra-orbital antigens of our patients. The exact mechanism involved awaits further studies of the interaction of IVIG with the more antigen-specific mechanisms associated with TED. At this time, however, we believe that providing active TED is present, IVIG presents a logical first line of therapy for the condition.

Summary

Eight women with thyroid eye disease (TED) were treated with three monthly intravenous infusions of 2 g/kg of pooled and concentrated IgG (Intragam, Commonwealth Serum Laboratories, Melbourne, Australia). Five of the women had previously failed to respond to immunosuppressive and anti-inflammatory regimens, involving in two cases the use of Cyclosporin A and orbital irradiation. Seven of the eight women (whose ages ranged from 40 to 72 years) had a satisfactory response to therapy with IVIG. The eighth responded to gamma globulin and Cyclosporin A. The mechanism of action whereby IVIG induced these changes is unknown, but may involve the regulation of humoral and cell-mediated immune reactions to extra-orbital antigens. A significant fall in the level of thyroid stimulating immunoglobulins (TSIG) measured by bioassay, and antibody to the receptor for thyroid stimulating hormone (TSH-R) may suggest immune manipulation *via* an anti-idiotypic influence on a damaged regulatory loop. We believe IVIG may provide an effective treatment beneficial for the management of this serious problem, free of the significant side-effects inherent in most of the currently utilized regimens.

References

1. Atkinson, S., Holcombe, M. and Kendall-Taylor, P. Ophthalmopathic immunoglobulin in patients with Graves' ophthalmopathy. *Lancet* ii: 374–376; 1984.
2. Hollows, F. Thyroid eye disease (TED)—a current understanding. *Aust. J. Ophthalmol.* 9: 239–249; 1981.
3. Hollows, F. C. and Beaumont, P. Thyroid eye disease and its relationship to the long-acting thyroid stimulator. *Trans. Aust. Coll. Ophthal.* 1: 37–43; 1969.
4. McKenzie, J. M. and McCullagh, E. P. Observations against a causal relationship between the long-acting thyroid stimulator and ophthalmopathy in Graves' disease. *J. Clin. Endocrinol. Metab.* **28**: 1177–1182; 1968.
5. Teng, C. S., Smith, B. R., Clayton, B., Evered, D. C., Clark, F. and Hall, R. Thyroid-stimulating immunoglobulins in ophthalmic Graves' disease. *Clin. Endocrinol.* **6**: 207–211; 1977.
6. Kendall-Taylor, P., Atkinson, S., and Holcombe, M. A specific IgG in Graves' ophthalmopathy and its relation to retroorbital and thyroid autoimmunity. *Br. Med. J.* **288**: 1183–1187; 1984.
7. Mahieu, R. and Winand, R. Demonstration of delayed hypersensitivity in retrobulbar and thyroid tissues in human exophthalmos. *J. Clin. Endocrinol. Metab.* **34**: 1090–1092; 1972.
8. Munro, R. E., Lamki, L., Row, V. V. and Volpé, R. Cell mediated immunity in the exophthalmos of Graves' disease as demonstrated by the migration inhibition factor (MIF) test. *J. Clin. Endocrinol Metab.* **37**: 286–292; 1973.
9. Kodama, K., Sikorska, H., Bandy-Dafoe, P., Bayly, R. and Wall, J. R. Demonstration of a circulating autoantibody against a soluble eye-muscle antigen in Graves' ophthalmopathy. *Lancet* ii: 1353–1356; 1982.
10. Kendall-Taylor, P., Holcombe, M. and Atkinson, S. Studies of ophthalmopathic IgG in 2 patients with Graves' ophthalmopathy. *Ann. Endocrinol. (Madrid)* t**44**: 83A; 1983.
11. Werner, S. C. Prednisone in emergency treatment of malignant exophthalmus. *Lancet* **2**: 1004–1006; 1966.
12. Apers, R. C., Oosterhuis, J. A. and Bierlaagh, J. J. Indications and results of prednisone treatment in thyroid ophthalmopathy. *Ophthalmologica* **173**: 163–167; 1976.
13. Brennan, M. W., Leone, C. R. and Janaki, L. Radiation therapy for Graves' disease. *Am. J. Ophthalmol.* **96**: 195–199; 1983.
14. Kelly, W., Longson, D., Smithard, D. *et al.* An evaluation of plasma exchange for Graves' ophthalmopathy. *Clin. Endocrinol.* **18**: 485–493; 1983.
15. Prummel, M. F., Maarten, P. H., Mourits, M. D., *et al.* Prednisone and

cyclosporine in the treatment of severe Graves' ophthalmopathy. *N. Engl. J. Med.* 321: 1353–1359; 1989.

16. Imbach, P., Barandun, S., D'Appuzzo, V. *et al.* High dose intravenous gammaglobulin for idiopathic thrombocytopenic purpura in childhood. *Lancet* i: 1228–1230; 1981.
17. Southgate, K., Creagh, J., Teece, M., Kingswood, C. and Smith, B. R. A receptor assay for the measurement of TSH receptor antibodies in unextracted serum. *Clin. Endocrinol.* 20: 539–548; 1984.
18. Kasagi, K., Konishi, J., Iida, Y. *et al.* A new in vitro assay for human thyroid stimulator using cultured thyroid cells: Effect of sodium chloride on adenosine 3′,5′-monophosphate increase. *J. Clin. Endocrinol. Metab.* 54: 108–114; 1982.
19. Dietrich, G., Rossi, F. and Kazatchkine, M. D. Modulation of autoimmune responses with normal polyspecific IgG for therapeutic use. In "Progress in Immunology" (Eds Melchers, F. *et al.*), Vol. VII, pp. 1221–1227. Springer-Verlag, Berlin; 1989.
20. Nilsson, I. M., Berntorp, E. and Zettervall, O. Induction of immune tolerance in patients with hemophilia and antibodies to factor VIII by combined treatment with intravenous IgG, cyclophosphamide and factor VIII. *N. Engl. J. Med.* 318: 947–950; 1988.
21. Kimberly, R. P., Salmon, J. E., Bussel, J. B., Crow, M. K. and Hilgartner, M. W. Modulation of mononuclear phagocyte function by intravenous gammaglobulin. *J. Immunol.* 132: 745–750; 1984.
22. White, W. B., Desbonnet, C. R. and Ballow, M. Immunoregulatory effects of intravenous immune serum globulin therapy in common variable hypogammaglobulinemia. *Am. J. Med.* 83: 431–436; 1987.
23. Engelhard, D., Waner, J. L., Kapoor, N. and Good, R. A. Effect of intravenous immune globulin on natural killer activity: possible association with autoimmune neutropenia and idiopathic thrombocytopenia. *J. Pediatr.* 108: 77–87; 1986.
24. Rotella, C. M., Zonefrati, R., Toccafondi, R., Valente, W. A. and Kohn, L. D. Ability of monoclonal antibodies to the thyrotropin receptor to increase collagen synthesis in human fibroblasts: an assay which appears to measure exophthalmogenic immunoglobulins in Graves' sera. *J. Clin. Endocrinol. Metab.* 62: 357–367; 1986.

The use of IVIG for the treatment of recurrent spontaneous abortion

C. COULAM, A. PETERS, J. McINTYRE and W. FAULK

Center for Reproduction and Transplantation Immunology, Methodist Hospital of Indiana, Inc., Indianapolis, Indiana, USA

Spontaneous abortion is the expression of products of conception prior to 20 weeks of gestation. It is the most common complication of pregnancy. Spontaneous abortion can occur sporadically or recurrently within individuals. Recurrent spontaneous abortion has been defined as three or more pregnancy losses and has been described as a syndrome (1). Recurrent spontaneous abortion (RSA) is the cause of childlessness in 2–5% of reproducing couples (2, 3).

While sporadic spontaneous abortions appear to be due to karyotypic abnormalities (4), the prevalence of abnormal chromosomal analyses among recurrent abortions is low (5). Recent reports suggest that immunologic mechanisms may play a role in the etiology of recurrent spontaneous abortion (6–13). Various forms of immunotherapy have been attempted in individuals thought to have an immunological mechanism associated with recurrent spontaneous abortion. Intravenous immunoglobulin (IVIG) has been used to treat women with a presumed autoimmune component associated with recurrent pregnancy loss (14–16). We now report the results of a pilot study conducted to observe the effect of IVIG on pregnancy outcome in women with a history of recurrent spontaneous abortion of an unknown etiology.

Immunotherapy with Intravenous Immunoglobulins
ISBN 0–12–370725–0

Materials and methods

Women with an obstetrical history of recurrent pregnancy loss with an unknown etiology were given the option of participating in the pilot study to observe the efficacy of IVIG therapy in maintaining pregnancy. All women had the following tests performed to eliminate any known cause of recurrent pregnancy loss: chromosome analysis, hysteroscopy, endometrial biopsy and luteal phase serum progesterone, and studies for autoantibodies including ANA, APA and APTT. Husbands also had chromosome analysis. In addition, HLA tissue typing and the presence or absence of maternal antipaternal lymphocytotoxic antibodies was determined for each couple.

Each woman received an intravenous infusion of immunoglobulin (Sandoglobulin®) 500 mg/kg during the follicular phase of the menstrual cycle when pregnancy was desired. The same infusion was repeated every 28 days until pregnancy was documented for 3 months. If pregnancy did not occur within 3 months, the patient is dropped from the study and replaced with another patient. Once conception was documented, the patient received a 500 mg/kg infusion every 28 days until delivery or until 36 weeks of gestation whichever is sooner.

The outcome of five pregnancies was studied. The time of gestation at delivery, the weight of the infant at birth, and Apgar scores were recorded. Any abnormalities at the time of newborn examination and physical examination at one month of age were noted.

Results

A total of seven women with recurrent spontaneous abortion were entered into the study. Five women achieved pregnancy. These five women had experienced a total of 23 previous pregnancies including 22 previous abortions (mean pregnancy per patient 4.7; range 2–9). One of these women had had a previous live birth, and shared three HLA antigens with her spouse. Another had six previous spontaneous abortions, no children, and shared no HLA antigens with her spouse. A third participant had nine spontaneous abortions, no children, and shared three HLA antigens with her spouse. The two remaining participants had no previous live births and displayed antipaternal lymphocytotoxic antibodies in their sera. All of these women had a diagnosis of unexplained recurrent spontaneous abortion.

The outcome of each pregnancy is summarized in Table 1. Four women delivered healthy infants between 35 and 40 weeks gestation.

One pregnancy resulted in a preterm birth of a 1844 g female who had no neonatal problems. The fifth pregnancy is currently ongoing at 10 weeks of gestation with ultrasonic evidence of normal fetal growth and fetal cardiac activity.

Table 1
Pregnancy outcome after treatment with IVIG in five women with recurrent spontaneous abortion

Patient	Weeks	Weight (g)	Sex	Apgar	Infant
1	38	3348	F	9	Healthy
2	35	1844	F	8	Healthy
3	39	3093	F	9	Healthy
4	40	3859	M	9	Healthy
5	10	Ongoing			+FHT

Discussion

The results of this pilot study indicate IVIG may be efficacious in preventing recurrent spontaneous abortions. The mechanisms by which IVIG exerts its effect are not known. Understanding these mechanisms is limited by lack of knowledge of the pathophysiology of abortion. Immunochemical data from normal human pregnancies have been used to build a pathophysiological basis for recurrent spontaneous abortions (17). This model suggests that if an aborting woman is genetically compatible for trophoblast antigens with her partner, she fails to produce antibody (Ab_1) to trophoblast antigen and thus fails to produce anti-idiotype antibody (Ab_2). In the absence of Ab_2, maternal allogeneic rejection reactions are not down-regulated (18), and innate killer cell response can reject the blastocyst. Similarly, if an aborting woman is a poor autoanti-idiotype producer and produces Ab_1 but not Ab_2, her cytotoxic Ab_1 could be transported into the placenta. In both of these scenarios the defect in normal maternal immunological response to the pregnancy allograft is lack of production of Ab_2.

In our laboratories we have been able to generate rabbit antibodies to human anti-idiotype to trophoblast lymphocyte cross-reacting (TLX) antigen (unpublished data). These rabbit antibodies can recognize antibodies contained in commercially available IVIG as Sandoglobulin® (unpublished data). We reasoned that if the defect in recurrently aborting women was the absence of Ab_2 and if we gave Ab_2

in the form of IVIG, we should be able to maintain pregnancies for this reason. The results of this pilot study suggest IVIG may be an efficacious treatment option for women with unexplained recurrent spontaneous abortion. A randomized placebo controlled trial is now necessary to test this suggestion.

Summary

Recurrent spontaneous abortion (RSA) is the cause of childlessness in 2–5% of reproducing couples. Recent reports suggest that immunological mechanisms may play a role in the etiology of some cases of RSA. Various forms of immunotherapy have been attempted in individuals thought to have an immunological mechanism associated with RSA. IVIG has been used to treat women with autoimmune and unexplained RSA with no demonstrable maternal lymphocytotoxic antibodies, with an overall success rate of 70–80%. We now report the results of a pilot study of five women with RSA who had experienced a total of 23 pregnancies with 22 RSAs (mean 4.7; range 2–9). Four of the women were primary aborters and one was a secondary aborter. One woman who had a previous live birth shared three HLA antigens with her spouse. One woman with six RSAs and no children shared no HLA antigens with her spouse and one woman with nine RSAs and no children shared three HLA antigens with her spouse. Two women with no previous live births displayed antipaternal lymphocytotoxic antibodies in their sera. All of these women had a diagnosis of unexplained RSA. These patients were treated with IVIG 500 mg/kg per month beginning prior to conception. Four patients have delivered successful pregnancies at 35–40 weeks gestation. One woman is pregnant at 10 weeks with ultrasonic evidence of fetal growth and fetal cardiac activity. The results of this pilot study suggest IVIG may be an efficacious treatment option for patients with unexplained RSA. A randomized placebo controlled trial is necessary to test this suggestion.

References

1. Strobino, B. R., Kuni, J., Shrout, P., Stein, Z., Susser, M. and Warburton, D. Recurrent spontaneous abortion: definition of a syndrome. *In* "Human Embryonic and Fetal Death" (Eds Porter, I. H. and Hook, E. B.), pp. 315–329. Academic Press, London; 1980.

2. Roman, E. Fetal loss rates and their relation to pregnancy order. *J. Epidemial Community Health* **38**: 29–35; 1984.
3. Mills, J. E., Simpson, J. L., Driscoll, S. G., Jovanovic-Peterson, L. *et al.* Incidence of spontaneous abortion among normal women and insulin-dependent diabetic women whose pregnancies were identified within 21 days of conception. *N. Engl. J. Med.* **319**: 1617–1622; 1988.
4. Hassold, T., Chen, N., Funkhouse, J. *et al.* A cytogenetic study of 1000 spontaneous abortions. *Ann. Hum. Genet.* **44**: 151; 1980.
5. Coulam, C. B. Unexplained recurrent pregnancy loss: epilogue. *Clin. Obstet. Gynecol.* **29**: 999; 1986.
6. McIntyre, J. A., Faulk, W. P., Nichols-Johnson, V. R. and Taylor, C. B. Immunological testing and immunotherapy in recurrent spontaneous abortion. *Obstet. Gynecol.* **67**: 169; 1986.
7. Unander, A. M. and Olding, L. B. Habitual abortion: Parental sharing of HLA antigens, absence of maternal blocking antibody, and suppression of maternal lymphocytes. *Am. J. Reprod. Immunol. Microbiol.* **4**: 171; 1983.
8. Gill, T. E. Immunogenetics of spontaneous abortions in humans. *Transplantation* **35**: 1; 1983.
9. McIntyre, J. A. and Faulk, W. P. Recurrent spontaneous abortion in human pregnancy: Results of immunogenetical, cellular and humoral studies. *Am. J. Reprod. Immunol. Microbiol.* **4**: 165; 1983.
10. Coulam, C. B., Moore, S. B. and O'Falon, W. M. Association between histocompatibility antigen and reproductive performance. *Am. J. Reprod. Immunol. Microbiol.* **14**: 54; 1987.
11. McIntyre, J. A., McConnachie, P. R., Taylor, C. S. and Faulk, W. P. Clinical, immunologic and genetic definitions of primary and secondary recurrent spontaneous abortions. *Fertil. Steril.* **42**: 849; 1984.
12. Faulk, W. P. and McIntyre, J. A. Trophoblast survival. *Transplantation* **32**: 1; 1981.
13. Mowbray, J. F. Genetic and immunological factors in human recurrent abortion. *Am. J. Reprod. Immunol. Microbiol.* **15**: 138; 1987.
14. Carreras, L. O., Perez, G. N., Vega, H. R. and Casavilla, F. Lupus anticoagulant and recurrent fetal loss: successful treatment with gammaglobulin. *Lancet* **2**: 393–394; 1988.
15. Francis, A., Freund, M., Daffos, F., Remy, P., Cuach, M. and Jacquot, C. Repeated fetal loss and the lupus anticoagulant. *Ann. Intern. Med.* **109**: 993–994; 1988.
16. Park, A., Maier, D., Wilson, D., Andreoli, J. and Ballow, M. Intravenous gammaglobulin, antiphospholipid antibodies and pregnancy. *Ann. Intern. Med.* **110**: 495–496; 1989.
17. Faulk, W. P. and McIntyre, J. A. Role of anti-TLX antibody in human pregnancy. *In* "Reproductive Immunology" (Eds Clark, D. A. and Croy, B. A.), p. 106. Elsevier, Amsterdam; 1986.
18. Suciu-Foca, N., Reemtsma, K. and King, D. W. The significance of the idiotypic anti-idiotypic network in humans. *Transplant. Proc.* **18**: 230; 1986.

Discussion

J. A. Schifferli
Could you specify to us the relation between your TA_2 and MCP (membrane cofactor protein) of complement?

C. B. Coulam
The monoclonal antibodies which recognize TA_2 or TLX, specifically H316, also recognize MCP. Monoclonal antibodies raised against MCP also recognize targets known to contain TA_2 or TLX at least on the placenta and on the lymphocytes. We have found TLX in seminal plasma. Antibodies to MCP do not recognize TLX expression in seminal plasma. More importantly, TLX activity was originally described as allotypic, causing cytotoxicity in chromium release assays. When our TLX antisera are absorbed with MCP this cytotoxic activity is not ablated. Therefore, there is some suggestion that MCP and TLX or TA_2 are closely related but are not identical.

Immunodeficiency in Down's syndrome

A. FERRANTE[1], L. J. BEARD[1], Y. H. THONG[2], V. VUDDHAKUL[2], B. ROWAN-KELLY[1], D. GOH[1], G. T. MAI[2], R. K. S. LOH[2], S. C. HARTH[2], C. PEARSON[1] and D. ROBERTON[1]

[1] Department of Immunology and University Department of Paediatrics, Adelaide Children's Hospital, South Australia
[2] University Department of Child Health, Mater Children's Hospital, South Brisbane, Queensland, Australia

Introduction

Down's syndrome (trisomy 21) is a chromosomal disorder characterized by a distinctive facies, mental retardation, abnormal dermatoglyphics, and skeletal and heart abnormalities. The incidence of this syndrome ranges from 1 per 1000 births in young mothers to 1 per 50 births in mothers more than 40 years of age. Increased susceptibility to infection and high risk of malignancies, especially leukemia are two of the many concerning manifestations of trisomy 21 (1–7). Infection is the leading cause of death in these patients (8). Down's syndrome patients present with deficiencies of both the humoral and cellular arm of the immume response (9–20) including deficiencies of phagocytic cell function (21–25). This has led to the concept that increased susceptibility to infection and malignancy may be a consequence of primary immunodeficiencies in trisomy 21. However, there is still no clear understanding of (i) whether the deficiencies found are actually responsible for increased susceptibility to infection, (ii) why there are

Immunotherapy with Intravenous Immunoglobulins
ISBN 0-12-370725-0

discrepancies in the types of immunodeficiencies reported, and (iii) the basis for the immunodeficiencies, and whether some are primary and others, secondary.

Studies excluding institutionalized Down's syndrome patients, taking into consideration the effect of age on the expression of an immunodeficiency, and avoiding testing of patients with infections may shed some light on the problems outlined. We have examined a group of non-institutionalized Down's syndrome patients for immunological competence by a variety of tests at a time when they were free from major infections.

Materials and methods

Clinical and normal subjects

Forty-six Caucasian patients with Down's syndrome, ranging in age from 6 months to 16 years were studied. All had a non-translocated trisomy 21 karyotype. None of the patients had been institutionalized. These were tested as outpatients at the time of study and were free of infections. A clinical examination was performed on all children by a pediatrician. The records of the patients were analyzed with regard to frequency and type of infection. A score system was used to assess the infection proneness of patients (Table 1). A score of >20 was considered by us to indicate increased infection proneness.

Serum from 292 healthy children from the general community and from immunization clinic attenders was used to establish age–normal percentile ranges for the immunoglobulin isotypes including IgG subclasses. Direct questioning and written questionnaires were used to ensure that controls were not excessively infection-prone according to the criteria in Table 1. Subjects with atopic disorders were excluded.

For cellular studies, healthy adult volunteers were used as control subjects due to ethical constraints in obtaining age-matched controls for venepuncture and since day-to-day variations in cellular studies led us to believe that the control cells were required to be run in parallel to those of patients. However, previously published reports have found no significant differences in proportions of CD3, CD4, CD8, B cells and in responses to phytohemagglutinin (PHA) pokeweed mitogen (PWM) and concanavalin A (ConA) and cytotoxicity of NK cells (26, 27) between children and adults.

Table 1
Assessment of infection-proneness

Condition	Score/episode
Recurrent suppurative bronchitis	10
Severe bacterial infection, e.g. lobar pneumonia	8
Other lower respiratory tract infection (e.g. cough and fever not asthma)	3
Severe coryzal infection (nasal discharge and obstruction not allergic)	2
Pharyngitis (localized pharyngeal inflammation with fever and constitutional disturbance)	2
Tonsillitis (infection localized in tonsils which are red and swollen, with fever and constitutional disturbance)	2
Otitis media (inflamed ear drum with pain and fever)	3
Sinusitis (sinus tenderness, purulent nasal discharge, radiological signs)	3
Bronchiectasis (chronic suppurative lung disease with dilatation of bronchi, cough and sputum)	20
Croup (hoarseness, harsh barking cough, stridor)	2
Bronchiolitis (cough, wheeze and tachypnoea with isolation of RSV)	3
Diarrhea (infective or presumed infective)	2

A score of >20 (over 12-month period) indicates increased infection-proneness.

Leukocyte preparation

Mononuclear leukocytes (MNL) and neutrophils were prepared by the rapid one-step method described by Ferrante and Thong (28). Heparin—containing blood from patients and control subjects—was layered onto Hypaque–Ficoll (d = 1.114) and centrifuged at 400 g for 30 min. The MNL and neutrophils were resolved into two distinct bands and were carefully removed and prepared for the studies.

Leukocyte phenotyping

The monoclonal antibodies recognizing T cells and T-cell subsets, OKT3 (anti-CD3), OKT4 (anti-CD4) and OKT8 (anti-CD8) were obtained from Ortho Diagnostic Systems Inc., NJ. The monoclonal antibody Leu 16 (anti-CD20) was used to identify B cells (Becton Dickinson Monoclonal Center, Mountain View, CA). The monoclonal Leu 11 (anti-CD16) was used to detect NK cells (Becton Dickinson). The FITC-antimouse IgG was obtained from Cappel, Malvern, PA,

USA. Cells bearing the above antigens were enumerated by flow cytometry using a FACS IV instrument (Becton Dickinson, Sunnyvale, CA), as previously described (27).

Lymphocyte proliferation

MNL were cultured in the presence of either PHA, PWM, ConA or formalin-fixed heat-killed *Staphylococcus aureus* essentially as previously described (27, 29). The degree of proliferation was assessed by pulsing cultures with ^{3}H–TdR after 3 days of culture and counting the radioactivity incorporated.

Measurement of cytokines

The polypeptide cytokines, tumor necrosis factor alpha (TNFα) and TNFβ were measured by an ELISA method (29, 20). This involved the use of cytokine-specific monoclonal antibodies and cytokine-specific polyclonal antisera. Recombinant human TNFα (rhTNFα) and rhTNFβ were used as standards. All these reagents were kindly provided by Dr G. R. Adolf, Ernst–Boehringer Institute, Vienna, Austria. Supernatants obtained from the above proliferation studies were evaluated for TNFα and TNFβ concentrations.

Natural killer cell activity

The NK cytotoxicity was evaluated by testing the ability of the MNL preparations to lyze the erythroid myeloid leukemia cell line K562 which has been labeled with $Na_2{}^{51}CrO_4$ at various ratios of effector cell:target cell (27).

Neutrophil functions

Neutrophil chemotaxis was measured by the migration-under-agarose method (31) using f-met–leu–phe as the chemotactic agent. Quantitative leukocyte iodination activity was measured by a semi-automated microassay method using ^{125}I-sodium iodide (31). This was measured both under conditions in which zymosan was opsonized with pooled human AB group serum or autologous serum. The bactericidal activity of neutrophils was measured by mixing leukocytes with *S. aureus* and incubating this with end-to-end mixing at 37°C. Viability of bacteria at different times was assessed by colony formation on agar (32). The hexose monophosphate (HMP) shunt activity of the neutrophils was assessed by measuring the release of $^{14}CO_2$ from (1–^{14}C)-L-glucose following stimulation with zymosan (31).

Complement measurements

Complement components C3 and C4 were quantitated by an immunochemical system (ARRAY, Beckman Instruments, Brea, CA). Complement activity was measured as total hemolytic complement using sheep erythrocytes sensitized with hemolysin (33).

Immunoglobulin measurements

Serum IgA, IgM and IgG were quantitated by the immunochemical method (ARRAY). IgG subclasses were measured by an ELISA using subclass–specific monoclonal antibodies and the WHO 67/97 as standard (34, 35). The assay was performed with the assistance of an automated workstation BIOMEK (Beckman, Palo Alto, CA). The monoclonal antibodies used were NL16 (Oxford, Unipath), HP6014, SJ33 and SK44 (Miles–Bioyeda) for IgG_1, IgG_2, IgG_3 and IgG_4 respectively. Normal age-related percentiles for IgG subclasses have been reported previously (35).

Statistics

The data was analyzed by either the Mann–Whitney U test or χ^2 test.

Results

Mononuclear leukocyte subpopulations

MNL from normal subjects and patients with Down's syndrome were studied for distribution of subpopulations. The results are summarized in Fig. 1. The proportions of T cells bearing the CD3 antigens were similar in the two groups. However, one individual in the Down's syndrome group showed a low (34%) CD3 proportions (normal range 48–88%). Data on CD4 and CD8 lymphocytes showed that patients had lower CD4 values compared to normal subjects. Only one patient was, however, found to have a value (20%) below our normal range (24–69%). Interestingly, the CD8 lymphocytes were increased in patients. Comparisons with our laboratory normal range for CD8 cells (9–46%) showed that all normal subjects were within

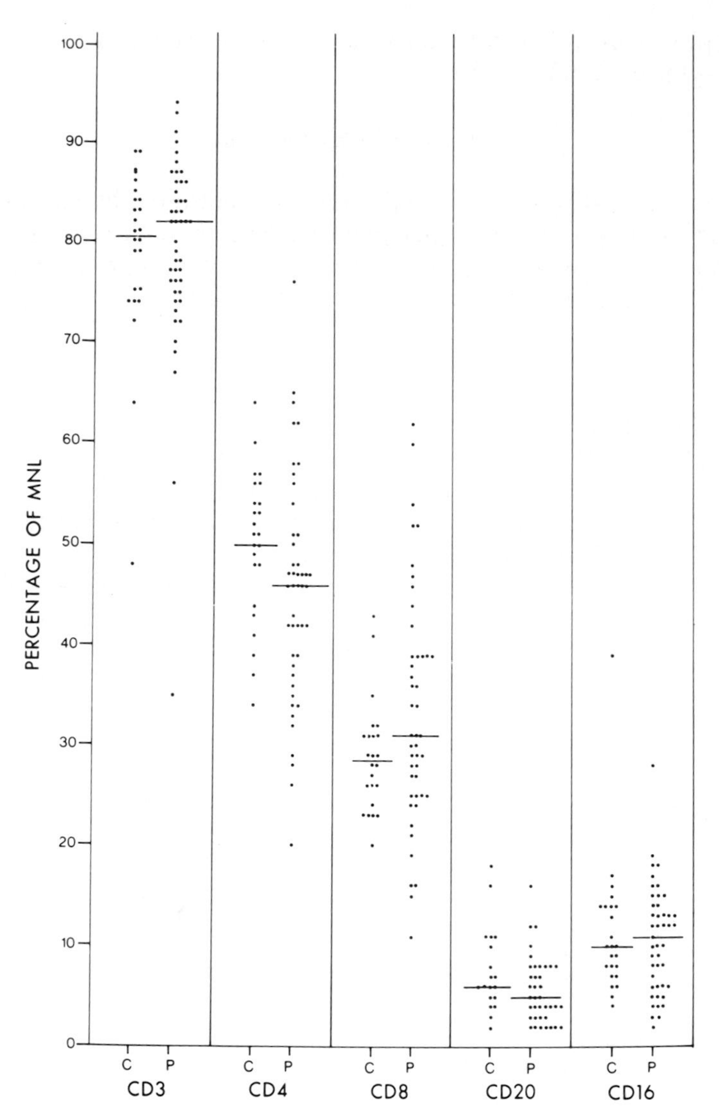

Figure 1. Leukocyte subpopulations in Down's syndrome subjects. [C] = control subjects; (P) Down's syndrome patients. The bar is the median.

the normal range but eight of the Down's syndrome subjects were outside (above) the range. This difference in the levels of CD4 and CD8 lymphocytes in Down's syndrome subjects was reflected in a lower CD4:CD8 ratio. For example, 4% of normal subjects had a ratio of <1 compared to 20% of the trisomy 21 group.

Essentially no differences were observed in proportions of B cells (CD20) and NK cells (CD16).

In vitro *lymphocyte function*

Lymphocyte function was examined by measuring the proliferative response of these cells to mitogens and their ability to produce the lymphokine TNFβ. Basal lymphoproliferation, as well as responses to PHA, ConA and *S. aureus* were similar in the two groups (Fig. 2).

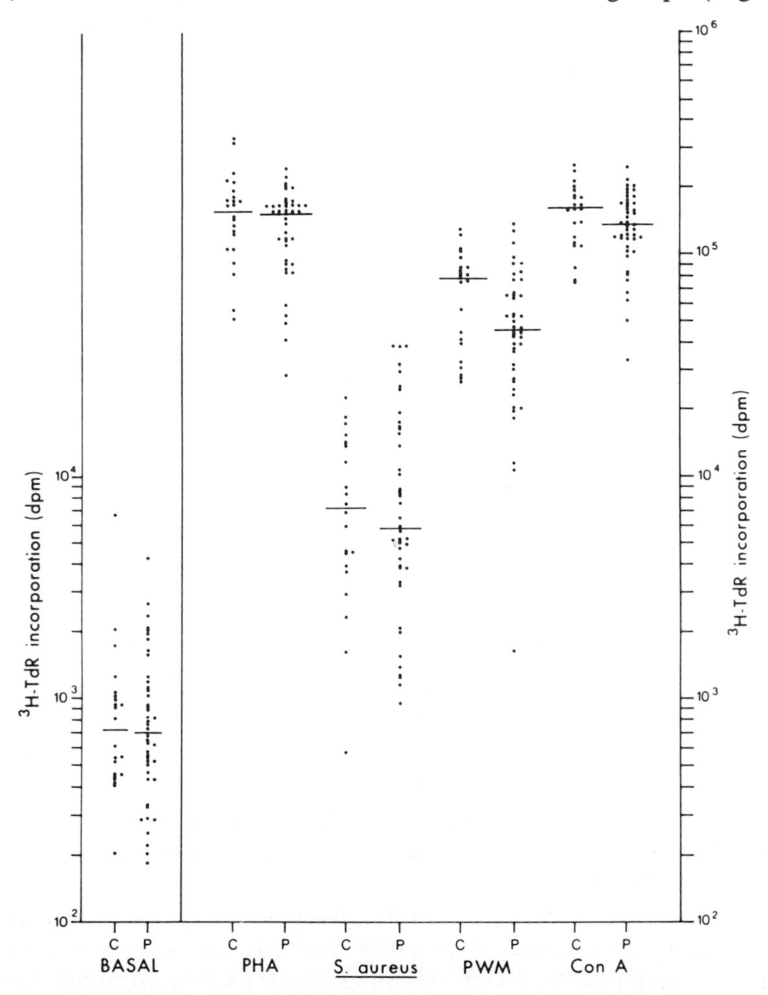

Figure 2. The lymphoproliferative response of cells from Down's syndrome subjects. (C) = controls and (P) = Down's syndrome patients. The bar shows the median.

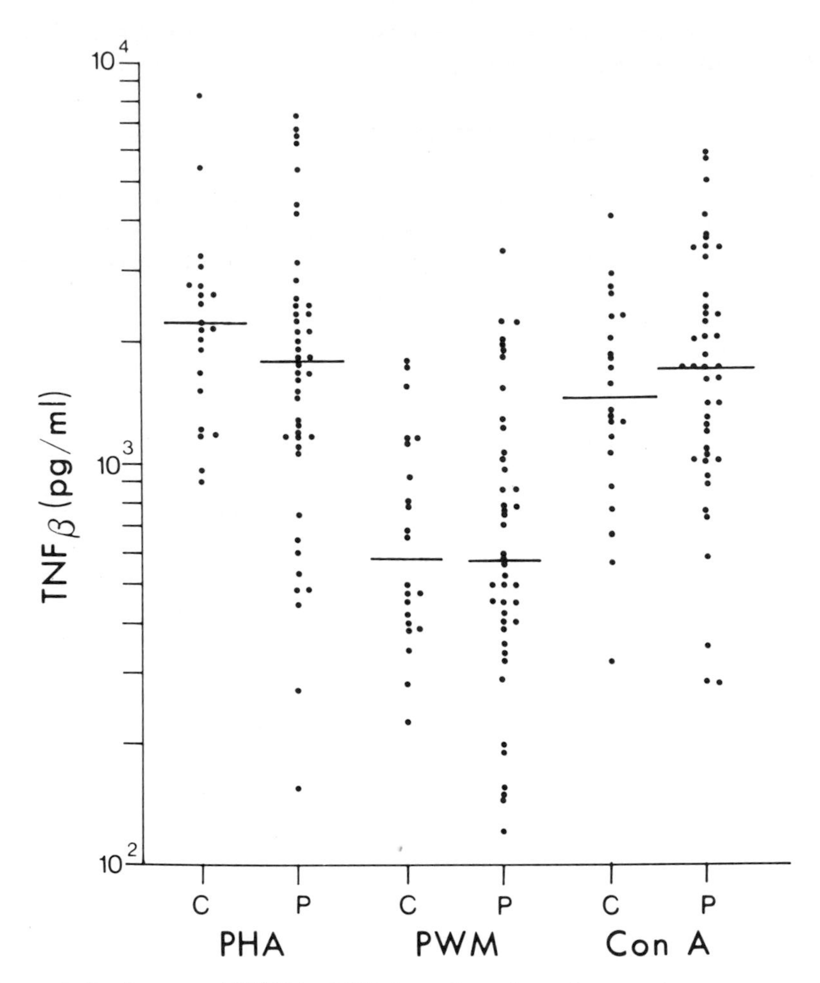

Figure 3. Production of TNFβ by MNL from Down's syndrome subjects in response to mitogens. (C) = control subjects and (P) = Down's syndrome patients. The bar is the median.

Only the proliferative response to PWM was significantly different (depressed in trisomy 21) ($P<0.05$). One patient showed a poor response to PWM.

Further investigations indicated abnormalities of T-cell function in some patients. A number of patients showed very poor production of TNFβ in response to PHA ($P<0.05$) and PWM, although normal cytokine responses to ConA were evident (Fig. 3).

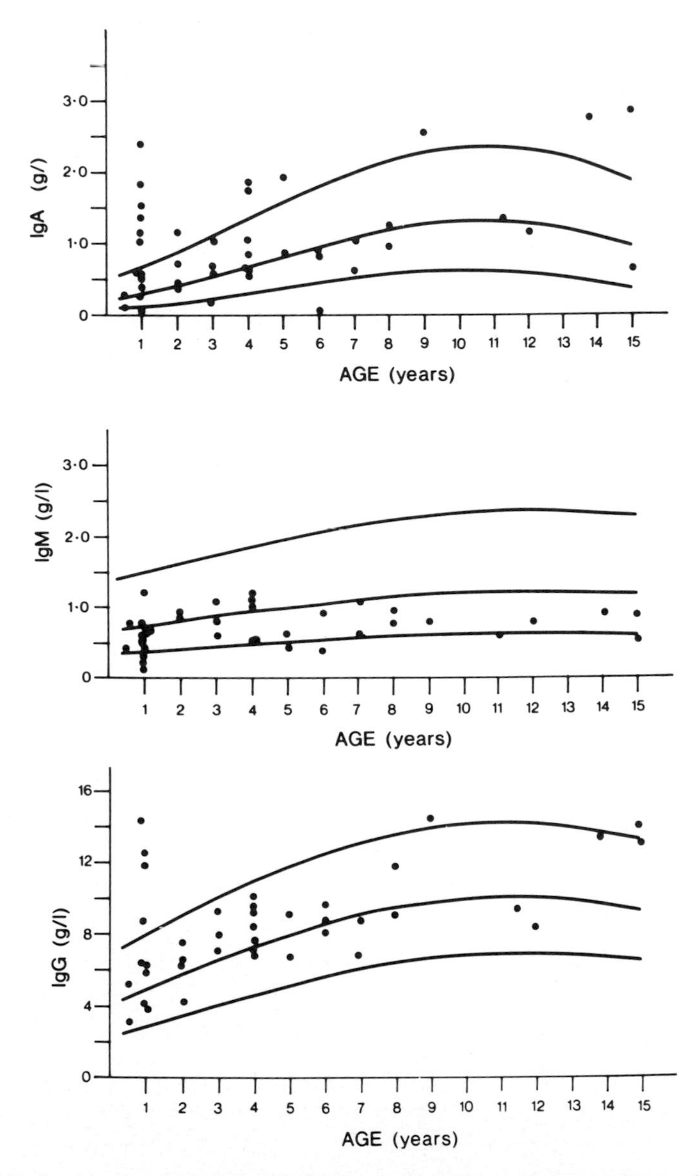

Figure 4. Serum immunoglobulin classes in Down's syndrome subjects. The solid lines represent the age-related 5th, 50th and 95th percentiles.

Serum immunoglobulin levels

Serum immunoglobulin abnormalities were quite evident in a significant proportion of the trisomy 21 subjects (Figs. 4 and 5; Table 2) relative to the 95th and 5th percentiles. A significant number of Down's syndrome subjects showed elevated IgA and IgG but significantly reduced IgM concentrations (Fig. 4, Table 2). Although the IgG concentration was increased in trisomy 21, IgG subclass deficiency was evident. A significant number of Down's syndrome subjects had reduced IgG_2 and IgG_4, but elevated IgG_1 and IgG_3 (Fig. 5, Table 2).

Natural killer cell (NK) cytotoxicity

Examination of Down's syndrome subjects for NK cytotoxicity showed that there was no difference at all ratios of effector:target cells from those of control subjects (Fig. 6). None of the subjects in

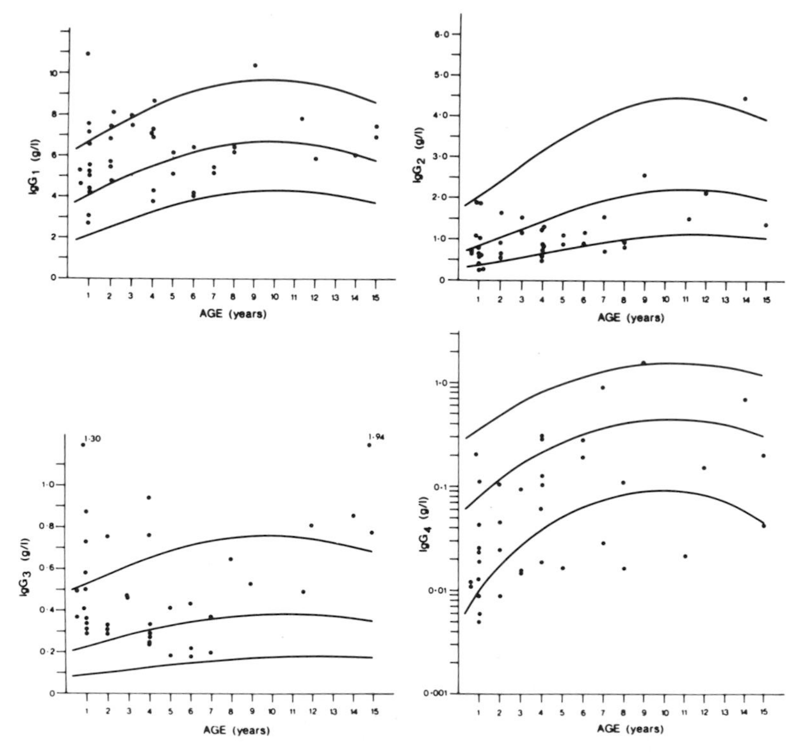

Figure 5. Serum IgG subclasses in Down's syndrome subjects. The solid lines represent age-related 5th, 50th and 95th percentiles.

Table 2
Numbers of patients with immunoglobulin isotype concentrations below or above the fifth percentile of age

Isotype	<P5	>P95
IgA	3	13****
IgG	—	7*
IgM	8**	—
IgG_1	—	8**
IgG_2	11***	1
IgG_3	—	13****
IgG_4	13****	1

χ^2: **** $P<0.005$, ***$P<0.01$, **$P<0.05$, *$P<0.1$

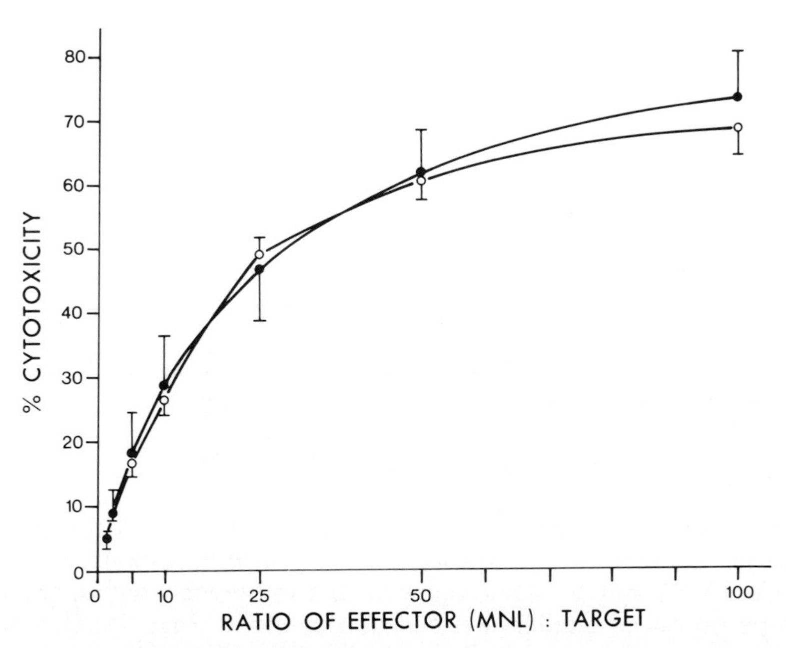

Figure 6. NK cell cytotoxicity in MNL from Down's syndrome subjects. (●) Down's syndrome subjects; (○) control subjects.

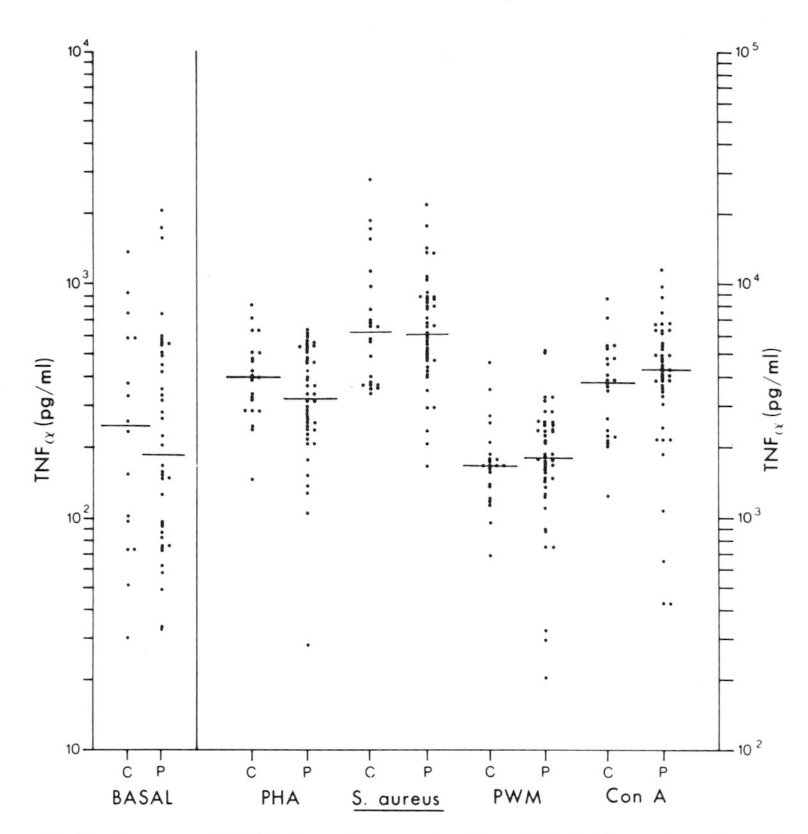

Figure 7. Production of TNFα by mitogen-stimulated MNL from Down's syndrome subjects. The bar represents the median.

the trisomy 21 group showed either depressed or increased NK cytotoxicity relative to our laboratory normal range.

Macrophage cytokine production

TNFα is mainly a product of stimulated macrophages. A comparison of MNL from the two groups to produce TNFα in response to PHA, ConA, PWM and *S. aureus* showed that individuals within the two groups produced similar levels of the cytokine (Fig. 7). However, there were a very few individuals in the trisomy 21 group who produced very low levels of TNFα.

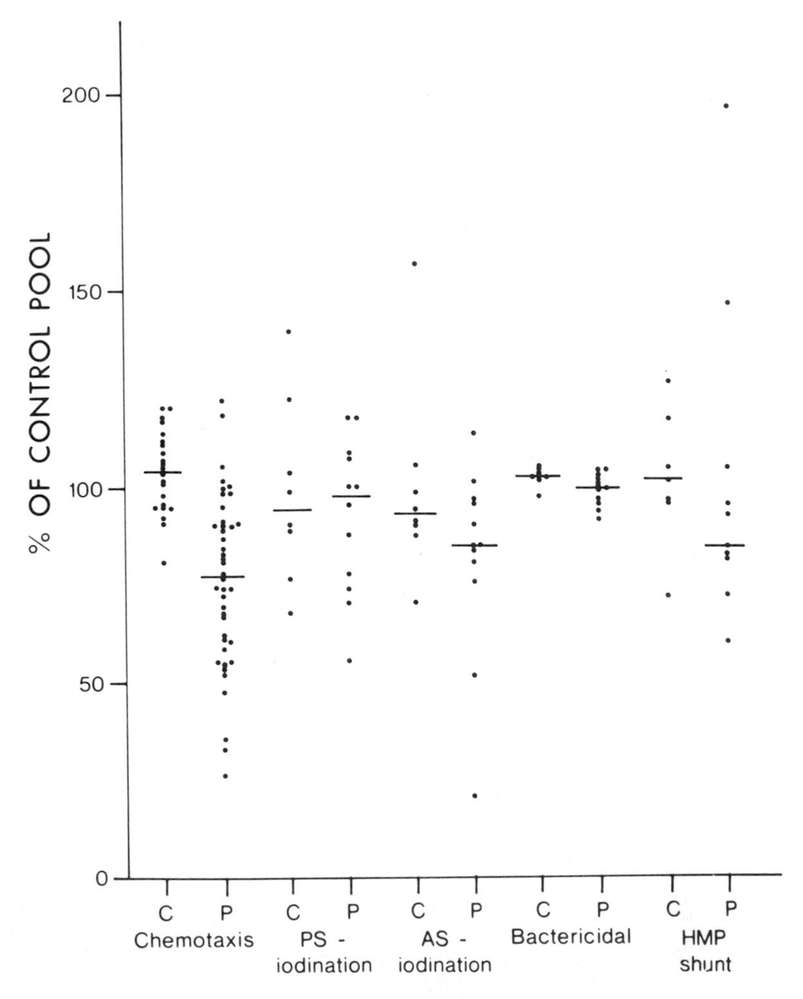

Figure 8. Neutrophil function in Down's syndrome subjects. The bars represent the median.

Neutrophil functions

Neutrophils from trisomy 21 subjects and control subjects were examined for a range of functions; chemotaxis, quantitative leukocyte iodination, bactericidal activity and hexose monophosphate (HMP) shunt activity. Subjects with Down's syndrome showed clear evidence of a chemotactic defect ($P<0.0001$) (Fig. 8). Almost all the trisomy 21 subjects gave values below the 50th percentile of the control subjects.

Table 3
Summary of immunological abnormalities in Down's syndrome

Leukocyte (%):	CD3	CD4	CD8	B cells	CD16
	N	D	I	N	N

Lymphocyte function:

Stimulus	Aggreg. +LFA–1	Prolif.	Ab	Cytok. TNFβ/IL–2		NK cyt.
None	I	N		N	N	N
PHA		N?		D	N	
PWM		D		D		
ConA		N		N		
S. aureus		N				
Anti–CD3		D				
TT		D	D		D	
Influenza		D	D		D	
PMA	I					

Immunoglobulins:

IgA	IgM	IgG	IgG_1	IgG_2	IgG_3	IgG_4
I	D	I	I	D	I	D

In vivo immune responses:

TT	Typhoid	φ×174	Influenza	Hepatitis B	PS
D	D	D	D	D(IgG_1)	D

Macrophages: TNFα production decreased
Neutrophils: Reduced chemotaxis, Normal bactericidal activity

Complement activity: Normal

Abbreviations: Aggreg. = aggregation; Prolif. = proliferation; Ab = antibody; Cytok. = cytokine; cyt. = cytotoxicity; TT = Tetanus toxoid; φ×174 = bacteriophage×174; PS = pneumococcal polysaccharide.
Scores: N = Normal; D = Decreased; I = Increased.

The quantitative leukocyte iodination reaction, bactericidal activity and the HMP shunt activity were similar in the two groups (Fig. 8). However, one patient showed a highly reduced iodination reaction in the presence of autologous serum and another a highly elevated HMP shunt activity.

Complement

Essentially no difference was observed between the Down's syndrome subjects and control subjects in concentration of C3 and C4, and in the hemolytic complement activity.

Discussion

A summary of immunological abnormalities, taking into consideration the results from our present study and those published previously, in trisomy 21 are presented in Table 3. In our extensive study, we present evidence that non-institutionalized Down's syndrome subjects display a range of immunological deficiencies. Since these subjects were tested when free from infection, it is unlikely that any of the parameters studied were secondary to infection. Interpretation of a number of previous studies has been confounded by factors such as institutionalization of patients and/or age-associated deficiencies. Nevertheless, it is likely that not all immunodeficiencies observed in trisomy 21 can be accounted for by institutionalization.

Our data showed that the proportions of T cells (CD3+) were normal in trisomy 21 which is consistent with a number of previous reports (9, 12, 14, 36–38). However, one child in our Down's syndrome group showed a disturbingly low percentage of T cells. This, considered with the findings discussed below, suggests that trisomy 21 subjects present as a group with a spectrum of immunodeficiencies. A consistent finding amongst Down's syndrome subjects is a decreased proportion of CD4+ T cells and increased proportions of CD8+ T cells (9, 12, 14, 36–39). This tendency towards decreased CD4+ cells and increased CD8+ cells in trisomy 21 was seen in our study. However, as a group these levels were not significantly different from controls. But again there were Down's syndrome subjects who showed concerningly low CD4+ and elevated CD8+ lymphocytes. The differences in CD4+ and CD8+ T cells of the two groups were reflected in a decreased CD4:CD8 ratio. For example, we found that 74% of Down's syndrome subjects were below the 50th percentile for the control subjects.

B cell proportions and numbers, similar to our findings, have been reported to be normal. We have also found that the cells bearing the CD16 antigen (highly toxic natural killer cells) were normal in trisomy 21. This was consistent with our observation that there were no differences in cytotoxicity mediated by NK cells between the two groups. Noble and Warren (38) also found no differences in NK cytotoxicity between trisomy 21 subjects and controls. In addition, their study showed that these cells from the two groups were equally sensitive to activation by interferon–γ.

We found very little difference in lymphocyte responses to mitogens as assessed by lymphoproliferation. This stands in agreement with some reports (9, 13, 39, 40) but in disagreement with others (9, 37,

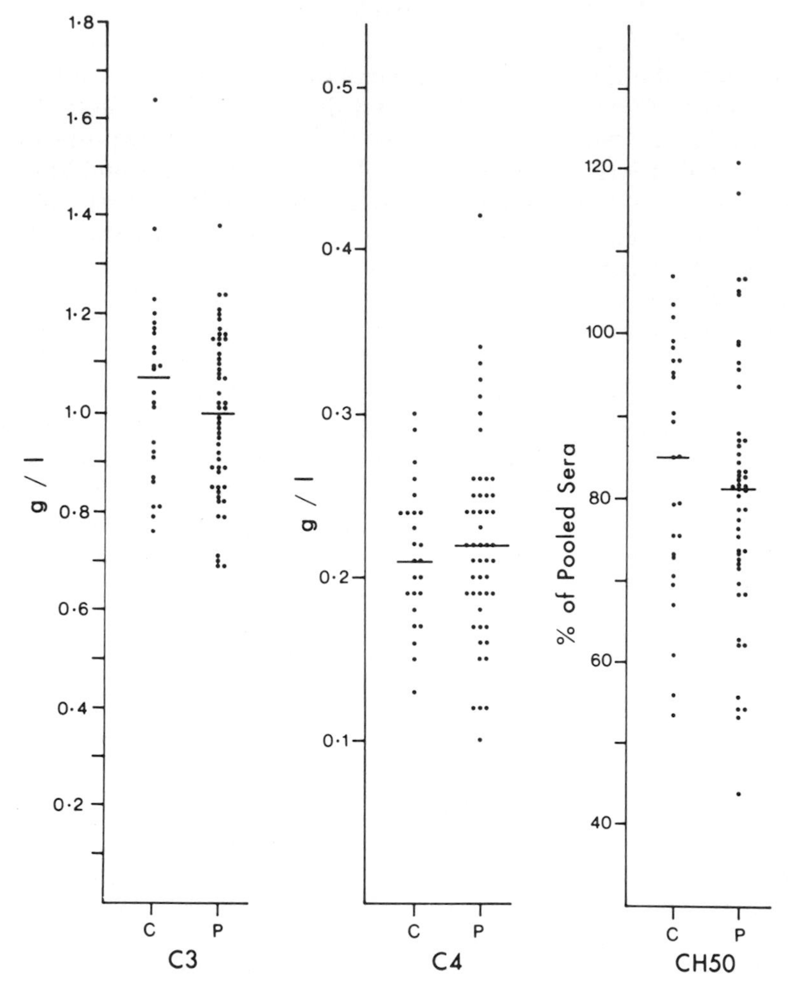

Figure 9. Serum levels of the complement components C3 and C4, and complement activity (CH_{50}) in Down's syndrome subjects. The bars represent the median.

41–43). The interesting finding from our results is that production of the lymphokine TNFβ in response to these mitogens is decreased in some Down's syndrome subjects. This was seen in response to PHA and PWM but not ConA. Production of another T-cell lymphokine IL–2 has been studied by Philip *et al.* (14) and Karttunen *et al.* (12). Both found normal production of IL–2 by lymphocytes from Down's syndrome subjects in response to PHA.

Although previous studies have documented an imbalance of

immunoglobulin classes, it has not been clear whether there is a significant increase in IgA and a significant decrease in IgM in trisomy 21 (37, 44, 45). Our data confirm that a significant number of Down's syndrome subjects show elevated IgG and establish that a significant number have increased IgA and significantly decreased IgM. Of major interest are our results which show that a significant number of trisomy 21 subjects have elevated IgG_1 and IgG_3 and depressed IgG_2 and IgG_4. This supports and extends our previous observations of IgG subclass deficiency in trisomy 21 (46). The deficiency in IgG_2 and IgG_4 in some Down's syndrome subjects could be responsible for increased susceptibility to bacterial infections (33, 46–51). IgG antibodies to viral antigens are predominantly distributed in the IgG_1 and IgG_3 isotypes. Although this stands at variance with the finding that the Down's syndrome patients show an increased susceptibility to viral infections, it is possible that the risk is in part a consequence of an "antibody deficiency syndrome" associated with an inability to make protective levels of IgG_1 and IgG_3 anti-viral antibodies. This was observed by Avanzini *et al.* (45). In this investigation Down's syndrome subjects had normal total IgG_1 but made decreased anti-hepatitis B antibodies in this isotype. Increased susceptibility to viral infection may also be associated with decreased production of TNFβ and also TNFα in some patients, since these cytokines are believed to play an important role in defense against viruses.

An impairment of the *in vitro* T-lymphoproliferative response to the bacterial antigen tetanus toxoid and a similar impairment of the response to influenza virus antigen has been described in trisomy 21 (14). The IL–2 production induced by these antigens was also significantly reduced. In addition, it was found that the IgG antibody response to these antigens was significantly depressed in Down's syndrome. Since others have found normal proliferative responses to staphylococcal, streptococcal and sendai virus antigens (52) and to purified protein derivative (39), it is possible that the inability to make antibodies in trisomy 21 is restricted to certain antigens.

Decreased *in vivo* antibody responses to a variety of antigens, tetanus toxoid (53), typhoid vaccine (53), bacteriophage ϕx174 (21), hepatitis B (45), influenza A (54) and different pneumonococcal polysaccharides (54) have been reported in Down's syndrome. Others have, however, described normal responses in Down's syndrome subjects to tetanus toxoid and hepatitis B vaccine (56, 57).

We found no evidence for a defect in neutrophil bactericidal activity, respiratory burst activity and leukocyte iodination activity in Down's syndrome subjects. The major finding was depressed neutrophil chemotaxis. Since the patients were free from infections at time of study, it is unlikely that the reduced chemotaxis can be attributed to infection-induced pathophysiologic factors. Over 93% of the trisomy 21 subjects had chemotaxis migration values below the 50th percentile for normal subjects. Chemotactic defects in Down's syndrome was also reported by Khan *et al.* (22).

We found no evidence suggesting that immunodeficiency is more prominent with an increase in age in trisomy 21. The high incidence of proneness to infection (approximately 80%) and high incidence of immunodeficiency (approximately 80%) is shown in Table 4. Both are obviously quite striking.

Table 4
Incidence of infection-proneness and immunodeficiency

	Infection-prone	Not infection-prone
Deficiency	32	6
No deficiency	5	2

Figures represent the number of Down's syndrome subjects with or without a deficiency

Our studies show that trisomy 21 subjects present as a heterogeneous group in relation to imbalances of immunological activities. However, the basis for the various immunological abnormalities is difficult to ascertain at present. In part the T lymphocyte associated deficiencies may be a consequence of abnormal thymuses in trisomy 21, and it has been suggested that a deficient expansion of T lymphocyte precursors occurs which leads to the generation of an inadequate T-cell repertoire (58). Both T-cell dependent and T-cell independent responses may be affected.

Others have observed an over-expression of the lymphocyte function-associated antigen, LFA–1, on lymphoblastoid cell-lines derived from patients with trisomy 21 which was associated with enhanced adherence (59). One interpretation of this is that the increased adherence could adversely affect leukocyte interaction and prevent cytotoxic T cells from damaging virus-infected cells.

Other adhesion molecules on leukocytes may also be increased in trisomy 21. For example, Rosner and Kozinn (44) found neutrophils from Down's syndrome subjects to have increased adherence. Perhaps this increased adherence may be the reason why the neutrophils show decreased movement.

Summary

Down's syndrome patients are at increased risk of infection and malignancies. A number of immunological abnormalities are evident in these patients, which are not associated with institutionalization. Many immunological functions are depressed but the type of immunodeficiency may vary within the group of trisomy 21 subjects. Our studies showed that there exists a high incident of immunodeficiency and increased proneness to infection in trisomy 21. Immunodeficiencies occur both in the cellular and humoral arm of the immune response, and in phagocytic cells such as neutrophils. The presence of both deficiencies of IgG_2 and IgG_4 as well as antibody deficiency to specific antigens in other IgG subclasses suggest that gammaglobulin replacement therapy needs a serious consideration in some of these patients.

Acknowledgement

We are grateful to Julie Hagedorn and Kathy Carman for dedicated technical assistance and to Dr G. Smith for referring patients. The work was supported in part by funds from the Channel 7 Children's Medical Research Foundation of South Australia, the Mayne Bequest Foundation (University of Queensland) and the University of Adelaide Research Grants.

References

1. Epstein, C. J. "The consequences of Chromosome Imbalance. Principles, Mechanisms and Models." University Press, New York; 1986.
2. Siegel, M. Susceptibility of mongoloids to infection. I. Incidence of pneumonia, influenza A and *Shigella dysenteriae*. *Am. J. Hyg.* **48**: 53–56; 1948.
3. Rosner, F. and Lee, S. L. Down's syndrome and acute leukemia: myeloblastic or lymphoblastic? *Am. J. Med.* **53**: 203; 1972.
4. Robinson, L. L., Nesbit, M. E. Jr., Sather, H. N., Level, C., Shahidi, N., Kennedy, M. S. and Hammond, D. Down syndrome and acute leukemia in children: a 10-year retrospective study from Children's Cancer Study Group. *J. Pediatr.* **105**: 235–242; 1984.
5. Miller, R. W. Neoplasia and Down's syndrome. *Ann. N.Y. Acad. Sci.* **171**: 637–644; 1970.
6. Krivit, W. and Good, R. A. Simultaneous occurrence of mongolism and leukemia. *Am. J. Dis. Child.* **94**: 289–293; 1957.

7. Scholl, T., Stein, Z. and Hansen, H. Leukemia and other cancers, anomalies and infections as cause of death in Down's syndrome in the United States during 1976. *Dev. Med. Child. Neurol.* **24**: 817–829; 1982.
8. Oster, J., Mikkelsen, M. and Nielsen, A. Mortality and life-table in Down's syndrome. *Acta Paediatr. Scand.* **64**: 322–326; 1975.
9. Burgio, G. R., Ugazio, A., Nespoli, L. and Maccario, R. Down's syndrome: A model of immunodeficiency. *Birth Defects* (Original Article series) **19**: 325–327; 1983.
10. Nair, M. P. N. and Schwartz, A. Association of decreased T-cell-mediated natural citotoxicity and interferon production in Down's syndrome. *Clin. Immunol. Immunopathol.* **33**: 412–424; 1984.
11. Leven, S., Schlesinger, M., Handdzel, A. *et al.* Thymic deficiency in Down's Syndrome. *Pediatrics* **63**: 1–4; 1979.
12. Karttunen, R., Nurmi, T., Ilonen, J. and Helja–Marjasurcel. Cell-mediated immunodeficiency in Down's syndrome: normal IL–2 production but inverted ratio of T cell subsets. *Clin. Exp. Immunol.* **55**: 257–263; 1984.
13. Bertotta, A., Arcangeli, C., Grupi, S., Marinelli, I., Gerli, R. and Vacarro, R. T cell response to anti-CD3 antibody in Down's syndrome. *Arch. Dis. Child.* **62**: 1148–1152; 1987.
14. Philip, R., Berger, A. C., McManus, N. H., Warner, N. H., Peacok, M. A. and Epstein, L. B. Abnormalities of the in vitro cellular and humoral responses to tetanus and influenza antigens with concomittant numerical alterations in lymphocyte subsets in Down's syndrome. *J. Immunol.* **136**: 1660–1667; 1986.
15. Seger, R., Buchinger, G. and Stroder, J. On the influence of age of immunity in Down's syndrome. *Eur. J. Pediatr.* **124**: 77–87; 1977.
16. Franceschi, C., Licastro, F., Paulucci, P., Masi, M., Cavicchi, S. and Zannotti, M. T. and B lymphocyte subpopulations in Down's syndrome. A study on non-institutionalized subjects. *J. Ment. Defic. Res.* **22**: 179–182; 1978.
17. Spina, C. A., Smith, D., Korn, E., Fahey, J. L. and Grossman, H. J. Altered cellular immune functions in patients with Down's syndrome. *Am. J. Dis. Child.* **135**: 251–255; 1981.
18. McMillan, B. C., Hanson, P., Golubjatnikov, R. and Sinha, S. K. The effect of institutionalization on elevated IgD and IgG levels in patients with Down's syndrome. *J. Ment. Defic. Res.* **19**: 209–223; 1975.
19. Burgio, G. R., Ugazio, A. G., Nespoli, L., Marcioni, A. F., Botelli, A. M. and Pasquali, F. Derangements of immunoglobulin levels phytohemagglutin responsiveness and T and B cell markers in Down's syndrome at different ages. *Eur. J. Immunol.* **5**: 600–603; 1975.
20. Lopez, V., Ochs, H. D., Tuline, H. C., Davis, S. D. and Wedgwood, R. J. Defective antibody response to bacteriophage $\phi \times 174$ in Down syndrome. *J. Pediatr.* **86**: 207–211; 1975.

21. Gregory, L., Williams, R. and Thompson, E. Leucocyte function in Down's syndrome and acute leukaemia. *Lancet* 1: 1359–1361; 1972.
22. Kahn, A. J., Evans, H. E., Glass, L., Shin, Y. H. and Almonte, D. Defective neutrophil chemotaxis in patients with Down's syndrome. *J. Pediatr.* 87: 87–89; 1975.
23. Barkin, R. M., Weston, W. L., Humbert, J. R. and Maire, F. Phagocytic function in Down's syndrome-I chemotaxis. *J. Ment. Defic. Res.* 24: 243–249; 1980.
24. Barkin, R. M., Weston, W. L., Humbert, J. R. and Sunada, K. Phagocytic function in Down's syndrome-II. Bactericidal activity and phagocytosis. *J. Ment. Defic. Res.* 24: 251–256; 1980.
25. Kretschmer, R. R., Lopez–Osuna, M., De la Rose, L. and Armendares, S. Leukocyte function in Down's syndrome quantitative N.B.T. reduction and bactericidal capacity. *Clin. Immunol. Immunopathol.* 2: 445–449; 1974.
26. Falcao, R. P., Ismael, S. J. and Donadi, E. A. Age-associated changes of T lymphocytes subsets. *Diag. Clin. Immunol.* 5: 205–208; 1987.
27. Ferrante, A., Davidson, G. P., Beard, L. J. and Goh, D. H. B. Alterations in function and subpopulations of peripheral blood mononuclear leukocytes in children with Portal Hypertension. *Int. Arch. Allergy Appl. Immunol.* 88: 348–352; 1989.
28. Ferrante, A. and Thong, Y. H. Separation of mononuclear and polymorphonuclear leucocytes from human blood by the one-step hypaque-ficoll method is dependent on blood column height. *J. Immunol. Methods* 48: 81–85; 1982.
29. Ferrante, A., Roberton D. M., Toogood I. and Giorgiou G. M. Normal tumor necrosis factor alpha (TNFα) but deficient TNFβ production in a patient with severe combined immunodeficiency. Abstracts of the Australian Society for Immunology, Adelaide, December 1989.
30. Ferrante, A., Seow, W. K., Rowan–Kelly, B. and Thong, Y. H. Tetrandrine, a plant alkaloid, inhibits the production of tumor necrosis factor alpha (cachectin) by human monocytes. *Clin. Exp. Immunol.* 80: 232–235; 1990.
31. Ferrante, A., Rowan–Kelly, B., Seow, W. K. and Thong, Y. H. Depression of human polymorphonuclear leucocyte function by anti-malarial drugs. *Immunology* 58: 125–130; 1986.
32. Ferrante, A., Harvey, D. and Bates, E. J. *Staphylococcus aureus* stimulated MNL conditioned medium increases the neutrophil bactericidal activity, and augments the oxygen radical production and degranulation in response to the bacteria. *Clin. Exp. Immunol.* 78: 366–371; 1989.
33. Beard, L. J., Ferrante, A., Oxelius, V.-A. and Maxwell, G. M. IgG subclass deficiency in children with IgA deficiency presenting with recurrent or severe respiratory infections. *Pediatr. Res.* 20: 937–942; 1986.
34. Ferrante, A. and Beard, L. J. IgG subclass assays with polyclonal

antisera and monoclonal antibodies. *Monogr. Allergy* 23: 61–72; 1988.

35. Beard, L. J., Ferrante, A., Hagedorn, J., Leppard, P. and Kiroff, G. Percentile ranges for IgG subclass concentrations in healthy Australian children. *Pediatr. Infect. Dis. J.* 9: S9–S15; 1990.
36. Bertotto, A., Gerli, R., Fabietti, G., Arcangeli, D. F., Branchi, S. and Vacarro, R. Immunodeficiency in Down's syndrome: analysis by OKT monoclonal antibodies. *Thymus* 6: 365–367; 1984.
37. Lockitch, G., Singh, V. K., Puterman, M. L., Godolphin, W. J., Sheps, S., Tingle, A. J., Wong, F. and Quigley G. Age-related changes in humoral and cell-mediated immunity in Down syndrome children living at home. *Pediatr. Res.* 22: 536–540; 1987.
38. Noble, R. L. and Warren, R. P. Analysis of blood cell populations, plasma zinc and natural killer cell activity in young children with Down's syndrome. *J. Ment. Defic. Res.* 32: 193–201; 1988.
39. Fowler, I., Hollingsworth, D. R. and Traurig, H. Response to stimulation *in vitro* of lymphocytes from patients with Down's syndrome. *Proc. Soc. Exp. Biol. Med.* 144: 475; 1973.
40. Epstein, L. B. and Epstein, C. J. T-lymphocyte function and sensitivity to interferon in trisomy 21. *Cell. Immunol.* 51: 303–318; 1980.
41. Rigas, D. A., Elsasser, P. and Hecht, F. Impaired *in vitro* response of circulating lymphocytes to phytohaemagglutinin in Down's syndrome: dose and time response curves and relation to cellular immunity. *Int. Arch. Allergy Appl. Immunol.* 5: 600; 1970.
42. Burgio, G. R., Ugazio, A. G., Nespoli, L., Marcioni, A. E., Bottelli, A. M. and Pasquale, F. Derangements of immunoglobulin levels, phytohaemagglutinin responsiveness and T and B cell markers in Down's syndrome at different ages. *Eur. J. Immunol.* 5: 600–603; 1975.
43. Whittingham, S., Sharma, D. L. B., Pitt, D. B. and Mackay, I. R. Stress deficiency of the T lymphocyte system exemplified by Down syndrome. *Lancet* 1: 163–166; 1977.
44. Rosner, F. and Kozinn, P. J. Leucocyte function in Down's syndrome. *Lancet* ii: 283–284; 1972.
45. Avanzini, M. A., Söderström, T., Wahl, M., Plebani, A., Burgio, G. R. and Hanson, L. A. IgG subclass deficiency in patients with Down's syndrome and aberrant hepatitis B vaccine response. *Scand. J. Immunol.* 28: 465–470; 1988.
46. Loh, K. S., Harth, S. C., Thong, Y. H. and Ferrante, A. Immunoglobulin G subclass deficiency and predisposition to infection in Down syndrome. *Pediatr. Infect. Dis. J.* (In press.)
47. Oxelius, V.-A. Chronic infections in a family with hereditary deficiency of IgG2 and IgG4. *Clin. Exp. Immunol.* 17: 19–27; 1974.
48. Beck, C. S. and Heiner, D. C. Selective immunoglobulin G4 deficiency and recurrent infections of the respiratory tract. *Am. Rev. Respir. Dis.* 124: 94–96; 1981.

49. Hammarström, L. and Smith, C. I. E. IgG deficiency in healthy blood donor. Concomitant lack of IgG2, IgA and IgE immunoglobulins and specific anti-carbohydrate antibodies. *Clin. Exp. Immunol.* **51**: 600–604; 1983.
50. Beard, L. J. and Ferrante, A. Aspects of Immunoglobulin replacement therapy. *Pediatr. Infect. Dis. J.* **9**: S54–S61; 1990.
51. Ferrante, A., Beard, L. J. and Feldman, R. G. IgG subclass distribution of antibodies to bacterial and viral antigens. *Pediatr. Infect. Dis. J.* **9**: S16–S24; 1990.
52. Funa, K., Anneren, G., Alm, G. V. and Bjorksten, B. Abnormal interferon production and NK responses to interferon in children with Down's syndrome. *Clin. Exp. Immunol.* **56**: 493–500; 1984.
53. Siegel, M. Susceptibility of mongoloids to infection II Antibody responses to tetanus toxoid and typhoid vaccine. *Am. J. Hyg.* **48**: 63–73; 1948.
54. Gordon, M. C., Sinha, S. K. and Carlson, S. D. Antibody responses to influenza vaccine in patients with Down's syndrome. *Am. J. Ment. Defic.* 75: 391–399; 1971.
55. Nurmi, T. Disturbed immune functions associated with chromosome abnormalities. Academic dissertation. University of Oulu, Oulu, Finland; 1982.
56. Griffiths, A. W. and Sylvester, P. E. Mongols and nonmongols compared in their response to active tetanus immunization. *J. Ment. Defic. Res.* 11: 263–266; 1967.
57. Troisi, C. L., Heiberg, D. A. and Hollinger, F. B. Normal immune response to hepatitis B vaccine in patients with Down's syndrome. *J. Am. Med. Assoc.* **254**: 3196–3199; 1985.
58. Larocca, L. M., Piantelli, M., Valitutti, S., Castellino, F., Maggiano, N. and Musiani, P. Alterations in thymocyte subpopulations in Down's syndrome (Trisomy 21). *Clin. Immunol. Immunopathol.* **49**: 175–186; 1988.
59. Taylor, G. M., Haigh, H., Williams, A., D'Souza, S. W. and Harris, R. Down's syndrome lymphoid cell lines exhibit increased adhesion due to the over-expression of lymphocyte function-associated antigen (LFA–1). *Immunology* **64**: 451–456; 1988.

Part VI
Closing remarks

Maximizing the therapeutic potential of intravenously administered immunoglobulin G

JOHN M. DWYER

Department of Clinical Immunology, the Prince Henry Hospital of the University of New South Wales, Sydney, Australia

Introduction

As is usual with our IVIG meetings, 3 days of intensive scientific discussion leaves one excited by the new information provided, and frustrated at the lack of progress in some of the problem areas. Thus we have heard of the amelioration of severe steroid-dependent asthma and the minimizing of fetal wastage accomplished by gammaglobulin therapy, but we still don't know if patients with acute sepsis will benefit from a combination of antibiotics and IVIG. We still await the definitive decision on the ability of IVIG to prevent serious infection in patients with multiple myeloma or severe thermal trauma. All of these problem areas were previously discussed in Interlaken in 1985, and we would have expected an answer by now. Specific comments on this conference can be divided between its two major themes: immunodeficiency, and immunomanipulation.

Immunotherapy with Intravenous Immunoglobulins
ISBN 0–12–370725–0

Immunodeficiency

Immunology is all about specificity. While we heard of antibodies with broad specificity being produced transiently by the immature immune system (Cooper) those products of our communities' collective antigenic experience, found in pooled gammaglobulin, are totally restricted to specific antigenic determinants. Thus it is surprising that insufficient attention continues to be given to antigen specificity in passive protection strategies. While it is clear that most hypogammaglobulinemic patients will be well managed if trough levels of serum IgG are not allowed to fall below normal values, optimum management for the more difficult patient requires attention to the concentration, affinity and half-life of immunoglobulins reactive against troublesome organisms. Individual variability in the catabolism and/or consumption of total IgG, IgG subclasses, and specific antibodies was emphasized by a number of speakers (*Wedgwood, Ferrante, Nadler*). Nothing clears a limited amount of antibody from serum more efficiently than antigen arising from infection. Dosage, frequency of administration of IVIG and strategies for preventing mid-cycle infection need to be individualized for many.

Although companies providing IVIG products are loath to supply serological profiles on each batch of gammaglobulin produced, the clinical problems discussed at this meeting make such a request from clinicians more than reasonable. A standardized profile detailing antibody titers for the 20 most common organisms likely to trouble patients receiving IVIG would facilitate therapy and research. For viral serology, the titers of neutralizing antibodies are required.

Despite 10 years of discussion, the potential for producing hyperimmune globulin by capitalizing on regionally specific serological profiles has not been realized. If donors from one collection area have higher than normal titers to, for example, group B *Streptococcus*, why not hold some of this serum for a neonatal product rather than diluting its potential in the larger pool?

The excellent discussions on the role of IVIG in the management of the premature infant and the septic neonate suggest that definitive recommendations are close. Clearly in countries with advanced neonatal medical and nursing skills, mortality in neonatal nurseries is so low that it is difficult to produce an improved outcome with any strategy. Better antibiotics used more skilfully will undoubtedly restrict the need for IVIG in neonates. The major advances to be expected in the near future will come from clear guidelines for the identification of the high-risk infant most likely to benefit from IVIG.

Clearly, lives will be saved by using the product in selected infants (*Baker, Fischer*). More attention needs to be placed in the future on immunizing mothers during pregnancy, especially against those important community organisms to which she has not made an adequate antibody response, as well as to hospital-based organisms. Packaging 12% IVIG in small volumes would be an important practical and cost-effective advance.

A number of delegates expressed their concern at the experimental design being utilized to examine the benefit of IVIG in hypogammaglobulinemic patients with B-cell malignancies. A double-blind format dictates that all patients receive the same dose of IVIG. Preliminary data (*Chapel and McLennan*) suggest that, understandably, attained levels of IgG vary, and some patients who, despite therapy, become septicemic had less than satisfactory levels of IgG. Such trials are only likely to give conclusive results if the defect thought likely to contribute the susceptibility to infection is corrected. Not "blinding" the physicians who would adjust dosage to achieve a satisfactory steady-state concentration of IgG seems a preferable approach.

There seems little doubt that severely immunosuppressed patients have less trouble with cytomegalovirus infection (CMV) of their lungs and intestinal tract if given IVIG. However, the dosage required, the duration of therapy and the role for IVIG in prophylaxis rather than treatment seems unclear. Here again, the use of batches which are not standardized in terms of neutralizing antibody to CMV may pose a significant problem. Measuring CMV titers by an ELISA technique may not provide values which correlate with neutralizing activity. Batch-to-batch variability and brand variability have been noted.

Desirable advances for the future would see a concentrated IVIG preparation made from a selected donor (e.g. the mother of a child with an ECHO virus encephalitis) who could provide a specific antibody not found in the pooled products. Clearly, the future will involve the administering of IVIG in combination with antibiotics, antiviral agents and cytokines to maximize host defense.

Preliminary data (*Nadler*) indicated that commercial amounts of a stable human monoclonal antibody could be generated. The efficacy of such antibodies against CMV and hepatitis B await clinical trials. Already a cautionary note was sounded after phase I studies of toxicity. Viral mutants with reduced affinity for a specific monoclonal antibody presented after a number of months of therapy. Initial killing will need to be efficient, and monoclonal "cocktails" may be required. This is particularly likely to be true for bacterial opsonization and killing.

Ultimately, satisfactory progress will see an ever-decreasing role for pooled polyspecific IgG products. Molecularly engineered and monoclonal antibodies should play increasingly important roles, while genetic engineers should cure a number of patients with primary and severely immunodeficient states. There is no such thing as a patient with absolute agammagloblinemia. Patients with both congenital X-linked and acquired hypogammagloblinemia secrete at least trace amounts of immunoglobulin, indicating that the structural genes are present.

Immunomanipulation

The list of diseases attributed to immunopathology and improved by therapy with IVIG continues to expand. New data were presented on the treatment of thyroid eye disease (*Dwyer*), rheumatoid arthritis (*Corvetta*), polyneuropathies (*Vermeulen*), inflammatory bowel disease (*Ochs*), and vasculitis (*Lockwood*). Favored as the mechanism most likely to explain their observations were Fc receptor blockade, and T- and B-cell manipulation by id–anti-id complexes. In reality, many simultaneously operative manipulations may be needed for a clinical response.

Many studies suggest that pooled IgG contains a considerable repertoire of $F(ab')_2$ idiotypes capable of binding to autoantibodies. Of much interest was the report that IVIG contains antibodies able to block two autoantibodies capable of binding to different glycoproteins on the surface of platelets (*Berchtold*). A major question concerns the idiotypic specificity of those apparently naturally occurring and *not* disease-associated antibodies probably involved in the maintenance of tolerance to self. Evidence presented strongly suggests that disease-associated autoantibodies are not recognized by these normal network autoantibodies. If this is the case, disease-regulating anti-idiotypic antibodies would only be controlled by a minority of donors to a pool. Presumably they would have recovered from an autoimmune disease, or be in remission (*Kazatchkine*). The finding that anti-idiotypic antibodies to disease-associated autoantibody may be polyspecific, *i.e.* capable of binding via $F(ab')_2$ to a number of autoantibodies, suggests a potential product from the molecular engineer.

A number of delegates indicated that immunomanipulation requires intact IgG: did this not suggest that anti-idiotypic binding may be less important than some theorized? Fc determinants would be expected to play a vital role even in any anti-idiotypic effect, as without Fc the half-life of the anti-idiotypic antibodies would be too short, and id–anti-id complexes would not bind to regulatory T cells: an interaction likely to be of major importance. Of course, the demonstration that $F(ab')_2$ from IVIG can bind autoantibody does not mean that such binding is all-important *in vivo* (*Gelfand*).

The concept and preliminary data suggesting that Tallergic responses (*Dwyer*) can produce immunopathology and be manipulated by IVIG is likely to be of considerable importance. The inadequately disciplined release of T-cell lymphokines, and perhaps additional cytokines from cells under T-cell control, could produce a spectrum of pathology just as excessive amounts of IgE can lead to disease. Contact sensitivity, toxic shock syndrome, Kawasaki's disease, inflammatory bowel disease, atopic dermatitis and chronic fatigue syndrome represent significant problems likely to be caused by Tallergy. It seems convenient therefore to divide allergic responses into Tallergic and Ballergic varieties. The demonstration that subjects with chronic fatigue syndrome may benefit from IVIG represents the first double-blind placebo-controlled trial to suggest a therapeutic approach to this difficult problem.

In general, there are still too many anecdotal reports of one or two cases of various diseases partially responding to IVIG. The product is very expensive, and local distributors of IVIG (often financially independent subsidiaries of a parent company, and of course hospital pharmacies) are finding it increasingly difficult to fund large controlled trials. It would seem prudent to have centralized protocols for various autoimmune diseases agreed upon by an international committee, perhaps working with the International Union of Immunological Societies (IVIS). This would facilitate the speedy and orderly collection of multicenter data which may soon provide much-needed answers. Primary questions to be asked should always include: Does it work? How well does it work when compared to other therapy? What is the minimum dose which will achieve a beneficial result? Is this a cost-effective approach to management?

As with the management of immunodeficiency, autoimmune disease will no doubt be best managed by combining a number of therapies. Plasma exchange using IVIG to replace normal IgG, down-regulate autoantibody production and protect normal B-cell clones from subsequent therapy with *e.g.* cyclosporin A, may prove to be of special benefit in a number of conditions. A library of disease-associated idiotypes needs to be collected and compared. A "super" polyspecific anti-id may revolutionize therapy.

Summary

The most exciting developments at this meeting, if explored to realize their full potential, could see the demise of IVIG therapy within 15 years. In the meantime, extensive coordinated research with the product should enable us to tell the molecular biologist which tools we need produced to supply better and cheaper therapy. For now, we should be grateful that for many conditions, suffering is already being minimized by a remarkable, fascinating, yet poorly understood re-organization of a distilled immunological network.

Part VII
Abstracts of poster sessions

PRIMARY IMMUNODEFICIENCY

X-Linked agammaglobulinemia: a comparison of different immunoglobulin substitution schemes in the therapy of 29 patients

JOHANNES LIESE[1], UWE WINTERGERST[2], PETER KLOSE[1], KLAUS D. TYMPNER[1] and BERND H. BELOHRADSKY[2]

[1] Städtisches Krankenhaus München-Harlaching, [2] Universitäts-Kinderklinik-München, Lindwurmstr. 4, D-8000 München 2, FRG

X-Linked agammaglobulinemia (XLA) is due to a B-cell differentiation failure with markedly decreased immunoglobulin levels leading to an increased susceptibility to severe bacterial infections. Treatment of XLA consists in regular immunoglobulin substitution. Between 1965 and 1989 a total of 29 patients with XLA were treated with different immunoglobulin substitution schemes. The data were analyzed retrospectively to evaluate the dose regimen providing the best clinical long-term results.

According to the quantity of substituted immunoglobulin, patients were divided into three groups: an intramuscular immunoglobulin (IMIG) (100 mg/kg/3 weeks), an intravenous immunoglobulin (IVIG) low-dose (200 mg/kg/3 weeks) or high-dose (600 mg/kg/3 weeks) substitution group. The time before substitution was started served as a control. The following parameters were evaluated: serum IgG level, side effects, days in hospital caused by infections, frequency of infections, pulmonary function tests, complications of chronic infections and disease-related death. Patients receiving IVIG high-dose substitution had fewer days in hospital and a substantial reduction of bronchitis, pneumonias, ear–nose–throat and bacterial CNS infections compared with patients receiving lower doses of immunoglobulins. This effect became even more evident when regular substitution was started before the fifth year of life. Chronic pulmonary disease and bronchiectasis did not occur so far in both IVIG substitution groups. Six out of 18 patients older than 10 years have symptoms of chronic encephalitis. The course of this complication could not be improved either by IVIG low-dose or high-dose substitution. Treatment of chronic "encephalitis" remains a major problem in XLA.

Differences in supportive therapeutic measures, such as prophylactic antibiotic treatment and regular physical therapy certainly influence the results of this retrospective study. Nevertheless we recommend high-dose IVIG substitution for children with XLA to achieve normal immunoglobulin levels and fewer infectious complications. Only a prospective study can give a more relevant answer to the best dose regimen. However, such a study in a rare disease such as XLA, may be difficult to conduct.

Evaluation of clinical and immunological parameters in children with primary humoral immunodeficiency treated with intravenous immunoglobulins

C. BARBIERI, V. RAGNO, R. GERARDI, L. BUSINCO

Dept of Paediatrics, University "La Sapienza", Rome, Italy

We have treated seven children aged 10–21 years (median age 13) affected by agammaglobulinemia or severe hypogammaglobulinemia with IgG serum levels lower than 100 mg% with i.v. gammaglobulin (Sandoglobulin®) at the dose of 300–400 mg/kg/3 weeks for 7 years. The children suffered from severe and recurrent bacterial infections, mainly of the respiratory tract, leading to chronic tissue damage. They had been previously treated with i.m. gammaglobulins (0.8 ml/kg/3 weeks) for 2 years, but their serum IgG values were never higher than 75 mg%. Pulmonary function has been tested in all the children who collaborated actively (5 children) studying the following parameters: CVF, FEV 1, PEF, MEF, FER at 25% and 50%. All the patients showed a significant clinical improvement during the treatment with IVIG in comparison to the IMIG. They reached, on average, 800 mg% of IgG serum level. Minor adverse reaction (chills, fever, abdominal pain) were observed only in one child. Lung function tests in four children reached and sometimes overcame 100% of predicted values and were perfectly included in normal values.

Hypogammaglobulinemia in children with pneumonia

K. MANTALENAKI-LAMBROU, O. MORALOGLOU, O. KANARIOU, T. LIAKOPOULOU, F. PSHYCHOU, P. NICOLAIDOU, P. VLACHOU and C. KATTAMIS

Immunology and 1st Pediatric Department of Athens University, "Aghia Sophia" Children Hospital, Athens, Greece

This study aimed to investigate deficiencies of serum immunoglobulins in children admitted to hospital for pneumonia. Serum levels of IgG, IgG_1, IgG_2, IgG_3, IgG_4, IgA, and IgM were evaluated.

Within 24 h of admission immunoglobulin levels were tested in 129 randomly selected children aged 3 months to 14 years (64 boys, 65 girls). IgG, IgA, IgM were determined by nephelometry, while IgG subgroups by radial immunodiffusion with monoclonal antibodies.

Twenty children (15%) had low immunoglobulin levels: IgG 13/129, IgA 4/129, IgM 1/129, IgGIgA 1/129, IgAIgM 1/129. Additionally, 10/129 had low IgG subgroups. IgG subgroups were found low in 40 children with normal levels of total IgG, IgA and IgM, IgG_2 25/129, (10 with 0 levels) IgG_3 1/129, IgG_4 7/129, IgG_1IgG_2 1/129, IgG_2IgG_3 2/129, IgG_2IgG_4 6/129.

From the hypoglobulinemic children, 19/129 were younger than 2 years, 13/129 between 2–5 years and 30/129 older than 5 years.

As almost half of the investigated children with pneumonia (62/129) were found with low immunoglobulin levels, it is suggested that the therapeutic administration of IVIG will most probably reduce the hospitalization days.

Rapid infusion of Sandoglobulin® in patients with primary humoral immunodeficiency

RICHARD I. SCHIFF, REBECCA H. BUCKLEY and DEBRA SEDLAK

Duke University Medical Center, Durham, North Carolina, USA

The dose of IVIG used for the treatment of immune deficiency has been increased to 400 mg/kg for most patients, and the doses used for diseases such as autoimmune thrombocytopenia is 1 g/kg per dose. Such large doses create problems with regard to the volume infused as well as the time commitment. Current recommendations for preparations licensed in the US range from 0.4–3.3 mg/kg/min for Gammagard®, to 0.5–4.0 mg/kg/min for Gamimune-N®, to 15–60 mg/min (not weight determined) for Sandoglobulin®. The rate for Sandoglobulin® equates to approximately 3 mg/kg/min for a 50-kg patient. Sandoglobulin® is provided as a lyophilized powder that does not contain NaCl, which is in the diluent fluid. Thus, it is possible to reconstitute Sandoglobulin® at concentrations higher than the 3–6% currently recommended.

In order to determine the practicality of infusing Sandoglobulin® at much higher rates of infusion and concentrations, we studied 16 patients with primary disorders of humoral immunity. All patients had a history of receiving IVIG on a regular schedule without adverse reactions. In the first portion of the study the concentration of Sandoglobulin® was increased from 6 to 12% to determine whether that would be tolerated. In the second portion the flow rate was increased to 5 mg/kg/min and if no reactions occurred, the time of each successive infusion was decreased by 10 min until infusions were completed in 15–20 min or vasomotor reactions occurred.

Thirteen of the 16 patients completed the study, having received 8–14 infusions. Six patients achieved reaction-free rates >15 mg/kg/min (30.6, 24.2, 16.2, 26.9, 25.8, and 24.2), and the others ranged from 7.1 to 12 mg/kg/min. In several of the patients, venous access was the limiting factor. Infusion times were below 30 min in 7 patients, with 4 completing infusions in 15 min. There were 14 reactions in 159 infusions in this group, but only 4 infusions were interrupted and none were not completed. Most consisted of fever and chills, and often occurred at the end or after the infusion. Three patients were not able to complete the study, having received 2, 3, and 6 infusions. There were 8 reactions in 11 infusions with 2 interrupted and 3 incomplete. Only one patient had a severe reaction with shaking chills and circumoral cyanosis at the end of the infusion which was given at 3.67 mg/kg/min, but he resolved with only infusion of normal saline.

In conclusion, 13 of 16 patients were able to achieve infusions rates of Sandoglobulin® as much as 10 times the standard rates now recommended. Adverse reactions occurred in 8.8% of the infusions in this group, but none were severe enough to prevent completion of the infusion. Three patients dropped from the study due to adverse reactions. Infusion times for doses of 400 mg/kg were as short as 15 min, but difficult venous access limited some patients from reaching these rates. Thus, rapid infusion of 12% solutions of Sandoglobulin® are practical in the majority of patients with immune deficiency and can greatly decrease the inconvenience to the patient and improve efficiency in the physician's office.

NEONATAL INFECTIONS

IgG subclasses in critically ill premature infants treated with intravenous immunoglobulins

V. PUCCIO, M. SOLIANI, L. BONI, A. BIANO, F. PUNCUH, L. BRUNELLI, M. L. MASSONE, S. FOSSA and P. CORNAGLIA-FERRARIS

Gaslini Research Children's Hospital, Genoa, Italy

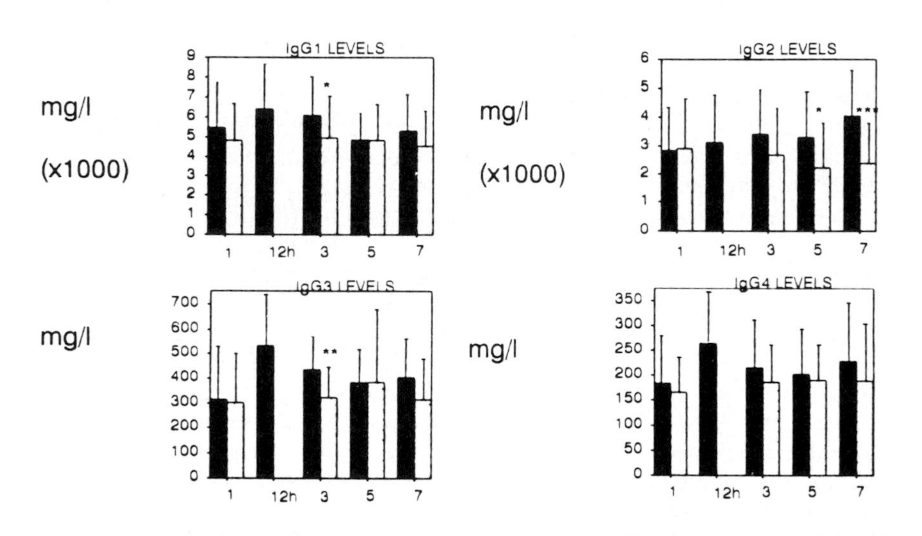

Group 1: ▬ Gest. age 31 ± 3 wks. Birth weight 1315 ± 364 g. Apgar 1': 3.7 ± 2.2; Apgar 5': 6.6 ± 3.3. Ded./total 4/25. Septic./total 3/25.

Group 2: ▭ Gest. age 31 ± 2.4 wks. Birth weight 1455 ± 361. Apgar 1' 5 ± 2.3; Apgar 5' 7 ± 1.8. Ded./total 6/33. Septic./total 7/33.

IgG subclass serum levels have been evaluated in 58 critically ill premature infants (needing mechanical ventilation and intensive therapy). Twenty-five patients (group 1, black bars) were treated with antimicrobial chemotherapy (CT) associated with intravenous IgG (IVIG) (500 mg/kg as a single dose within 12 h from birth), while 33 (group 2, white bars) received only CT. IgG subclass serum levels were evaluated in both groups from day + 1 to + 7. After 2 h from the end of Ig infusion, only group 1 patients reached IgG subclass levels statistically not different from term neonates. IgG_1 and IgG_3 levels were significantly higher in group 1 only at the 3rd day, while IgG_2 became significantly higher at the 5th and 7th postnatal day. IgG_4 serum levels never reached a statistical difference. Results suggest that the dose of IVIG administered in the present study, allowed IgG serum levels similar to term neonate only 12 h after infusion. Moreover, a different kinetic pattern from each IgG subclass is suggested. Clinical correlations between gestational age, birth weight, degree of RDS, infection prophylaxis and IgG subclasses will be presented and discussed. (* $P < 0.05$; ** $P < 0.02$; *** $P < 0.01$).

Use of intravenous immunoglobulin in the prevention of sepsis in very low birth weight infants

B. VAN OVERMEIRE and P. VAN REEMPTS

Neonatal Intensive Care Unit, University Hospital Antwerpe, Belgium

Newborns and especially prematures and infants of very low birth weight (< 1500 g) are immunologically immature. The incidence of sepsis is very high in this group of infants, and ranges from 1 to 30% in neonatal intensive care units.

We evaluated the prophylactic effect of intravenously administered immune globulin (IVIG) on the occurrence of infection in very low birth weight infants.

Of the 98 infants initially enrolled, 87 were randomly assigned to either IVIG (39) or no prophylactic treatment (48). The two groups were comparable by gestational age, birth weight, non-infectious complications and intensive care manipulations.

Serum was drawn shortly after birth for serum IgG determination. Within 12 h of birth, those infants assigned to treatment received 500 mg of IVIG. This dose was repeated for 6 consecutive days. Thereafter one dose a week was administered for 3 more weeks. After a period of 28 days IgG serum levels were determined again.

IgG levels were significantly higher ($P < 0.001$) in the treated group after 28 days. There was, however, no difference in the outcome between the two groups: in the treated group the incidence of infection was 21.8%, in the non-treated group 22.2%.

We conclude from these data that prophylactic administration of IVIG cannot prevent infections in VLBW infants, despite a significant sustained increase of IgG levels in most cases.

A control trial of I.V. immunoglobulins for the prevention of nosocomial infections in very low birth weight neonates

S. PHOTOPOULOS, O. MARALOGLOU, A. MANDALENAKI and M. XANTHOU

Neonatal Intensive Care Unit and Immunology Dept, "Aghia Sophia" Children's Hospital, Athens, Greece

It is well known that the deficiency in host defense mechanisms of very low birth weight neonates is due partly to their very low immunoglobulin levels at birth. In order to reduce nosocomial infections we tried the i.v. administration of immunoglobulins very soon after birth. In 45 VLBW neonates (body weight < 1500 g) IVIG were started within 48 h of birth. A daily dose of 0.5 g Sandoglobulin® was given for 6 consecutive days. Thirty-two comparable neonates who did not receive IV immunoglobulins served as controls. Serum immunoglobulins levels of the 45 neonates before the administration of immunoglobulin were 425 ± 132 mg% and rose to 1550 ± 305 mg% after the completion of therapy, six days later. The half-life of the administered immunoglobulins was found to be 21.7 days. Of the 45 neonates who received immunoglobulins 8 (18%) developed nosocomial infections at postnatal mean age of 24, 3 days, while 12 (38%) out of thirty two neonates without immunoglobulins developed infection at a mean post-natal age of 10 days ($P < 0.05$). From our results it can be seen that the prophylactic administration of IV immunoglobulins helps in preventing nosocomial infections and that a further administration of immunoglobulins is advisable around the third week of postnatal age.

Postnatal prophylaxis of infections in preterm neonates: effect of IVIG on the rate of endogenous IgG production

F. KANAKOUDI, V. DROSOU, P. PRATSIDOU, G. PARDALOS and A. ANDEROU

1st Dept of Pediatrics, University of Thessaloniki and Neonatal Unit, Ippocration Hospital of Thessaloniki, Greece

In this prospective study, serum immunoglobulin levels (IgG, IgA, IgM) and IgG subclasses of 66 preterm neonates (GA ≤ 34 weeks) were measured longitudinally from birth to 12 months of age. The neonates were randomly divided into two groups comparable for gestational age and birth weight. Group A consisted of 33 newborns who received prophylactically IVIG (0.5 g/kg). 13/33 infants in this group had a birth weight (BW) of less than

Table 1 Mean serum IgG concentrations (g/l) at different ages in the study and control groups

	Groups of preterm neonates	n	Time of IgG measurement					
			1^{st}d	1^{st}m	3^{rd}m	5^{th}m	7^{th}m	12^{th}m
A_1	BW < 1500 g	13	6.5	6.36*	3.54	4.33	5.78	6.96
B_1	BW < 1500 g	11	5.7	3.37*	2.74	4.06	5.71	7.67
A_2	BW > 1500 g	20	7.70	7.58**	3.35	4.37	4.99	7.75
B_2	BW > 1500 g	22	7.11	4.17**	2.66	3.93	5.11	7.87

* $P = 0.003$, ** $P < 0.0001$.

1500 g ($\bar{x} = 1283 \pm 101$, group A_1) and 20/33 had a BW of 1500–2000 g ($\bar{x} = 1787 \pm 115$, group A_2). Group B consisted of 33 neonates who did not receive IVIG and served as the control group. 11/33 infants in this group had a BW of less than 1500 g ($\bar{x} = 1276 \pm 118$, group B_1) and 22 had a BW of 1500–2000 g ($\bar{x} = 1776 \pm 152$, group B_2). The results of subsequent measurements of IgG concentration in the above groups are summarized in Table 1.

Comparison of the mean IgG values between the groups A_1–B_1 and A_2–B_2 showed that the IgG concentration during the 1st month of life was significantly higher in groups A_1 and A_2 than in the control groups B_1 and B_2 ($P < 0.005$). However, during the following months, no significant difference was found in the mean IgG levels between the study and control groups ($P > 0.05$). Similar results were obtained regarding measurements of IgG subclasses. These findings suggest that administration of IVIG for revention of neonatal infections in preterm infants (BW 1000–2000 g) does not influence the rate of endogenous production of IgG and consequently the duration or severity of normal hypogammaglobulinemia of infancy.

IVIG therapy in preterm neonates with high risk of infection at birth

R. CEREZO, R. FIGUEROA and J. RODAS

Newborn Intensive Care Unit, IGSS, Guatemala City, Guatemala

One hundred preterm neonates of less than 1500 g with high risk of infection were managed and studied at the intensive care unit of IGSS, Guatemala. They were randomly assigned to two groups: group A (50 patients) receiving 0.5 g/kg/4 days of IVIG plus antibiotics, and the control group B (50 patients) receiving antibiotics only. Both groups were alike for other variables and received the supportive care necessary for their condition. The percentage of positive blood cultures in group A was 16%, and in the control group was

12%. Even though in the group treated with Sandoglobulin® and antibiotics we found a higher percentage of positive blood cultures, we were able to show a reduction in mortality, which was statistically significant ($P < 0.05$) when compared to the control group. No side effects were observed in patients treated with IVIG in the follow-up period.

From our study, we recommend the use of IVIG plus antibiotics in patients with suspected sepsis, or in preterm neonates at risk of infection with very low levels of IgG at birth.

The effect of single-dose i.v. human gammaglobulin on the serum immunoglobulin levels of premature infants, below 2000 g

M. A. AKŞİT, C. SANDIKLI, Z. KILIÇ, F. AKŞİT and N. AKGÜN

Neonatology Unit of Anadolu University Teaching and Training Hospital, Medical Faculty, Eskişehir, Turkey

A single dose, 500 mg/kg, i.v. human gammaglobulin (Sandoglobulin®), was given to 15 premature infants which were below 2000 g. The newborn infants were between 31–37 weeks of gestational age (average 33.4 weeks), 1400–1900 g in weight (average 1686.6 g), 10 were appropriate for gestational age (AGA), 5 were small for gestational age (SGA) and all were below the age of 4 days at the infusion date. Six mothers had prenatal problems during pregnancy, 12 of 15 newborn infants had infections but only 5 died due to sepsis neonatorum; 2 also had respiratory distress syndrome (RDS) apart from sepsis.

Serum immunoglobulin levels were determined by radial-immunodiffusion. Samples were taken before the infusion, then 15 minutes after the infusion and on day 4 and day 7 afterwards. Average immunoglobulin levels were as follows: (1) before the administration ($n = 15$); IgG: 718.8 mg/dl, IgM: 19.77 mg/dl, IgA: 0 mg/dl; (2) 15 min after infusion ($n = 15$); IgG: 1156.3 mg/dl, IgM: 27.91 mg/dl, IgA: 14 mg/dl; (3) after 4th day ($n = 9$); IgG: 1008.22 mg/dl, IgM: 40.41 mg/dl, IgA: 13.12 mg/dl; (4) after 7th day ($n = 5$); IgG: 799 mg/dl, IgM: 45.02 mg/dl, IgA: 10.5 mg/dl.

When we compared the values in the infants, according to their previous serum immunoglobulin levels and after 15 min of i.v. gammaglobulin perfusion, IgG and IgA values were significantly increased ($P < 0.01$, $P < 0.05$ respectively). At the 4th day, only IgM levels were remarkably high ($P < 0.05$). But, at the 7th day, all immunoglobulin titers were the same as pre-administration levels.

Although immunoglobulin levels were not significantly higher at the 7th day after infusion than the first level, it seems that IgG levels were near the base line, IgM levels gradually increased up to 2.3-fold, IgA levels were the same as the 15 min level.

Sandoglobulin® is a human gammaglobulin. We encountered the effect not only on IgG, but also on IgM and IgA. For vital support immunoglobulins are not the sole factor but an important one. Antibiotics are also a prime factor in the treatment of sepsis neonatorum, but not the only one to return newborn infants to life.

Oral monomeric IgG administration in necrotizing enterocolitis (NEC) prevention

FRANCA BENINI, MARIELLA SALA and F. F. RUBALTELLI

Pediatrics Department, University of Padua, Italy

Necrotizing enterocolitis is one of the major causes of morbidity and mortality in LBW preterm neonates. We evaluated the efficacy of oral monomeric IgG administration on its prevention. In a randomized clinical trial, we studied 100 newborns of birth weight of less than 1500 g and gestational age of less than 34 weeks for whom breast milk from their mothers was not available. According to the protocol used, 500 mg IgG, divided in 5 doses, were given per os for the first 2 weeks of life. None of the 50 treated infants developed NEC during the period of oral administration. In the control group, we had 4 cases of NEC during the first 2 weeks of life. One of these died of NEC, but the other three newborns had a favorable disease course. One of the treated infants developed NEC 2 days after the cessation of oral prophylaxis. This newborn didn't need surgery and didn't have early or late complications. The number of preterm infants studied up to now has been limited. However, it is close to statistical significance ($P = 0.14$). It seems that the oral monomeric IgG administration could prevent the development of NEC in LBW infants.

Decreased extrinsic viral resistance (EVR) of neonatal neutrophils

R. L. ROBERTS, B. J. ANK, H. H. ZHU and E. R. STIEHM

UCLA Department of Pediatrics, Los Angeles, California, USA

Neutrophils are essential for preventing bacterial infection but their anti-viral properties have not been established. We investigated the ability of Percoll-isolated neutrophils to inhibit viral replication using an EVR technique. Cultured Vero cells infected with herpes simplex I virus (HSV) were exposed to neutrophils for 18 h at 37°C. The neutrophils and infected Vero cells were removed from the plates, then frozen and thawed (× 3) to lyse the intact cells. The number of viral particles were assayed by the ability of the lysate to form viral plaques in another Vero cell monolayer. Normal adult neutrophils reduced the log number of plaques by 1.036 ± 0.175 ($n = 13$) when pre-activated with phorbol myristate acetate (PMA) which was allowed to bind to neutrophils at 4°C (100 ng/ml) followed by washing to remove unbound PMA. Neonatal neutrophils from cord blood were only able to reduce the plaques by 0.523 ± 0.213 log ($n = 5$) under the same conditions. Eosinophil-enriched cell populations caused a greater reduction in plaques, while neutrophils from patients with chronic granulomatous disease were much less effective than normal neutrophils. These results are similar to those obtained with a new EVR assay using HSV-infected CEM cells in suspension as targets.

These results indicate that different granulocyte populations have a wide range of antiviral activity and that neutrophil treatment of viral diseases may be appropriate in certain situations, particularly in the newborn.

HIV INFECTION

Infections in children with HIV infection treated with intravenous immunoglobulin (IVIG) and zidovudine (AZT)

P. D'ARGENIO, G. CASTELLI GATTINARA, B. LIVADIOTTI, M. CANIGLIA and L. ELIA

Ospedale Bambino Gesù IRCCS, Rome, Italy

A variety of serious infections are frequent in HIV-infected patients. Bacterial infections are particularly frequent in children despite the finding of significant hypergammaglobulinemia, while antibody responses are functionally impaired. This study points out the type and frequency of treatment before and during AZT–IVIG treatment in 10 HIV-infected children, followed for more than 6 months. All the children were vertically infected and have evidence of HIV infection: 6 of them responding to the CDC AIDS criteria. Patients simultaneously received 400–600 mg AZT/m^2 per day perorally and 400 mg IVIG/kg/month, starting at a mean age of 14.5 months (range 3–38) and followed for a mean period of 15.5 months (range 6–36). During the 145 person-months observation period before treatment the 10 children showed 27 infectious episodes: 11 bacterial (7 pneumonia, 1 sepsis, 1 parotiditis); 11 mycotic (10 persistent oral candidiasis, 1 oesophagitis); 3 viral (herpetic infections); 2 protozoal (*Pneumocystis carinii* pneumonia). Since the start of this treatment children were followed for a total period of 155 person-months, showing relevant reduction in number (12) and seriousness of infections: 5 bacterial infections (4 pneumonia, 1 pulmonary abscess); 4 mycotic (persistent oral candidiasis); 2 viral (CMV hepatitis, herpetic infection); 1 protozoal (*Pneumocystis carinii* pneumonia—patient who died).

In conclusion our preliminary study seems to indicate clinical benefit of this treatment for symptomatic HIV-infected children.

A random study of the IVIG role in the treatment of adult patients with ARC and AIDS

N. MONGIARDO, V. BORGHI, C. MUSSINI, F. PELLEGRINO and B. DE RIENZO

Department of Infectious and Tropical Diseases, University of Modena, Italy

Even though some authors have suggested that patients infected by human immunodeficiency virus (HIV) could receive some benefits from therapy with human intravenous immunoglobulins (IVIG) at high doses, no controlled study has been done, yet. There are some theoretical assumptions for this treatment. Low IgG_2 serum levels, insufficient antibody response against neo-antigens in spite of a polyclonal activation of B cells, recurrent bacterial infections of the respiratory tract by capsulated organisms have been documented in HIV patients. The granulocytopenia induced by zidovudine (AZT) could be itself an indication for IVIG therapy.

Eight HIV-positive patients (5 ARC, 3 AIDS), 7 male and 1 female, mean age = 34 years (range 27–48), randomly enlisted among 85 patients in therapy with AZT, have been treated with the following therapy: human intact IVIG at the dose of 300 mg/kg every 15 days for 6 months and AZT at the dose of 600–1000 mg/day. The control group for the clinic observations was made up of 77 patients in therapy only with AZT, and 6 among these patients were random–enlisted to constitute the control group for the IgG subclass assay.

At the end of the study there was no significant statistical difference between patients treated with IVIG and the control group in the incidence of infections: bacterial ($P = 0.1$); viral ($P = 0.2$); protozoal ($P = 0.6$). Mycotic infections were significantly fewer in the control group ($P = 0.006$). In the group of treated, no patients with ARC developed AIDS, while in the control group 3 patients with ARC developed AIDS. Cell-mediated immunity didn't show any alteration in the treated group, while important and significant alterations have been observed in IgG subclass assays between the two groups before and after the treatment.

This study, in spite of the low number of treated patients and the short observation period, shows that IVIG therapy in adult patients with ARC and AIDS does not seem to be a determinant factor in the prevention of opportunistic infections, nor of bacterial infection, even if under treatment a positive modification of the humoral immunologic pattern could be documented. It is possible that also in the bacterial infections of adult HIV patients cell-mediated immunity could play a role of primary importance.

Intravenous immunoglobulin for treatment of HIV-infected adult patients

F. PUPPO, S. ROGNA, A. TORRESIN, R. RUZZENENTI, A. FARINELLI and F. INDIVERI

ISMI, Cattedra di Metodologia Clinica 1, University of Genova, Genova, Italy

Human immunodeficiency virus type 1 (HIV)-infected patients often develop a functionally ineffective hypergammaglobulinemia associated with imbalancement in IgG subclasses, autoantibodies and circulating immune complex. Intravenous immunoglobulin (IVIG) treatment in pediatric AIDS seems established. We treated with IVIG (200 mg/kg) 15 HIV-positive hypergammaglobulinemic subjects. Each patient received from 10 to 30 IVIG infusions at weekly intervals. Half of the IVIG infusions were coupled with plasma exchange to remove immunoglobulin excess, autoantibodies and immune complexes. IVIG treatment was well tolerated and major toxicities were not recorded. In all patients we observed a prompt clinical amelioration, weight gain and resolution of fever and infections, when present. A better survival rate and natural course of HIV infection was observed in IVIG-treated patients as compared with an untreated historical control group. The follow-up is, however, at present too short to draw any definitive conclusion.

In 5 patients the serum opsonizing activity against bacteria by polymorphonuclear cells from healthy donors was also evaluated. The impaired opsonizing activity of HIV-positive sera was significantly increased following IVIG treatment. We suggest that IVIG associated with plasma exchange is a useful supportive treatment for HIV-positive hypergammaglobulinemic adult patients.

TOLERABILITY AND SAFETY

Long-term safety and tolerability of Sandoglobulin® for intravenous use

M. A. HANY[1], A. RYAN[2], J. FARRANT[2] and A. D. B. WEBSTER[2]

[1] *Kinderspital Zürich, Switzerland;* [2] *Clinical Research Centre, Harrow, UK*

We studied a large group of patients (54) having been treated i.v. with immunoglobulin (Sandoglobulin®) either at home or in the hospital environment. They were monitored over a mean period of 33.8 months. The mean frequency of i.v. application was every 2.07 weeks. A total of 3816 infusions were given. The mean dose was 0.226 g/kg body weight.

Since other preparations have had to be abandoned during initial clinical trials after they were found to transmit non-A non-B hepatitis viruses, we monitored liver enzymes with regard to safety.

The patients also returned a questionnaire asking about the tolerability of the intravenous infusions and the nature of any immediate or delayed reaction.

In conclusion, using liver enzymes as a parameter for ongoing hepatitis, we had to examine any patient with altered liver enzymes (ALAT, alkaline phosphatase, gGT) in order to look for any alternative cause for their pathology. The five cases with alterations could be explained reasonably by causes other than hepatitis (e.g. lymphoma, bowel disease). We conclude, therefore, that no hepatitis was transmitted. Only a small number of patients were prone to reactions, and most of these were mild. None of the reactions were significant enough to stop home therapy.

High-dose intravenous IgG treatment is responsible for a transient impairment of renal function in patients with renal diseases

J. A. SCHIFFERLI, H. FAVRE, P. IMBACH[1], U. NYDEGGER[2], K. DAVIES[3] and M. LESKI

Division de Néphrologie, Hôpital Cantonal Universitaire, Genève, Switzerland, [1] Zentrallabor des Blutspendedienstes SRK, Bern; [2] Hämatologisches Zentrallabor, Inselspital, Bern, Switzerland; and [3] Department of Medicine, RPMS, Hammersmith Hospital, London

Recent reports have suggested that therapy with high-dose intravenous (i.v.) IgG may be beneficial in patients with nephrotic syndrome due to membranous or lupus nephritis.

To evaluate these preliminary observations, we started an open trial of high-dose IVIG therapy in nephrotic patients with glomerulonephritis. The six patients included to date demonstrated a transient rise in plasma creatinine whilst receiving IgG (0.4 g/kg/day for 5 days). The highest rise was observed in a patient with impaired renal function: pretreatment creatinine 293 μmol/l, post-infusion: 650 μmol/l, 2 weeks later: 295 μmol/l). Clearance studies were performed before and immediately after treatment in three of these patients who received two series of infusions. The increase in plasma creatinine was attributable exclusively to a modification in tubular transport of creatinine in two of these patients, while in the third, a fall in glomerular filtration rate was also observed.

Two other patients (with pre-existing renal impairment, but without nephrotic syndrome) are also described, in whom a transient and reversible rise in plasma creatinine occurred directly following IVIG therapy for idiopathic thrombocytopenic purpura, and acquired factor VIII deficiency, respectively. The latter became transiently oliguric.

These observations suggest that high-dose IVIG infusion can produce short-lived perturbations in renal function in patients with heavy proteinuria or pre-existing renal impairment.

Safety of intravenous immunoglobulins: a prospective multicenter non-comparative open-label trial to exclude the risk of transmission of non-A, non-B hepatitis

P. AFFENTRANGER, B. A. PERRET and P. IMBACH

Central Laboratory, SRC Blood Transfusion Service, Bern, Switzerland

The safety of intravenous immunoglobulin (IVIG) preparations in relation to a possible transmission of non-A, non-B hepatitis (NANBH) is difficult to ascertain. In fact some clinical centers have reported that experimental lots of IVIG transmited NANBH.

The aim of the study was to demonstrate that pH 4-treated IVIG (Sandoglobulin®) does not transmit NANBH. Five batches of IVIG were prepared and distributed to the five collaborating clinical centers. With one exception each of the centers received IVIG from one batch only. 81 patients with primary immunodeficiency were enrolled.

After a 4-week evaluation period 68 patients (41 adults and 27 children) were eligible. Treatment consisted of three infusions of 200 mg IVIG/kg body weight at 2-week interval. During the treatment period and the following 20 weeks the patients were monitored at regular time intervals (biweekly during the first 12 weeks and then in 3–4 week interval). Liver function tests (ALAT, ASAT, GGT, AP, bilirubin) as well as an examination especially aimed at hepatitis symptomatology were performed.

All of the 68 patients completed the study. None of the patients had clinical signs of hepatitis and the monitoring of the liver function tests revealed no liver dysfunction during the whole study period.

In conclusion, this study supports the safety of pH 4-treated IVIG manufactured by the Central Laboratory of the Swiss Red Cross Blood Transfusion Service in relation to NANBH transmission.

SECONDARY IMMUNODEFICIENCY

Use of intravenous immunoglobulin (IVIG) in patients with multiple trauma

C. MANCINI[1], C. NAZZARI[1], G. RAPONI[1], M. T. LUN[1], F. FILADORO[1], M. ANTONELLI[2] and R. A. DE BLASI[2]

[1] *II Cattedra di Microbiologia Università "La Sapienza", Roma, Italy;*
[2] *Istituto di Anestesiologia e Rianimazione Università "La Sapienza", Roma, Italy*

Patients with multiple trauma often develop bacterial infections during their hospital stay. Those treated in intensive care units may have an infection rate approaching 20%. The development of infections represents a serious hazard to patients' well-being and is responsible for a loss of patient care time together with increasing cost in their hospital stay. The rare occurrence of bacterial infections in healthy individuals indicates that a disruption in host defense precedes infection. One of the most important host defense mechanisms concerns the opsonization of microorganisms: deposition of specific antibodies and activated complement factors on the bacterial membrane. IVIG, gained from pooled serum of normal donors, has been shown to contain opsonic activity against a number of clinical isolate Gram-positive and Gram-negative bacteria. We tested in a randomized double-blind study the efficacy of IVIG, associated with conventional antibiotic therapy, in the prevention of infections in patients with multiple trauma. Inclusion in the study required the presence of two or more long-bone fractures with or without cranial and/or thoracic trauma. Patients treated with 2 g × 4 of piperacillin, were divided in two groups: one receiving 250 mg/kg of IVIG on the 1st and 7th day from the admission and another receiving sterile saline as placebo. Sera were collected 1 h before and 24 h after each IVIG administration. Serum opsonic activity was tested by measuring phagocytosis by neutrophils from healthy individuals of radiolabeled *Escherichia coli* ATCC 25922 opsonized in IVIG treated patients' sera and compared to that of patients with antibiotic only. Also, C3 complement fraction and total IgG and IgM concentration was determined.

The effectiveness of prophylactic intravenous immunoglobulin on the incidence of septicemia in leukemic children

S. GRAPHAKOS, J. PANAGIOTOU, E. VRACHNOU, V. KITRA, S. POLYCHRONOPOULOU, K. MANDALENAKI and S. HAIDAS

Department of Haematology, Immunology and 1st Department of Pediatrics, Athens University, "Aghia Sophia" Children's Hospital, Athens, Greece

Since March 1989, 39 leukaemic children on induction, remission or consolidation chemotherapy have been randomized to receive (19 patients, group A) or not to receive (20 patients, group B) intravenous immunoglobulin 0.4 g/kg body weight every 15 days for 3 months. There was no difference between the two groups on the duration of neutropenia (group A: 27.8 ± 17.7 days; group B: 23.4 ± 13.0 days) and the duration of febrile episodes (group A: 7.3 ± 5.5 days; group B: 8.4 ± 7.4 days). However, patients receiving immunoglobulin had significantly fewer episodes of septicemia during the 4-month observation period, with 1 (5.2%) patient in group A having 1 episode compared to 7 (35%) patients in the control group. Two patients died in group B (1 from septicemia). Eight (72.7%) types of organisms isolated from blood cultures were Gram-positive cocci while 3 (27.3%) were Gram-negative bacteria. None of the patients experienced complications with the immunoglobulin infusion.

Although the group of patients is low, these results suggest that the administration of IVIG may be effective in decreasing the incidence of septicemia in leukemic children receiving intensive chemotherapy.

Treatment of Gram-negative septic toxic diseases with an immunoglobulin preparation containing IgG, IgM and IgA: A prospective randomized clinical trial

I. SCHEDEL, U. DREIKHAUSEN, B. NENTWIG, M. HÖCKENSCHNIEDER, M. RAUTHMANN and S. BALIKCIOGLU

Department of Clinical Immunology, Medical University of Hannover, FRG

In a clinical study, 55 patients with septicemia were randomly allocated to two groups. One group of patients received a commercially available immunoglobulin preparation containing high titers of IgG, IgM and IgA antibodies specific for endotoxic determinants during the first 3 days after inclusion in the study. The other group did not receive any immunoglobulin preparation. During the observation period of up to 6 weeks after the beginning of clinically apparent septicemia, death related to the septic process occurred in one out of 27 patients who received immunoglobulin. By comparison, nine patients of the control group ($n = 28$) died during this period (chi square test: $P < 0.01$).

Within the first 48 h after onset of the clinically apparent septic process significantly elevated activity of circulating endotoxin and simultaneously decreased specific IgG-serum titers to lipid A were detected in the group of patients who did not survive.

Prophylaxis and treatment with IVIG in acute leukemic patients with severe sepsis

U. DI PRISCO[1] and C. SGUOTTI[2]

[1] *Dept of Hematology, University of Modena, Italy;* [2] *Sandoz, Milan, Italy*

In patients with hematologic malignancies cytoreductive and radiation therapies cause moderate to severe immunodeficiencies involving both cellular and humoral mechanisms. As a result, they are more susceptible to infections which, according to recent reports, are the cause of death in more than 70% of patients with acute leukemia.

A historical comparative study in infected neutropenic patients with acute leukemia was carried out to evaluate the efficacy of IVIG (Sandoglobulin®) plus antibiotics vs. antibiotics alone (historical group). The IVIG group was composed of 30 patients (13 ALL and 17 AML), each of whom received IVIG 0.4 g/kg on the first day of clinical evidence of infection and for a further 3 days. Patients with severe infections received additional administration on the 5th and the 8th day. There were no differences in the age, body weight, sex or disease status between the two groups. Survival was 80% (24/30 patients) in the IVIG group vs. 60% (18/30 patients) in controls (historical group). Moreover, the IVIG group had a shorter median period of infection, shorter duration of fever and fewer days of hospitalization. In order to prevent the development of infections, IVIG was administered to a further group of 30 patients at risk for sepsis (12 ALL and 18 AML) at a dose of 0.2 g/kg/day for 7 days every fortnight for 3 cycles. Survival in this group was 95%. There was also a reduced incidence of severe sepsis (5/30, 17%). These results suggest that there is a benefit from long-term prophylaxis with IVIG although further studies need to be undertaken to confirm our data.

IVIG treatment in the well-being of cancer patients (preliminary results)

M. J. HADJIHANNAKIS, CH. KOUFOS, D. LOUFA, CH. PAPADEMETRIOU and KAT. KONIAVITOU-HADJIYANNAKI

Cancer Unit, Physiological Pathology Dept Medical School, Athens University, Laïkon Hospital, Athens, Greece

Cancer patients were entered into a randomized trial for prophylaxis and treatment with i.v. immunoglobulin (Sandoglobulin®). Nine patients are at present under study, with the following criteria: (1) fever resistant for at least 5 days in triple antibiotic regimen; (2) uncontrolled pain (neo DV paraneoplasmatic); (3) cachexia-anorexia; (4) weakness; and (5) thrombopenia.

Treatment protocol was 24 g Sandoglobulin® infused on day 0 within 8–10 h; the same dose was repeated on day 30.

In all cases fever disappeared on day 5 onwards. There was analgesia present from day 4, while there was a remarkable increase of appetite, decrease in cachexia and weakness, and increase in body strength. There was an obvious well-being of patients within 6–10 days after treatment, continuing for 30 days at least in 3 patients who had already had a second Sandoglobulin® dose. So far, the laboratory findings on day 10 after the first infusion are: (1) increase in thrombocyte count (9/9); (2) decrease in ESR (5/9); and (3) positive Mantoux test (3/9) (prior to treatment negative Mantoux 9/9).

At the moment, and in view of further analysis, IVIG treatment looks very promising in our efforts to enhance the well-being of cancer patients.

High dose of intravenous immunoglobulins in patients receiving bone marrow transplant

V. ZOLI, N. PETTI, F. BLANDINO, A. DE BLASIO, L. DE ROSA, A. MONTUORO, L. PACILLI, L. PESCADOR, A. PESCAROLLO and A. DE LAURENZI

Divisione di Ematologia, Ospedale di San Camillo, Rome, Italy

Infectious complications are a crucial point in the management of transplant patients. The most frequently isolated bacterial and mycotic agents are:

Pseudomonas a., *Staphylococcus* and *Candida*. Interstitial pneumonia due to CMV is a frequent and often fatal complication of bone marrow transplantation. Several studies suggest that prophylaxis with high-dose IVIG can prevent infections after marrow transplantation. From 1985 to 1989 we included the high-dose IVIG in the prophylactic schedule of 62 patients who had received an allogeneic (BMT) or autologous bone marrow transplant (ABMT) or autologous blood stem cells transplant (ABSCT) (16 BMT, 39 AMBT, 7 ABSCT). Conditioning regimens were: Cy + TBI (29 patients); Cy + MLP + TBI (7 patients); Cy + BCNU + VP16 (18 patients); BuCy (7 patients); MLP + Cy (1 patient). High doses of IVIG were given 300/500 mg/kg on day − 7 and 200 mg/kg on days + 8, + 16, + 24, + 32, + 40 and monthly for 6 months. Trimethoprim–sulfamethoxazole, acyclovir and oral adsorbable antibiotics were also administered. After the transplant we observed 3 FUO, 6 bacterial infections (4 *E. coli*, 1 *Pseudomonas a.* and 1 *Staphylococcus* sepsis) and 3 systemic mycosis (*Aspergillus*, *Candida a.*, *Mucor mycosis*). Interstitial pneumonia occurred in only 1 ABMT patient with delayed hematological recovery and in 1 BMT patient with grade 4 aGVHD. We conclude that the high-dose IVIG during the pre- and post-transplant period is well-tolerated and an effective prophylaxis in our patients with significant risk factors such as TBI (36/62 patients) and aGVHD (8/16 patients).

Oral IgG administration in marrow transplant recipients

A. BOSI, S. GUIDI, E. DONNINI, R. SACCARDI, A. M. VANNUCCHI, R. FANCI and P. ROSSI FERRINI

BMT Unit, Dept of Hematology, University of Florence, Italy

In an attempt to decrease the incidence of gastroenteritis as well as systemic infections in patients undergoing marrow transplantation for leukemia or lymphoma, oral immunoglobulins (Sandoglobulin®) were administered according to the protocol of Tutschka *et al.* (*Blood* 1987, 70: 1382–88). Twenty-one consecutive patients were consecutively enrolled into the study. Patient characteristics: mean age 30 years (range 9–57); diagnosis: ALL 5, ANLL 11, CML 4, NHL 1; transplant: allogenic 7, autologous 14; sex: M 14, F 7. All patients received IgG 50 mg/kg/body weight p.o. reconstituted with NaCl 0.9% in 4 divided doses, starting at day + 2 until + 28. Only two patients missed more than a single day's administration of IgG due to nausea: so 19 patients were evaluable. Two patients experienced grade I (WHO) diarrhea, one grade II lasting for 6 days; however, the search for a bacterial agent was negative in any instance. Three patients developed documented bacteremia; the days with fever > 38°C were 4.6 (range 0–16) in the whole patient population.

In our experience oral treatment with immunoglobulins may have a role in preventing systemic infections and gastroenteritis. A randomized study to determine the effectiveness of this treatment is underway at our institution.

AUTOIMMUNITY

IG-induced sustained remission of a steroid-refractory recurrent ITP in an adult patient

BRUNO ROTOLI, FEDERICO CHIURAZZI and LIDIA SANTORO

Division of Hematology, 2nd Medical School, University of Napoli, Italy

High-dose IVIG is an effective (although often transient) treatment for acute idiopathic thrombocytopenic purpura (ITP), while it rarely benefits chronic adult ITP. Since the mechanism of action of IVIG is unknown, it is still unclear what relationship exists between response to prednisone and response to IVIG; in our hands, refractoriness to prednisone (i.e. absence of any platelet increase following 1–2 mg/kg body weight for 2 weeks) is usually associated with poor (absent or transient) response to IVIG. We recently observed a patient who did not follow such an empirical rule. F. P., male, 47 years old, was suffering from recurrent ITP, having had two previous episodes at ages 24 and 40, with very low platelet count and severe bleeding tendency, in both cases controlled by prednisone 100 mg/day. Since there was a suspicion of drug hypersensitivity, the patient had not been given any drug over the last 7 years. Severe mucocutaneous bleeding tendency suddenly reappeared in April 1989; platelets were absent in peripheral blood and increased numbers of megakaryocytes were observed in the bone marrow. Prednisone 100 mg/day for 2 weeks was totally ineffective. High-dose IVIG (Sandoglobulin® 30 g/day for 5 days) was given as a preparation for splenectomy. On the 7th day platelet count was 152 000; on the 11th 195 000. No further treatment was given, and we decided to wait for an initial fall of platelets before performing splenectomy. After 9 months, platelet counts are still > 200 000.

We conclude that high-dose IVIG can be effective in adults with recurrent ITP even when there is evidence of absolute refractoriness to steroids, and that the response can be sustained.

High-dose intravenous gammaglobulin in adults with chronic thrombocytopenic purpura

M. COLOMBI, A. DELLA VOLPE, R. MOZZANA, M. CARDILLO and G. LAMBERTENGHI-DELILIERS

Istituto di Scienze Mediche-Università di Milano, Milan, Italy

We report our experience of the use of high-dose IVIG in 18 adults with chronic idiopathic thrombocytopenic purpura (ITP) (M/F: 7/11) aged 18–76 years (median 28 years). All patients had been previously treated with prednisone; four of them had also received other treatments (2 danazol, 1 danazol and azathioprine, 1 danazol and splenectomy). High-dose IVIG treatment (Sandoglobulin®), 400 mg/kg/day × 5 days, was started 5–132 months after diagnosis because of low platelet (plt) count (2000 to 62 000/μl; median 15 000/μl) or severe corticosteroid side effects. One patient discontinued the IVIG treatment for side effects on the second day; 5 patients also received boosters. Thirteen responders (patients at least tripling initial plt values) showed increases in plt count from the third day of therapy with plt peaks ranging from 45 000 to 470 000/μl (median 167 000/μl). However, this increase was transient in most cases and only 6 patients had a prolonged improvement: 2 maintaining more than 100 000 plt/μl for longer than 2 months after treatment, one of whom received 4 weekly boosters. Five patients showed no response.

Another 3 patients (not included in the above series) were treated with the same dosage of IgG for 3 days before splenectomy. Plt counts rapidly increased to safe levels and all of them underwent surgery without any bleeding complications. High-dose IVIG was well tolerated and boosters did not significantly increase overall length of response.

High-dose IVIG may be useful in ITP when a rapid increase in plt count is needed as in bleeding emergencies or before splenectomy.

Successful CAVB surgery on a patient with chronic ITP after extracorporeal removal of immunoglobulins and high-dose IVIG therapy

J. G. KADAR, P. GRIEB, N. SCHWICK, H. H. HILGER, E. R. DEVIVIE and H. BORBERG

Department of Medicine I and III, Department of Cardiac Surgery, University of Cologne, Cologne, FRG

The patient, a 64-year-old diabetic male with the classic criteria of chronic autoimmune thrombocytopenia (platelet count < 10 G/l, elevated PaIgG and typical bone marrow smear), presented for invasive studies for severe angina pectoris. The ITP was not previously treated. To enable coronary arteriography a platelet count of at least 40 G/l was required. Steroids were not indicated due to his diabetes, thus selective immunadsorption using tryptophan–Heparin–agarose columns (3 times qd, 100% of plasma volume processed per session) combined with immunomodulative therapy (IVIG, 0.4 g/kg body weight qd × 5) was initiated. Coronary arteriography, performed after the platelets had increased to 43 G/l, indicated the need for bypass surgery. The platelet count subsequently decreased. To allow surgery, IVIG (0.4 g/kg body weight × 7 days) was again administered, increasing the platelet count to 51 G/l. On the day of surgery, one single donor platelet concentrate was given, raising his platelet count to 81 G/l. Bypass surgery (CABG × 3), requiring the heart–lung machine, was performed without any bleeding complications. After the operation, the platelet count steadily increased (> 300 G/l) and Dipyridamol (50 mg/day) was necessary to actively prevent thromboembolic complications. Subsequently, during this same hospitalization, a prostatectomy became necessary and was performed without any further hematologic support. Again no bleeding complications occurred. Sixty days after bypass surgery, the PaIgG was found to be considerably reduced, demonstrating remission. Ninety days after the bypass surgery the platelet count was 147 G/l and continues to remain at adequate levels.

Immunological evaluation of patients with idiopathic thrombocytopenic purpura treated with high doses of intravenous immunoglobulins

H. TRINDADE, H. CARVALHO, J. CAIXINHA, I. ABREU, J. M. CAETANO and L. ROSADO

Serviço de Imunologia de Faculdade de Ciências Médicas, Universidade Nova de Lisboa, Serviço de Hematologia Infantil, Hospital D. Estefânia, Lisbon, Portugal

The assessment of several immunological data was performed on a group of six children bearing the diagnosis of ITP, and undergoing therapy using high doses of intravenous immunoglobulins. The study was performed on 3 different days: day 0, 10 and 45 after the administration.

The results obtained showed a rise of serum immunoglobulins on the 10th day (IgG, IgA and IgM) with normal levels of IgA and IgM by the 45th day as well as circulating immunocomplexes in all patients before and until the end of the study.

The hemolytic capacity of the serum (CH50) and the C3 levels were not altered by the therapy, although a sharp drop in C4 values was noticed on day 10.

The cellular immunity study did not show any significant alteration in lymphocyte count on peripheral blood with markers CD3, CD4, CD8 and HLA/DR, in any of the days of the study. The test on lymphoblastic transformation by T mitogens points out an increased response 45 days after the beginning of administration of high doses of immunoglobulins. The response to mitogens is altered mainly in the long term (45th day) and this was statistically significant for ConA. This suggests an activation of suppressing/cytotoxic T cells.

Our results point to a possible modulatory role of IVIG by interfering with induction/suppression mechanisms besides Fc blockade, protective action of platelet lining and release of sequestered platelets.

Acute autoimmune thrombocytopenia in childhood: which therapeutic options?

P. MATOS, J. BARBOT, L. VALE, E. COIMBRA, M. CAMPOS, B. JUSTIÇA, and B. VALENTE

Department of Hematology and Pediatrics. H. Santo António Oporto, Portugal

We have studied 39 patients under the age of 11 years old, with clinical and laboratorial criteria of ITP. Eighteen were not treated and 21 were treated either with prednisone (12) or IVIG (9).

The mean time of hospitalization was: 12.8 days for patients not treated; 17.9 days for patients treated with prednisone; and 6.4 days for patients treated with IVIG. Patients treated with prednisone showed a remission rate of 83%. Patients treated with IVIG had a remission rate of 55%.

Some patients may benefit from an expectant attitude and when they have a favorable clinical course no treatment should be given. Therapeutic options in patients with a more aggressive clinical course (hemorrhagic syndrome) can be corticosteroids, which induce a better remission rate but have more side effects and longer hospitalization time, or IVIG, which has no side effects, needs a shorter hospitalization but shows a lower remission rate.

The lower remission rate with IVIG could be explained by the criteria of admission to the treatment or perhaps by an expectant attitude before treatment. These attitudes will be discussed.

Intravenous gammaglobulin as a therapeutic tool in treatment of immune thrombocytopenic purpura in children

S. ARONI, A. VAZAIOU, H. PLATOKOUKI, A. MITSIKA, C. MANDALENAKIS and A. KONSTANTOPOULOS

Haemophilia Unit and First Dept of Pediatrics, Athens University, St Sofia's Children's Hospital, Athens, Greece

Several reports have demonstrated that repeated courses of IVIG therapy may achieve a permanent reversal of thrombocytopenia in a proportion of children with the acute or chronic form of the disease and it has been postulated that if given to every child at the onset of symptoms it might influence the progression to chronicity. We have analyzed the findings from a $4\frac{1}{2}$-year follow-up study of 27 children with ITP (acute ITP = 12, chronic ITP = 15 children) who were treated with IVIG infusions at some stage of their illness. The therapeutic schedule used was 0.4–1 g/kg/day IVIG (Sandoglobulin®, Sandoz) for 3 consecutive days and thereafter one or more boosters if the platelet count fell to $< 30 \times 10^3/\mu l$. Indications for treatment were: (1) acute and massive bleeding, (2) chronicity of disease prior to splenectomy, (3) emergency surgery, and (4) platelet count $< 10 \times 10^3/\mu l$. Twenty-three of 27 patients (85%) responded to IVIG therapy.

The response was independent of previous response to corticosteroid administration. A rapid increase of platelet count to normal values and 2–3-fold increase in serum IgG was observed after the first 3 days course of IVIG. Eleven of 12 (91.6%) children with acute ITP and 6/15 (40%) with chronic ITP were cured. The curative effect of IVIG in children with chronic ITP was related to the number of courses given.

The incidence of side effects was 8.8% and mainly consisted of fever, headache and vomiting. None of the patients developed non-A, non-B hepatitis or HIV antibodies.

Conclusions: Intravenous gammaglobulin appears to be: (a) a useful therapeutic tool for the acutely bleeding child; (b) an ideal therapy for preparing a child for emergency surgery; and (c) an alternative to splenectomy for the child with chronic ITP.

Intravenous gammaglobulin in patients with antiphospholipid antibodies and thrombocytopenia

M. GALLI, S. CORTELAZZO and T. BARBUI

Department of Haematology, Ospedali Riuniti, Bergamo, Italy

Antiphospholipid antibodies (APA), namely lupus anticoagulant (LAC) and anticardiolipin antibodies (ACA) are autoantibodies directed against negatively-charged phospholipids. Their presence is associated with thrombosis, repeated abortions and thrombocytopenia. Recently, we and other authors reported that APA may be transiently suppressed by infusion of high-dose gammaglobulin (IVIG) and in one case an idiotype–anti-idiotype mechanism has been demonstrated. We have extended our experience by evaluating the effect of IVIG infusion in 4 patients with APA and thrombocytopenia and by investigating the idiotype–anti-idiotype interaction between IVIG and APA by *in vitro* studies. IVIG (Sandoglobulin®) infusion (0.4 g/kg/day for 5 days) was followed by a transient disappearance of LAC activity and normalization of platelet count in 1 patient: 1 week later LAC activity was present again and platelet count returned to pretreatment value within 1 month. Also in another case a transient reduction of LAC activity was documented. Plasmatic ACA levels remained unchanged in all cases. *In vitro* studies were performed using total IgG fractions of the 4 patients, which showed LAC activity in an activated partial thromboplastin time (aPTT). 25 μl of IgG (0.5 mg/ml) were incubated with 25 μl of increasing concentrations of IVIG and 100 μl of normal plasma. After 1 h at 37°C and overnight at 4°C, an aPTT was performed on these mixtures. A dose-dependent inhibition (up to 50%) of LAC activity was observed when the molar ratio between patients' IgG and IVIG was between 1:20 and 1:50 (mg:mg, w:w). Our findings indicate that Sandoglobulin® infusion may be useful in patients with APA and thrombocytopenia since the risk of hemorrhage might be reduced by increasing platelet count and the adverse risk of thrombosis might be lowered by decreasing LAC activity.

Intravenous immunoglobulin therapy in rheumatoid arthritis

K. HELMKE[1], H. HATZ[1], H. BECKER[2] and G. MITROPOULOU[2]

[1] *IV Medizinische Abteilung, Rheumatologie-Klinische Immunologie, Akademisches Lehrkrankenhause München-Bogenhausen, FRG;* [2] *Medizinische Klinik III und Poliklinik, Justus-Liebig-Universität, Gießen, FRG*

Thirteen patients with rheumatoid arthritis were treated with intravenous immunoglobulin (IVIG). In 6 patients clinical results were impressive, although lasting responses could be achieved in only 3 patients. Immunological studies on 11 patients showed that this treatment was immunomodulating, since the immunoregulatory T-cell ratio (CD4/CD8) decreased following therapy by reducing CD4-positive cells *in vivo*. By use of anti-μ antibodies as a B-cell specific mitogen, IVIG-treatment was seen to suppress early processes of B-cell activation. In parallel to these cellular effects, IVIG led to a reduction in the levels of polyethylenglycol-precipitated circulating immune complexes as measured by laser nephelometry.

Use of high-dose intravenous immunoglobulin in rheumatoid arthritis: a pilot study of 7 patients

B. TUMIATI, A. BELLELLI and M. VENEZIANI

2nd Department of Medicine, Rheumatology Section, Ospedale S. M. Nuova, Reggio Emilia, Italy

High-dose (400 mg/kg) intravenous gammaglobulin (IVIG) was administered monthly for 6 months to 7 patients with severe rheumatoid arthritis (RA). Age ranged from 23 to 67 years and the disease had been active for 1–6 years. The functional stages were 2 in 5 cases and 3 in 2 cases. All patients failed treatment with NSAIDs and corticosteroids prior to IVIG treatment and in 3 of the cases gold and/or methotrexate had been ineffective.

A 50% improvement of Ritchie index was obtained in 6/7 patients, morning stiffness was reduced from greater than 2 h to less than 30 min in 6/7 patients. Swollen joints and Lee index improved in all patients. ESR did not show any change but RCP improved in 6/7 patients.

The drug was discontinued in 1/4 patients initially treated with corticosteroids, the dose reduced in 2 and remained unchanged in the other patients. Two patients were withdrawn from the study. One for no compliance; one for proteinuria. Renal biopsy showed a type 2 membrano-proliferative glomerulonephritis.

The study of lymphocyte subpopulation showed an increase of $CD20^+$ and $CD3^+$ cells, no significative variation in CD4, CD8 and CD4/CD8 lymphocyte rates and a significant increase in $2H4^+$ T cells without changes in $4B4^+$ subpopulation.

IVIG improves the clinical and laboratory features of patients with severe RA. The major problem in the use of IVIG therapy is the cost, but we think that they can find their place in well-selected patients with RA.

A randomized prospective controlled trial is underway to further determine the efficacy of IVIG in RA.

Effect of high-dose intravenous gammaglobulin on peripheral T-cell subsets from systemic onset juvenile arthritis patients

B. GONZALEZ, C. SEPULVEDA, C. GODOY, R. SALAZAR and C. RODRIGUEZ

Hospital L. Calvo Mackenna and Hospital Clínico Universidad de Chile, Santiago, Chile

The aim of this study was to determine the clinical status and peripheral T-cell subset evolution in 5 systemic onset juvenile arthritis (SOJA) patients treated with high-dose intravenous gammaglobulin (IVIG). The demonstration of important changes at these levels is relevant to support new therapeutic uses of IVIG.

The mean age was 7.2 years (range 2–14) and mean time of evolution was 3.14 years (range 0.9–9). In all patients previous treatment with NSAIDs and systemic steroids had failed. IVIG was administered at a dose of 400 mg/kg daily, for 3 consecutive days. T-cell subsets were determined by indirect immunofluorescence with monoclonal antibodies OKT3, OKT4 and OKT8 before treatment, and at 15 and 30 days after.

Three children presented important clinical improvement concomitantly with significant changes in the T-cell subsets. These patients had a decrease in the CD4/CD8 ratio (− 44.7%) due to an increase in the CD8 lymphocytes (+ 195%) ($P < 0.10$ Wilcoxon T). The two patients who showed no clinical response had an increase in the CD4/CD8 ratio (+ 60.6%), due to a decrease in the CD8 subset (− 40.5%).

These data suggest that IVIG may be helpful in SOJA patients who show an increase in the CD8 subset with this treatment. More children must be studied to confirm these findings.

Treatment of patients with rheumatoid arthritis (RA) with anti-CD4 monoclonal antibodies

W. J. PICHLER, CH. HERZOG, CH. WALKER and W. MUELLER

Institute for Clinical Immunology, University of Bern, Bern, and Dept of Rheumatology, University of Basel, Basel, Switzerland

Eight patients with severe arthritis were treated for 7 days with daily 10 mg anti-CD4 antibody (VIT4 or MT151). No side effects were observed. A partial or complete remission of RA was induced in 7 patients, which lasted between 3 weeks and 12 months. Laboratory parameters were not changed. However, the treatment induced a drastic fall of circulating T cells, mainly of the $CD4^+$ $CDw29^+$ subset, which lasted for 8–10 h. After 24 h, before the next treatment, the lymphocyte values were normalized again. Six of 8 patients developed a weak anti-mouse Ig response. Five of 8 patients had a transient skin anergy ("multitest") during treatment. Functional analysis of *in vivo* antibody-coated $CD4^+$ cells revealed an intact proliferative response, suggesting that mainly the altered cell distribution contributes to the impaired immune response. We conclude that mouse anti-CD4 monoclonal antibody (MoAb) treatment is well-tolerated and that the cellular immunological changes observed are short-lasting. The low incidence of side effects may justify further clinical studies to evaluate the clinical efficacy of such treatment.

Efficacy of high-dose intravenous gammaglobulin in 27 myasthenic patients

M. LOMBARDI, G. PICCOLO, A. ERBETTA and V. COSI

Neurologic Institute C. Mondino, University of Pavia, Italy

Intravenous gammaglobulin treatment has proved effective in myasthenic patients. Previous studies usually deal with a small number of cases. The present report includes 25 females and 2 males, 11–78 year old (mean 39), disease duration 2–232 months (mean 79). Twenty-one patients were thymectomized. All patients were affected by autoimmune generalized myasthenia gravis diagnosed on the basis of clinical, pharmacological and electrophysiological criteria. Nineteen patients had been in a stationary phase for at least 6 months; eight patients were in acute onset or relapsing phase. The clinical severity was graded according to Oosterhuis' global clinical classification myasthenic severity (OGCCMS): the baseline score was $\geqslant 3$ in 24 out of 27 patients. All patients were treated with Sandoglobulin® 0.4 g/kg body weight i.v. on five consecutive days. The clinical outcome was classified as "improved" or "unchanged" according to strict criteria on the basis of OGCCMS score before and 6, 12, 21, 28, 60, 180 days after the treatment. No side effects were noted. Seventeen patients (63.0%) improved, while the other

10 classified as unchanged even if a slight or short-term improvement had been observed in four cases. In eight cases (29.6%) the improvement lasted more than 180 days. The stationary patients did better (68.4%) than acute or relapsing ones (50.0%).

In conclusion high-dose intravenous gammaglobulin treatment is a safe and useful tool in the management of selected myasthenic patients.

MISCELLANEOUS

Induction of IgG subclasses by human T-helper clones

C. DEMBECH, I. QUINTI[1], E. CIMIGNOLI, N. ALBI, A. TERENZI, R. GALANDRINI and A. VELARDI

Dept of Medicine, University of Perugia, Italy; [1] Division of Clinical Immunology University of Rome, Italy

The contrasting IgG subclass distribution patterns for B cells ($IgG_2 > IgG_1$) and serum or plasma cells ($IgG_1 > IgG_2$) suggests that regulatory controls for IgG subclass expression may vary according to B-cell differentiation. In order to gain information on this issue, we established 256 $CD4^+$ T-cell clones and, following pre-activation with PHA, we cultured them with B cells. Interestingly, $CD4^+$ helper clones induced a single subclass or combinations of two subclasses, with negligible production of the others. The most frequent patterns of IgG subclass production were in the order: IgG_1, IgG_2, IgG_1 and IgG_2 together, IgG_3, IgG_4. The relative distribution of the observed subclass-specific helper effects was remarkably similar to the subclass distribution observed in the serum or among peripheral lymphoid tissue plasma cells, i.e. $IgG_1 \approx 60\%$, $IgG_2 \approx 30\%$, $IgG_3 \approx 5–10\%$, $IgG_4 \leqslant 5\%$. Since the IgG subclass distribution at the B-cell level is $IgG_2 > IgG_1$ ($\approx 50\%$ and $\approx 40\%$ respectively) the data suggest that a major factor responsible for the preferential induction of IgG_1, as opposed to IgG_2, antibodies, during B-cell proliferation and differentiation, is represented by the relative predominance of T cells capable of delivering IgG_1-specific, as opposed to IgG_2-specific, helper effects.

High-dose intravenous gammaglobulin in children with intractable epilepsy

A. ETZIONI, M. YAFFE, S. POLLACK, N. ZELNIK, A. BENDERLY and Y. TAL

Dept of Pediatrics and Clinical Immunology, Rambam Medical Center and Dept of Pediatrics, Bnai Zion Medical Center, Faculty of Medicine, Technion, Haifa, Israel

We have studied 8 children (mean age 6.5 years) with intractable epilepsy of various etiologies. Conventional anti-epileptic drugs did not improve their condition and the effect of high-dose gammaglobulin (Sandoglobulin® 200 mg/kg/3 week repeated after 4 weeks) was observed. Clinical, electroencephalographic and immunological studies were performed before and after therapy. T-cell subsets were found to be in the normal range with normal CD4/CD8 ratio. No autoantibodies were detected. Immunoglobulin G, A and M were normal in the serum and no case of IgG subclass deficiency was found. No change was observed post-therapy apart from increase in IgG. In 3 children a marked improvement was noted both in the clinical and the EEG findings. Two stopped all other medication and are currently on monthly injections of i.v. gammaglobulin. In 2 other cases a partial response was noted. No improvement was observed in the other 3 cases. We conclude that although the mechanism is still obscure, high doses of gammaglobulin may have a beneficial effect in a significant number of children with intractable epilepsy.

Quantitation of anti-A and anti-B IgG antibodies in therapeutic i.v. immunoglobulin by indirect ELISA

J. P. BUCHS and U. E. NYDEGGER

Central Laboratory of Hematology, University Hospital, and Regional Red Cross Blood Transfusion Center, Bern, Switzerland

An indirect ABO-ELISA was applied to quantitate anti-blood group A and B IgG antibodies present in seven commercial intravenous immunoglobulin G (IVIG) preparations. The capturing antigen was substance A or B fixed to polystyrene microtiter plates. Bound anti-A and anti-B were revealed with mouse monoclonal anti-human isotype-specific antibodies detected in turn by goat anti-mouse alkaline phosphatase-conjugate. The data obtained with the IVIG preparations were compared to the data obtained with anti-A and anti-B IgG affinity purified on Biosynsorb® and results were expressed as μg specific anti-A/anti-B per g total IgG present in the respective IVIG. In six preparations in which anti-A was detectable, the lowest/highest concentrations of specific anti-A IgG found were 0.32/2.4 μg/g total IgG; thus one molecule specific anti-A IgG was found per 4.1–31 $\times$ 10^5 total IgG molecules. In the seven preparations the anti-B IgG levels varied from 0.44 to

13.37 μg/g total IgG. The titer strength achieved by the same preparations in a hemagglutination test (HAT) varied 8-fold and regression analysis between ELISA and HAT results was significant ($P < 0.05$) for anti-A. It is likely that the higher sensitivity of ELISA and its direct measurement of antibody binding to antigen account for the wider scatter of ELISA results which makes this test suitable for quality control of IVIG.

Modulation of complement by intravenous IgG (IVIG): immediate effect of IVIG administration on levels of C1q, C1r and C1s in hypogammaglobulinemic patients

P. J. SPÄTH, H. ENGLER,* R. SCHERZ, L. MEYER-HÄNNI and A. MORELL

Central Laboratory, Swiss Red Cross Blood Transfusion Service, Bern, Switzerland

C1 levels may be diminished in patients with hypo- or agammaglobulinemia without a clear-cut diminution of total complement hemolytic activity. Replacement therapy normalizes C1 levels within days. C1 is a pentamolecular complex composed of $C1qC1r_2C1s_2$. A reduced turnover of C1q after normalization of IgG levels in such patients was suggested to cause rise of C1 levels. This study addressed two questions with respect to the effect of IVIG administration on C1 levels: (1) is the rise of C1 restricted to C1q alone or are the two other subcomponents C1r and C1s involved too? and (2) is the effect an immediate one or not? Sixteen patients with primary humoral immunodeficiency who did not receive intravenous or intramuscular IgG for more than 6 months were infused with IVIG. Before the first infusion 6 of these patients presented with C1q concentrations below 60% of normal and 4 had levels of C1s or C1r below the lower limit of the normal range, i.e. below 70% and 75%, respectively. Hemolytic activity of the complement system, when assessed by activation via the classical pathway, was apparently not reduced in these patients. Circulating immune complexes, which could have accounted for depressed C1 levels were not observed when assessed by the fluid-phase C1q binding assay. An initial amount of 9–15 g of IgG, administered within 7–9 h, was followed by a rise in concentrations of all three C1 subcomponents by a factor of 1.05–1.5. A rise by factors 2–2.5 of C1q, C1r and C1s was seen in a patient where the initial IgG infusion time had to be prolonged to 30 h because of a severe inflammatory reaction.

We conclude that in hypogammaglobulinemic patients reduced levels of C1q can be associated with reduced levels of C1r and C1s. A rise of circulating IgG by 3.2–5.1 g/l may provoke an immediate rise of all subcomponents of C1. Furthermore, following IgG infusion the pattern of increase in an individual patient was similar for circulating C1q, C1r and C1s.

IVIG inhibits IL-6- but not TNF-α-production *in vitro*

J. ANDERSSON and U. ANDERSSON

Dept of Immunology, Stockholm University, Stockholm, Sweden

The effects of IVIG addition on *in vitro* induced monokine production were studied. Individual peripheral blood monocytes, which produced IL-6 and TNF-α after *in vitro* stimulation were identified by cytokine-specific monoclonal antibodies and immunofluorescence technique (method in *Eur. J. Immunol.* 1989, 19:1157). Lipopolysaccharide (LPS) or *Borrelia burgdorfferi* spirochetes were used to induce TNF-α and IL-6 production in cultures. Peak synthesis occurred 2.5 h after initiation of the cultures in the majority of the monocytes but not at all in lymphocytes. IVIG preparations (Gammagard® or Sandoglobulin®, 6 mg/ml) were added 0.5 h prior to LPS or *Borrelia* exposure and were kept present during the whole culture period. Cultures without IVIG were used as controls.

IL-6 was produced by 64 ± 8 or 71 ± 9% of the monocytes after LPS or *Borrelia* stimulation, respectively. A significant reduction of the number of IL-6-producing monocytes was noted in the IVIG supplemented cultures ($P < 0.003$). In these cultures 24 ± 12 or 29 ± 12% of the monocytes made IL-6 in response to LPS or *Borrelia*. In contrast TNF-α synthesis was not inhibited by IVIG. LPS or *Borrelia* induction resulted in 47 ± 18 or 69 ± 7% TNF-α producing cells versus 48 ± 9 or 59 ± 3% cells in IVIG-supplemented cultures.

These experiments ($n = 12$) indicate down-regulation of IL-6 but not TNF-α production by IVIG. We consider direct antigen neutralization as an unlikely explanation for the divergent effects observed on monokine production after IVIG addition.

IVIG modulation of *in vitro* tumor necrosis factor and neopterin production

J. E. DORAN

Central Laboratory, SRC Blood Transfusion Service, Bern, Switzerland

We have examined the ability of i.v. immunoglobulin (IVIG) to modulate the activation state (as measured by neopterin) and tumor necrosis factor (TNF) production of THP-1 cells, cultured human monocytes derived from buffy coats, or whole-blood preparations stimulated with lipopolysaccharide (LPS). THP-1 cells or freshly prepared monocytes were suspended in serum-free media. Cells were incubated in the presence or absence of human recombinant interferon gamma (IFN) for 18–24 h, at which time IVIG was added to the cells and incubation continued for 2 h. Lastly, LPS was added to the cells, and supernatants harvested at various times. The whole-blood system utilized heparinized blood incubated with IVIG and LPS for a period of 6 h when supernatants were harvested. Tumor necrosis factor was measured using an immunoassay (Medigenix®) or bioassay (L929 cell lysis); neopterin was measured by immunoassay (Henning, Berlin).

TNF production in the THP-1 and buffy model systems is time-dependent, and dependent on both IFN activation and the amount of LPS used as the secondary stimulus. We have found a linear relationship between IFN and neopterin production, and a near linear relationship of neopterin and TNF. In the absence of exogenous LPS, virtually no TNF and neopterin were produced, indicating that both of these signals may be required to "activate" the THP-1 cells. In the presence of IFN, IVIG dose dependently augmented both TNF and neopterin production in LPS-stimulated cultures. In the absence of IFN, TNF but not neopterin was stimulated by IVIG. These stimulatory effects were only seen in the isolated cell systems; whole-blood preparations were not further stimulated by IVIG. We hypothesize that these differences may be related to the serum-free conditions used in the isolated cell systems, where Fc receptor interactions may be promoted to an extent not seen in the more physiologic milieu.

Anti-IgE autoantibodies in intravenous immunoglobulin preparations (IVIG)

S. MIESCHER, M. VOGEL, C. RITTER, E. JAROLIM, M. BÄTTIG, A. L. DE WECK and B. M. STADLER

Institute of Clinical Immunology, Inselspital, Bern, Switzerland

IVIG preparations contain autoantibodies to IgE. There is at present only limited information available on a potential *in vivo* role of such autoantibodies. However, anti-IgE autoantibodies have interesting *in vitro* functions. There seem to exist two distinguished biological entities among purified autoantibody preparations. We found, on the one hand, antibodies capable of triggering histamine release from human basophils and, on the other hand, antibodies which inhibited sensitization with IgE. Similarly, antibodies were found which either removed cytophilic IgE from CD23-positive cells, or enhanced binding to these cells.

Anti-IgE autoantibodies seem to form immune complexes with IgE and thereby inhibit accurate IgE determinations. The immune complexes are also mitogenic for human mononuclear cells, suggesting that anti-IgE antibodies might play a regulatory role in the formation of IgE.

In order to study whether a relationship exists between epitope specificity and function of anti-IgE antibodies, we have generated different recombinant IgE peptides, suitable for mapping of both properties. We found elevated levels of anti-IgE antibodies in sera from atopic blood donors, but also occasionally in healthy donors. High levels of anti-IgE antibodies were also detected in sera of asthmatic children. Highest levels were found so far in patients non-successfully treated by hyposensitization. Thus, anti-IgE autoantibodies contaminating IVIG might influence the biological properties of these therapeutic agents.

IgG antibodies to factor VIII in the plasma from healthy individuals

M. ALGIMAN[1], G. DIETRICH[2], U. NYDEGGER[3],
M. D. KAZATCHKINE[2] and Y. SULTAN[1]

[1] *Hôpital Cochin, Paris, France;* [2] *Hôpital Broussais, Paris, France;*
[3] *Inselspital, Bern, Switzerland*

Natural autoantibodies against a variety of self-related antigens are present in normal human sera. In a study designed to investigate the presence of anti-factor VIII antibodies in IVIG, we found that the plasma of 17% (85/500) of healthy male and female blood donors contained factor VIII neutralizing activity as assessed by the ability of heated plasma to inhibit factor VIII activity in a reference pool of normal human plasmas. Factor VIII neutralizing activity was expressed by IgG and $F(ab')_2$ fragments prepared from plasmas with inhibitor activity. Anti-factor VIII activity in normal plasmas ranged between 0.4 and 2 BU/ml. Mean factor VIII levels did not differ between normal individuals with or without anti-factor VIII antibodies, suggesting that antibodies from a given donor may react differently with autologous and allogeneic factor VIII. The latter hypothesis was confirmed in assays of anti-factor VIII containing IgG from healthy donors on a pool of normal plasmas and on each plasma constitutive of the pool. These observations demonstrate the presence of natural autoreactive and/or alloreactive IgG antibodies to factor VIII in the plasma from healthy individuals.

Cloning of the V-gene segments of the neuroblastoma-binding antibody CE7 reveals a novel V_κ gene family. Construction of a mouse/human chimeric antibody

H. AMSTUTZ, C. KYD and J.-J. MORGENTHALER

Central Laboratory SRC Blood Transfusion Service, Bern and Th. Kocher Institute, University of Bern, Bern, Switzerland

Our monoclonal antibody CE7-$\gamma_1/_\kappa$ recognizes a 190-kilodalton glycoprotein on the cell surface of neuroblastoma cells. It binds strongly to all neuroblastoma cell lines and tissues tested so far and only weakly to adrenal medulla. No binding was detected to any other normal or neoplastic tissue. We have identified the functionally rearranged variable gene segments by Southern analysis with J-probes. The relevant gene segments were isolated from phage libraries. Analysis of the sequences shows that the CE7-V_H gene is a new member of the J558 gene family. The CE7-V_κ sequence is unique insofar as the highest homology to a known V_κ gene (v-16 germline gene) is of only 73.5%. It therefore represents a novel V_κ gene family which we are currently characterizing. Chimeric genes have been constructed with these mouse V-segments and human constant region genes for γ_1 and κ chains in pSV2-derived plasmid vectors. They were transfected into SP2/0 cells by electroporation and among the G418 resistant clones those producing human γ_1 and κ chains were selected. By ELISA we could demonstrate that functional chimeric antibodies are assembled which bind to the human neuroblastoma cell line IMR-32 with properties identical to those of the original CE7. A chimeric antibody of this specificity should be useful for tumor imaging and eventually for therapy.

Study of immunological aspects of therapy resistant childhood epilepsy. Effects of therapy with intravenous immunoglobulin

B. G. M. VAN ENGELEN[1], P. F. W. STRENGERS[2], W. O. RENIER[1] and C. M. R. WEEMAES[3]

[1] *Center of Pediatric Neurology, St Radboud Hospital, University of Nijmegen, Nijmegen, the Netherlands;* [2] *Central Laboratory of The Netherlands Red Cross Blood Transfusion Service, Amsterdam, The Netherlands;* [3] *Institute of Pediatrics, St Radboud Hospital, University of Nijmegen, Nijmegen, The Netherlands*

High-dose intravenous immunoglobulin (IVIG) has been used successfully in the treatment of various immune-mediated diseases. Intramuscular immunoglobulin and IVIG therapy have also been tried by several groups in so-called "therapy resistant childhood epilepsy (TRE)" on the hypothesis that immune mechanisms may play a role in triggering or maintaining this severe form of epilepsy. We have performed a prospective study in 10 patients with West or Lennox epilepsy, enrolled between January 1989 and January 1990. Criteria for entrance in the study were severe therapy-resistant epilepsy (West syndrome or Lennox Gastaut syndrome), age between 6 months and 5 years, normal cranial CT-scan and normal cerebrospinal liquor, no therapeutic reaction on conventional therapy with anti-epileptica, and no therapy of ACTH or steroids during the last 6 weeks before start of IVIG therapy. Patients had no infections or other serious diseases or syndromes other than epilepsy, so-called idiopathic types of West or Lennox epilepsy. Each patient received IVIG 400 mg/kg body weight during 5 consecutive days and then 400 mg/kg body weight once every 2 weeks during 3 months. The IVIG was produced from plasma of more than 3000 Dutch blood donors by ethanol fractionation, treated at pH 4 with low concentration of pepsin.

Nine out of ten treated patients had a strong reduction in the frequency of seizures. Eight patients had a reduction of more than 50% of the pretreatment number of seizures. One child had no reaction in the beginning after IVIG therapy, but is without any seizure 4 months after therapy. One child had clinically no improvement at all. Eight patients showed better contact with the environment, as controlled by parents and psychologists. Motor functioning was also improved. In all but one tested patients the Denver test showed improvements of mental and motor function.

All children had a 1 h EEG before and after the IVIG therapy. The EEGs of nine children were studied "blind" by two independent neurologists. All EEGs after IVIG therapy showed an acceleration of background activity and a reduction of spike wave discharges of more than 30%. No changes were found in immunological parameters such as immunoglobulin levels (except a raise of IgG after therapy) number of T cells, T4/T8 ratio, lymphocyte stimulation *in vitro*. Before treatment all patients showed no IgG subclass deficiency.

The etiology of TRE is still unknown, but a dysregulation of the immune system may play a role. Although the study will continue until in total 20 patients with TRE are admitted, our clinical and electrophysiological data suggest that high-dose IVIG seems to be beneficial in a substantial number of patients with TRE.

We intend to compare the final results of this group with those from 100 conventionally treated TRE patients which have been studied during the last few years.

Intravenous immunoglobulins (IVIG) treatment of IgG k monoclonal gammopathy of undetermined significance (MGUS) – associated chronic inflammatory demyelinating polyradiculoneuropathy (CIDP)

C. BESANA, E. GORLA, R. NEMNI, U. DEL CARRO, G. S. ROI, M. PIROVANO, R. FINAZZI, C. CERIZZA and C. RUGARLI.

Istituto Scientifico San Raffaele. Università di Milano, Italy

A 56-year-old male patient with a severe IgG k MGUS-associated polyneuropathy has been treated with IVIG. A plasma exchange was not completed because of early cardiac arrest, and steroid treatment was started (February 1988). A 4-month partial remission ensued. Prednisone 1.2 mg/kg/day was ineffective on relapse (November 1988), and in January 1989 the patient developed staphylococcal pneumonia while still on prednisone. MGUS was stable. He had complete lower limbs adynamia and severe upper limb hyposthenia with acral hypo-paresthesias. Clinical manifestations, EMG, CSF and neural biopsy were consistent with Barohn's criteria (*Arch. Neurol.* 1989; 46:878) for CIDP. Taking into account the known efficacy of IVIG on CIDP, a single dose of 300 mg/kg was tried. A definite transient improvement of muscle strength was observed. We slowly tapered the steroid and thereafter treated the patient with repeated courses of IVIG, starting with 400 mg/kg/day, every 5 days for 4 weeks, and studied the relation between dosage, dose intervals and disease manifestations. Treatment has been very effective. The patient is able to walk and normal daily performances have been resumed with some difficulty. Clinical improvement started soon after each IVIG course, lasting less than 4 weeks. Standardized follow up of muscle strength by means of isokinetic dynamometry (CIBEX II, Lumex Inc., New York) has been more sensitive than EMG. Cost/efficacy analysis suggests the optimal schedule to be a 4-day course of 400 mg/kg/day every 3 weeks. To our knowledge this is the first report of effective IVIG treatment of MGUS-associated CIDP.

Intravenous immunoglobulin in multiple sclerosis: four cases report

A. ANANIA, G. CASCIO, M. M. VERNEY and C. RICCI

Clinica Medica B, Università di Torino, Italy

Multiple sclerosis (MS) is a chronic CNS immunological disorder in which the target is myelin. On the basis of improvement obtained with intravenous immunoglobulin (IVIG) in patients with rheumatoid arthritis (RA), auto-immune hemolytic anemia (AHA), we directed our interest toward patients who have different autoimmune disorders, such as MS. An agent able to block the RES, especially when this is activated, and saturate the receptor of the Fc fragment of macrophages, succeeds in down-regulating the aggressive effect of macrophages and the associated autoantibodies. This observation led us to undertake the treatment of subacute forms of MS with polyvalent human antibodies.

A 49-year-old female patient (O.MG.) affected with MS from the age of 26 has been treated with IVIG for 24 months. She received 150 mg/kg monthly. The clinical picture (paresthesias of the tongue and of the face) has improved and the relapses have become less frequent.

A young male MS patient (T.M.) aged 29 years who has been sick for 4 years was treated with ACTH. After remission, he started a monthly IVIG 150 mg/kg treatment which is continuing successfully. This patient has parethesias of the lower limbs and unstable walk which periodically relapses. At the moment he is well and for the past 2 years he has had only few relapses.

Our third patient is a young male university student aged 26 (A.N.) whose MS onset took place 3 years ago. He had ataxia and was first treated with a large dose of cortisone which led to relief of the symptoms as well as to hypogammaglobulinemia. Since then he has been treated monthly with IVIG 150 mg/kg and a subjective improvement has been observed. However, the patient is also being treated with azathioprine 100 mg/day. Thus, the above IVIG treatment must be considered only as a collateral therapy.

The fourth MS patient (D.A.), a man of 48 years, has been treated with IVIG for only 10 months. He had bad lower limb troubles and during these 10 months no further acute attacks have occurred. The main immunological finding in all the four patients is the high CD4:CD8 ratio which has not been modified because of the IVIG treatment.

The humoral defect in drug-induced hypogammaglobulinemia

E. TOUBI[1], J. FARRANT and A. D. B. WEBSTER

Clinical Research Centre, Harrow, Middlesex, UK; [1] Bnai Zion Medical Center and Faculty of Medicine, Technion-Israel Institute of Technology, Haifa, Israel

Gold compounds, D-penicillamine and sulfasalazine are well known anti-inflammatory drugs, widely used in rheumatoid arthritis (RA). One of the rare side effects of these drugs is hypogammaglobulinemia, the mechanism of which is still not clear. Defects in mitogen-induced proliferation of lymphocytes, monocyte-chemotaxis inhibition and defects in B-cell functions are documented in these patients. In our study we wanted to examine the effect of gold and sulfasalazine on the capacity of human peripheral blood non-T mononuclear cells to synthesize immunoglobulins. Two groups of non-T mononuclear cell preparations were examined. One was from 10 normal volunteers, the second from 3 RA patients in whom transient hypogammaglobulinemia developed under gold or sulfasalazine therapy. Flow cytometry using CD19 and surface IgM showed that the "non-T" preparation from the peripheral blood of both-mentioned groups, contained B cells in the range of 30–40% of the cells. The non-T cells (40 000/well) were cultured in 20 μl hanging drop cultures in 60–well Terazaki plates (Falcon) in the presence of different combinations of interleukins or anti-IgM beads with or without gold or sulfasalazine. After 7 days the cultures were assessed for total IgM and IgG in ELISA assay. Both gold and sulfasalazine inhibited IgM and IgG synthesis in a dose-related manner. In the RA group the inhibition was much more severe than in the control volunteers group. This study shows that these drugs are capable of inhibiting the differentiation of B cells, suggesting that the therapeutic efficacy of these drugs in RA is partly due to the reduction of antibody titers. One of our patients needed to be given i.v. gammaglobulin due to recurrent chest infections.

Therapeutic approach of cryoglobulinemia by high-dose immunoglobulins

T. BERNEY and S. IZUI

Département de Pathologie, Centre Médical Universitaire de Genève, Geneva, Switzerland

A murine IgG_3 mAb, clone 6–19, derived from unmanipulated autoimmune MRL-*lpr*/*lpr* mice, is a rheumatoid factor specific for IgG_{2a} and is able to generate cryoglobulins via non-specific IgG_3 Fc–Fc interaction. Intraperitoneal passive transfer of ascites containing the 6–19 mAb into BALB/c mice induces remarkable pathology characterized by skin leucocytoclastic vasculitis and acute glomerulonephritis associated with cryoglobulinemia. Since IgG_3 interact with each other, we have determined whether non-cryoprecipitating IgG_3 mAbs were able to inhibit the cryoprecipitation of 6–19 mAb and the development of related tissue lesions. *In vitro*, the cryoprecipitation of 6–19 mAb was completely inhibited by a 4-fold excess of a non-cryoprecipitating IgG_3 (9–23–106) mAb derived from MRL-*lpr*/*lpr* mice. Cryoprecipitation of five other IgG_3 mAbs was similarly inhibited by the 9–23–106 mAb, and two other non-cryoprecipitating IgG_3 mAbs inhibited the cryoprecipitation of 6–19 mAb. *In vivo*, pretreatment of BALB/c mice with 9–23–106 mAb totally prevented the development of skin vasculitis, and markedly reduced the glomerulonephritis induced by the 6–19 mAb. The cryoglobulin formation was greatly diminished in 9–23–106 mAb-treated mice, although their 6–19 mAb serum levels and rheumatoid factor activities were comparable to those of control mice. These results suggest a possible implication in high-dose immunoglobulin treatment for cryoglobulin-associated vascular diseases in man.

IVIG contain anti-idiotypes against a cross-reactive immunodominant idiotype of a thyroglobulin (TG) autoantibody directed against a specific disease-associated epitope of human TG

G. DIETRICH[1], M. PIECHACZYK[2], B. PAU[2] and M. D. KAZATCHKINE[1]

[1] *Inserm U 28, Paris, France;* [2] *Faculté de Pharmacie, Montpellier, France*

IVIG contain anti-idiotypes against idiotypic determinants expressed by autoantibodies (aAbs) from patients with a variety of autoimmune diseases. We have shown that IVIG recognize a cross-reactive α-idiotype (Id) on human anti-thyroglobulin (TG) aAbs that was defined by a rabbit anti-Id termed anti-T44. $F(ab')_2$ fragments from IgG of 9 patients with autoimmune thyroiditis and of 5 healthy donors were chromatographed on sepharose-bound $F(ab')_2$ fragments from IVIG. The T44 Id was expressed on IgG that bound to IVIG from 8 of 9 patients. In contrast, IgG from normal individuals that bound to IVIG–Sepharose did not express the T44 Id. A small amount of the T44 Id was also expressed on the fraction of IVIG that bound to itself upon affinity chromatography. The present study demonstrates that the expression of the T44 Id is strongly associated with the recognition by anti-TG aAbs of a specific epitope on human TG. The epitope specificity of anti-TG aAbs was investigated using a competitive ELISA with a panel of 15 mice mAbs that define 6 antigenic regions (I–VI) on human TG. All aAbs from patients showed a restricted specificity towards a single antigenic region termed region II. Anti-TG aAbs from healthy individuals did not recognize domain II. $F(ab')_2$ fragments from patients' IgG that were not retained on Sepharose-bound IVIG lost their reactivity with domain II of TG. The results show that aAbs from patients with autoimmune thyroiditis, which express the T44 cross-reactive Id, recognize a specific epitope on the TG molecule. IVIG contain anti-Id antibodies directed against an immunodominant disease-associated cross-reactive α-Id of human anti-TG aAbs with anti-domain II specificity.

A monoclonal anti-idiotypic antibody against the antigen-combining site of anti-factor VIII autoantibodies defines an idiotype that is recognized by IVIG

G. DIETRICH[1], P. PEREIRA[2], M. ALGIMAN[3], Y. SULTAN[3] and M. D. KAZATCHKINE[1]

[1] *Hôpital Broussais, Paris, France;* [2] *Institut Pasteur, Paris, France;* [3] *Hôpital Cochin, Paris, France*

We have suggested that the suppressive effect of IVIG on anti-factor VIII autoantibody activity was dependent on the presence in IVIG of specific anti-idiotypes against the autoantibodies (aAbs). The present study demonstrates that IVIG recognize an antigen-binding site-related idiotope of anti-factor VIII aAbs defined by a mouse monoclonal antibody (mAb) termed 20F2. mAb 20F2 was obtained by immunizing a mouse with affinity-purified anti-factor VIII $F(ab')_2$ fragments prepared from IgG of a patient with anti-factor VIII autoimmune disease. mAb 20F2 recognizes an overlapping epitope on the antigen-binding site of the patient's aAbs and the CH1 domain of IgG_1. Anti-γ1 CH1 reactivity was indicated by the capacity of mAb 20F2 to bind to human myeloma IgG_1 (κ or λ) and not to Fcγ1 fragments. Evidence for the anti-idiotypic specificity of mAb 20F2 included the ability of mAb 20F2 to neutralize anti-factor VIII activity of patient's aAbs and to specifically retain $F(ab')_2$ fragments with autoantibody activity on affinity columns. The idiotopic homogeneity of anti-factor VIII aAbs that were retained on Sepharose-bound mAb 20F2 was confirmed by the ability of mAb 20F2 to totally neutralize anti-factor VIII activity of this antibody fraction. IVIG inhibited anti-factor VIII activity of 20F2 idiotope-positive aAbs, thus indicating that IVIG recognize idiotypes containing the antigen-binding site-related 20F2 idiotope on patient's aAbs. These observations further support the concept of the presence in IVIG of anti-idiotypes against aAbs associated with autoimmune diseases.

Index

In this index IVIG is used as an abbreviation for intravenous immunoglobulin.